# THE MEDIEVAL HOSPITAL

# ReFormations

## MEDIEVAL AND EARLY MODERN

*Series Editors:*
David Aers, Sarah Beckwith, and James Simpson

# THE MEDIEVAL
# HOSPITAL

## LITERARY CULTURE
## AND COMMUNITY
### IN ENGLAND, 1350–1550

### NICOLE R. RICE

*University of Notre Dame Press*

*Notre Dame, Indiana*

Library of Congress Control Number: 2023930797

ISBN: 978-0-268-20511-9 (Hardback)
ISBN: 978-0-268-20513-3 (WebPDF)
ISBN: 978-0-268-20510-2 (Epub)

*For my family*

# CONTENTS

# FIGURES

ix

# ACKNOWLEDGMENTS

This book was developed with the support of many institutions and individuals. I hope to have remembered all of them below and apologize to any I have missed. A St. John's University summer research fellowship in 2015 and a research leave in Fall 2016 allowed me to begin surveying hospital-associated manuscripts and conceptualizing the project. I was privileged to receive an NEH Fellowship in 2018, which gave me crucial time to complete the bulk of research and writing. I thank St. John's University for providing ongoing support of my research, including a generous book subvention to offset production costs. For more than a decade, the English Department has given me a dynamic intellectual home full of generous colleagues. I am grateful to the New York Public Library and NYU Bobst Library for facilitating my research via the MARLI program.

Research on this project took me to numerous archives: I am grateful for the professionalism and kindness of their librarians. I spent many hours in St. Bartholomew's Hospital archive, whose staff (Clare Button, Dan Heather, Kate Jarman, Rachael Merrison) proved unfailingly helpful. I thank Laura Cracknell of Pembroke College, Oxford; Petra Hoffman of St. John's College, Oxford; Guy Mitchell of Gray's Inn; and Marc Statham and Paul Binski of Gonville and Caius College, Cambridge, for their assistance and answers to many follow-up requests. I am likewise indebted to the staff of Bristol Archives, Bristol City Council, Bristol Public Library, the British Library, Bodleian Library, Cambridge University Library, London Metropolitan Archives, the National Archives, York Archives and Local History, and York Minster Library. St. John's University Library interlibrary loan supplied me with countless obscure materials, and Dorothy McGovern assisted me in finding materials needed to finalize the book.

Conferences and seminars offered valuable chances to present work in progress. I am grateful to all the organizers and participants of these gatherings. They helped me to rethink my arguments, opened up new sources and ideas, and, above all, allowed me to connect with others interested in medieval hospitals and their cultural meanings. The Harvard Medieval Colloquium and the Victoria University Centre for Reformation and Renaissance Studies gave me places to present early work on the first chapter. I am grateful to the NYU Medieval and Renaissance Center and the Harlaxton Medieval Symposium for the opportunities to share work on medical texts and devotional manuscripts. The Early Book Society allowed me to present my work on Bristol manuscripts and on women at the reformed St. Bartholomew's. I was honored to speak on women at St. Bartholomew's at the Instituto de Historia at the Centro de Ciencias Humanas y Sociales. For welcoming me in Madrid, I thank Raúl Villagrasa-Elías, Cristina Jular, Fernando Mediano, and Salvatore Marino. While I was working on the book, Robert Hanning invited me to join the New York Meds, a lively seminar whose members welcomed me warmly and responded incisively to material from several chapters. I thank each of them for their kindness and rigor.

Many wonderful colleagues assisted this project at different points. Lisa Cooper and Tanya Pollard offered sage advice on fellowship proposals and support throughout. Mary Erler and Michael Sargent supported those proposals and helped at every stage: from reading chapters, to suggesting and lending sources, to answering last-minute calls for translation help. I am grateful to Jennifer Brown, an extraordinary coeditor, for reading the book manuscript multiple times and for helping me to stay sane while writing. Margaret Aziza Pappano and Matthew Sergi read the drama material with characteristic insight and made crucial suggestions for improvement. Margaret Connolly's astute reading helped me to improve the John Shirley discussion, and Julia Boffey's careful editing of the Harlaxton paper enabled me to envision chapter 4. I am grateful to David Aers, Sarah Beckwith, and James Simpson, the editors of the ReFormations series at University of Notre Dame Press, for sponsoring this project. I thank former editor Stephen Little, Editor-in-Chief Eli Bortz, and Managing Editor Matthew Dowd at UNDP for shepherding it to completion. The readers for UNDP offered extremely constructive feedback that helped immeasurably, and Scott Barker provided excellent copyediting. I take full responsibility for any remaining mistakes or infelicities.

I am grateful to generous colleagues who shared expertise, references, and advice to further this project. Many thanks to Marlene Hennessy and Kathryn Smith for their sound counsel on medieval images and equally for their friendship. For sharing work in progress on St. Bartholomew's Hospital,

I thank Caroline M. Barron. For helping me to decipher Mirfield's medical recipes, providing manuscript information, and inviting me to the med-med listserv, I thank Monica Green. For generously sharing his dissertation, I am indebted to Christopher Daly. For key references and materials, I am grateful to Lucy Barnhouse, Clifford Davidson, Tina Fitzgerald, Andrew Kraebel, Becky Krug, Steven Kruger, Esther Lewis, Daniel Sawyer, Claire Waters, and Sethina Watson. For help with transcribing and translating medieval Latin, I thank Maryanne Kowaleski and Shannon McSheffrey. I am grateful to Francely Rojas for research assistance and to Jamie Staples for stepping in to teach my course while I was on research leave.

I also wish to recognize several friends whose encouragement and good company have been vital over the past several years. Thank you to Tanya Agathocleous, Scott Combs, Marcy Engler, Meg Gay, Alfred Hiatt, Sahar Khan, Kathy Lubey, Leta Ming, and Jennifer Travis.

Portions of this book appeared in earlier forms in several places. A version of chapter 1 appeared as "The Feminine Prehistory of the York *Purification*: St. Leonard's Hospital, Civic Drama, and Women's Devotion," *Speculum: A Journal of Medieval Studies* 94, no. 3 (2019): 704–38. A short section of chapter 3 appeared as "Commemoration and Charity at the Medieval Hospital of St Bartholomew," in *The London Metropolitan Archives Newsletter*, May 2019. Part of chapter 4 appeared as "Devotional Reading and Display at St. Bartholomew's Hospital, London," in *Performance, Ceremony and Display in Medieval Britain: Proceedings of the 2018 Harlaxton Symposium*, edited by Julia Boffey, 176–92 (Donington: Shaun Tyas, 2020). I am grateful to the editors for permission to include previously published material here.

Most of all, I thank my family for their love and patience. This book is for you.

# ABBREVIATIONS

---

| | |
|---|---|
| BA | Bristol Archives |
| BL | British Library |
| *DIMEV* | *Digital Index of Middle English Verse.* https://www.dimev.net. |
| EETS | Early English Text Society ES: Extra Series OS: Original Series SS: Supplemental Series |
| *IMEP IX* | Eldredge, L. M. *The Index of Middle English Prose Handlist IX: Manuscripts in the Ashmole Collection, Bodleian Library, Oxford.* Woodbridge, Suffolk: D. S. Brewer, 1992. |
| LMA | London Metropolitan Archives |
| *MED* | *Middle English Dictionary.* https://quod.lib.umich.edu/m/middle-english -dictionary/dictionary. |
| *ODNB* | *Oxford Dictionary of National Biography.* https://www.oxforddnb.com. |
| *PL* | *Patrologia cursus completus series Latina.* 221 vols. Edited by J. P. Migne. Paris, 1844–1905. |
| *REED* | *Records of Early English Drama* |
| *REED: York* | *Records of Early English Drama: York.* 2 vols. Edited by Alexandra F. Johnston and Margaret Rogerson. Toronto: University of Toronto Press, 1979. |
| SBHB | Barts Health NHS Trust Archives and Museums |
| TNA | The National Archives (UK) |
| YML | York Minster Library |

# Introduction

*English Hospitals as Spiritual, Medical,
and Literary Communities*

The hospitals of late medieval England defy easy categorization. They were institutions of charity, medical care, and liturgical commemoration. At the same time, hospitals were cultural spaces sponsoring the performance of drama, the composition of medical texts, and the reading of devotional works. Such practices both reflected and connected the disparate groups — regular religious, ill and poor people, well-off retirees — that congregated in hospitals. In this book, I argue that hospitals constitute unique yet neglected sources for late medieval English literary and cultural history. Taking a new approach to literary history and its institutional contexts, I highlight hospitals as porous sites whose practices translated into textual engagements with some of urban society's most pressing concerns: charity, health, devotion, and commerce. Within these institutions, medical compendia treated the alarming bodies of women, and religious anthologies translated Augustinian devotional practices for lay readers. Looking outward, religious drama and socially charged poetry publicized and interrogated hospitals' caring functions within urban charitable economies.

The primary texts included in this study range from the canonical (the York play, John Lydgate's poetry) to the obscure (the *Breviarium Bartholomei*, Copland's *Hye Way to the Spyttell Hous*). Hospitals provided the auspices, audiences, and authors of such disparate literary works, propelling these texts into urban social life. Between about 1350 and 1550, English hospitals saw massive changes in their fortunes, from the devastation of the

Black Death, to various fifteenth-century reform initiatives, to the creeping dissolutions of religious houses under Henry VIII and Edward VI. In the heated decades of the 1530s and 40s, when religious regimes hinged upon rhetorical choices, public strategies of representation might translate into a hospital's demise or its survival. My study investigates how hospitals defined and defended themselves with texts, and in some cases reinvented themselves in the sixteenth century, using literary means to negotiate changed religious landscapes.

Historians of English hospitals, including Carole Rawcliffe and Miri Rubin, have offered detailed accounts of individual English hospitals and traced the late medieval histories of poor relief and medical care in which these institutions figured.[1] Literary historian Theresa Coletti has considered hospitals as sites for religious performance in the mass and liturgy and proposed the East Anglian hospital as a context for "devotional theater."[2] Some pioneering studies have investigated the copying and exchange of religious books at hospitals,[3] yet it remains true today, as Rawcliffe argued in 2002, that "the ownership and use of books by hospitals is . . . a neglected area of research."[4] To date there has been no book-length account of hospitals in relation to English literary and cultural practice. Rawcliffe has also noted that scholars have not always attended carefully to how hospital culture was constituted because so much artistic evidence of English hospital life was destroyed during the Dissolution years. Hospital cultural practices, she suggests, are due for a "radical reassessment."[5] I contribute to this reassessment by mapping the literary histories of three premodern English hospitals: St. Leonard's, York; St. Bartholomew's, London; and St. Mark's, Bristol. Founded in the eleventh, twelfth, and thirteenth centuries, respectively, by the later medieval period all were Augustinian institutions, located in England's three most populous cities. These hospitals are distinguished by well-documented histories and rich surviving archives. And although they shared certain liturgical and cultural assumptions, their differing resident populations, caring functions, and positions within their home cities made for distinct trajectories during the fraught centuries of my study.

The range of texts that I include in *The Medieval Hospital*—drama, history, medical treatise, poetry, devotional prose in Latin and Middle English—reflects the diversity of the three hospitals' populations and the range of their social interventions. Amid this variety, two important themes stand out: the influence of the Augustinian Order and its spirituality to the literary lives of the three hospitals, and the prominence of women within hospitals, as residents, patrons, and readers. I will suggest that a distinctive Augustinian approach to regulation, reading, and spirituality may have guided some of the canons in charge, influencing the construction of lay devotional practice and spiritual friendships within the three hospitals. Also crucial are the hospitals' roles as homes for women, manifesting differently in each case. Women were objects of intense concern and, in some cases, powerful agents within hospitals. Hospitals offered shelter to women at vulnerable stages of life and extremes of the social spectrum: destitute pregnant single women and affluent widows congregated at St. Bartholomew's. Within the hospital, texts were composed and copied to advise both groups. Nurses served as the primary caregivers at hospitals, and though they left few written records, at the sixteenth-century refoundation of St. Bartholomew's the matron became a figure of signal importance. Women, in a variety of roles and life stages, formed a constant object of hospitals' care and were central to their textual cultures.

The capacity of texts to define a hospital's place in the urban religious and charitable fabric became urgent in the sixteenth century, as hospitals became flashpoints in debates over charity, poverty, and vagabondage. Each house experienced a distinct Reformation history of dissolution, repurposing, or erasure from civic space and discourse. *The Medieval Hospital* develops an understanding of hospitals as institutions that were not simply suppressed but that reinvented themselves in the sixteenth century through varied literary means. Crucial to the study is a careful investigation of how texts figured in their Reformation histories, with results from virtually total disappearance (St. Leonard's), to refoundation as a secularized medical institution (St. Bartholomew's), to reinvention as a civic chapel (St. Mark's).

By constellating a novel combination of texts, writers, copyists, and readers, I hope to contribute in newly specific ways to recent work theorizing the hospital's role in late medieval Europe. Guy Geltner includes hospitals in the category of "semi-inclusive institutions" that, like brothels and prisons located within cities or at their borders, brought marginalized groups into productive proximity with broader urban populations: "Semi-inclusiveness offered no panacea for the myriad social problems afflicting medieval cities, but at the very least it promoted and reflected contemporaries' awareness of them. In this way, learning how to live alongside traditionally undesirable populations became part of a practical civic education."[6] Although most nonleprous hospital patients were not considered as "undesirable" as were prisoners or prostitutes, nevertheless they were overwhelmingly poor, sometimes pregnant or disfigured, and always vulnerable, whether children, disabled men, single women, or widows. Roberta Gilchrist emphasizes that English hospitals typically "catered for the general sick poor, and particularly for the most vulnerable groups within the life-cycle."[7] By resituating a range of texts that reflect upon this vulnerability in varied ways, I add the literary-cultural function to what historians have shown are the complex medical, spiritual, and social functions of hospitals.

In this introduction I describe the diversity of late medieval English hospitals' endeavors and populations, a diversity extended by a range of literary practices. First, I consider the many functions and varied residents of English hospitals. I then turn to the Augustinian canons, to consider how and why these religious became so closely linked with hospital administration. Finally, I introduce each of the three hospitals and suggest some of their overlapping yet distinctive qualities as sites for literary practice.

## RELIGIOUS, MEDICAL, AND SOCIAL FUNCTIONS

As Rubin notes, those expecting medieval hospitals to look like modern medical institutions will be disappointed. Their nonmedical activities, however, were varied: "They were venues for money-lending, liturgical practice and intercession, for pastoral work, a retirement-home for elderly and well-to-do burgesses, they could provide accommodation for clerics and students, and scope for speculation in the land market."[8] I put the limited textual vestiges of hospital medical practice into conversation with many of the practices Rubin mentions and with other practices, including the writing of history, the performance of drama, and the sharing of texts among lay and clerical members of the hospital community, many of whom did treat these institutions as a "retirement-home." By bringing these varied traditions to light, I emphasize the hospital's role as a cultural institution, uncovering the literary production arising in places that uniquely combined the alleviation of poverty, liturgical practice, medical care, and pastoral care (among other functions).

Defining the English medieval hospital is a tricky business given the great variety among these foundations and the changes that many underwent over their long histories. The term "hospital" (*hospitium, domus hos-*

*pitalis*) grounds these institutions in welcome but makes no reference to medical care.[9] Some English hospitals evolved from the monastic obligation to aid the poor and offer lodging to pilgrims, mandates reflected in monastic rules such as the *Regularis Concordia* and those of St. Benedict and Chrodegang of Metz.[10] One such example is Abingdon Abbey's hospital, which I highlight in chapter 2 as a site for the copying of John Mirfield's *Breviarium Bartholomei*.[11] Sethina Watson has shown that early English hospitals (founded ca. 1085–ca. 1200) were not generally religious communities; instead they were foundations of "sited alms" to support the poor and/or lepers. These early hospitals consisted of "a site, a designated form of alms and an endowment (regular, dependent, and often physical) to supply those alms."[12] The regular provision of alms was the essence of the endowment, and founders could assign these alms very precisely, including provisions for future income.[13] Hospital charters did not begin to appear in large numbers until circa 1180, as many founders saw in charters the opportunity to expand their hospitals' missions and create more elaborate institutions.[14] After about 1200, some English hospitals began to develop the characteristics of religious institutions, gaining chapels, coming under religious rules, and building more extensive compounds.[15] The three hospitals of this study were founded under varying auspices: by circa 1350 they all possessed chapels, religious communities, and a shared dedication to the Augustinian Rule to complement their essential mandate of caring for the poor.[16]

Although many later medieval English hospitals shared certain liturgical or pastoral characteristics with monasteries or priories, they remained distinctive in that they placed the works of mercy visibly at the center of their mission:[17]

> The medieval hospital was, in fact, the concrete expression, in bricks and mortar, of the Seven Comfortable Works, through the performance of which medieval men and women hoped to obtain 'health in body, grace in soul and everlasting joy'. The works in question, listed by Christ in St. Matthew's gospel (XXV, v. 32–36) were a constant theme of medieval preachers: feeding, clothing and giving drink to the poor, visiting prisoners, caring for the sick and sheltering the homeless were all charitable activities undertaken by hospitals, as, of course, was providing a proper burial for the dead, which took its inspiration from the Old Testament Book of Tobit.[18]

Hospitals might put these works into practice differently, welcoming various types of patients, including the chronically ill, retired priests, or lepers, but the outward-looking, charitable impulse was a constant.[19] Charity was expressed not only in the care of bodies as mandated by the Seven Works, and in the burial of those wishing interment on hospital grounds, but also through intercessory prayers for the souls of founders and benefactors.[20] In return for founding or donating to a hospital, late medieval benefactors might receive intercession through funeral prayers, special masses, or chantry services, as specified in numerous surviving wills and charters.[21] I discuss some of these in chapter 3, when I turn to wills as a type of hospital literature reflecting the charitable impulses and spiritual desires of laity connected to St. Bartholomew's.

Befitting the shared responsibility of securing intercession, it was not only the religious who prayed for the dead but sometimes also lay patients who were enjoined in specific terms to perform this work. "Through prayer, patients were supposed to help each other and, indeed, to assist their relatives and friends and people everywhere," states Edward J. Kealey.[22] The statutes of Ewelme almshouse, founded in 1440, required residents to perform a simplified yet rigorous daily round of Pater Nosters, Aves, and Creeds, numbering in the hundreds.[23] Embedded in the conception of the late medieval hospital was this clerical/lay cooperation in ritual practice, a unique form of charitable collaboration between religious and lay residents, and potentially between different configurations of rich and poor, young and old. Adam Davis argues that medieval hospitals embodied a continuum of care in which boundaries between personnel, those receiving care, and benefactors were sometimes porous. He insightfully depicts all of these agents as "bound up together in a social and spiritual web of mutual need, dependency, and assistance."[24]

The central metaphor of Christ as the spiritual physician, operative within late medieval Christianity as a whole, was animated in particular ways within hospitals. These institutions aimed to care for both body and spirit, understood as inextricable from each other. Some of the earliest extended treatments of *Christus medicus* appear in Augustine, who draws an analogy between Christ's passion and the bitter medicine of the physician: "Do not fear to drink. For to dispel your fear the physician drank first, that is, the Lord drank first the bitterness of the Passion."[25] Hence the logically related image of the priest as a spiritual physician with authority derived from Christ became familiar in a range of medieval religious texts, codified in a decree of the Fourth Lateran Council of 1215: "The priest shall be discerning and prudent, so that like a skilled doctor he may pour wine and oil over the wounds of the injured one. Let him carefully inquire about the circumstances of both the sinner and the sin, so that he may prudently discern what sort of advice he ought to give and what remedy to apply, using various means to heal the sick person."[26] The same council also banned clerics in major orders from surgery, among other activities involving bloodshed. Jeremy J. Citrome argues that even as priests were barred from operating on bodies, surgery became prevalent as an image for confession in pastoral literature after 1215: "Metaphors of surgery become the key rhetorical device through which subsequent pastoral writers explain spiritual health in this reinforced confessional context, and the surgeon, their foremost model for the perfect confessor."[27] Daniel McCann has also demonstrated the double valence of the *Christus medicus* image underpinning penitential practice, and, by extension, lay devotional reading in late medieval England. On the one hand, Christ's own sufferings are presented as curative for the penitent, as in the passage from Augustine cited above. On the other hand, Christ is a physician who must inflict wounds in order to heal.[28] In his study of the "therapeutic aspects of religious texts," McCann shows how vernacular devotional texts such as the *Prick of Conscience* and the *Penitential Psalms* function therapeutically "to evoke emotions intense enough to enable *salus animae*, or the health of the soul" in readers.[29] Although I will be looking at different texts from McCann, the concept of "soul-health" remains crucial throughout. In the space of the hospital, an institution focused on caring for the physically vulnerable while striving, through prayer, to bring spiritual health to its patrons and its diverse community, bodily and spiritual health were always intertwined. The priest's role as spiritual healer offering Christ's salutary suffering to the penitent became heightened and was textualized in diverse ways.

Although relatively few records survive from English hospitals of what we would today call medical care, hospitals played an important role in the late medieval health-care system.[30] During this period, most health care took place in the home, with women as the primary caregivers. Katharine Park notes that women served as "the first line of defense against illness and as those primarily entrusted, in the normative context of the home, with the ongoing management of health."[31] People with complex illnesses or injuries needing specialized care did not generally resort to hospitals: if they had the resources, they hired private doctors to come to their homes. Thus English hospitals with a mandate to care for sick patients were mainly serving those without such resources: the poor, the indigent, those shunned by family.

Although some hospital libraries contained medical texts, we have relatively few records of physicians attending the sick or injured in English hospitals prior to the sixteenth century.[32] Yet Roberta Gilchrist's recent archaeological work on hospitals and monastic infirmaries has uncovered "technologies of healing" that included "preventative care for the body, medical interventions such as surgery and bone-setting, the provision of prosthetics and specialist medicines."[33] Thus, limited recorded evidence for medical care in hospitals need not mean that such care was unavailable but rather that those providing it were not university-trained "physicians."[34] Carers were generally highly skilled nurses: I detail the extent of their activities in the next section.

Together with the care of their bodies, hospital patients received the spiritual comfort of seeing the mass daily and receiving confession and other sacraments. In the interest of promoting spiritual health, later medieval hospital architecture developed to enable patients to see the mass celebrated.[35] Large institutions for the sick poor (including St. Leonard's, York, and St. Bartholomew's, London) typically located a large open infirmary hall with a chapel just to the east, allowing patients to see the Eucharist elevated and listen to the service, even if they were too weak to rise from their beds. The building plans of these two hospitals were also fairly standard, employing central space such as a "close, cloister, quadrangle or courtyard as their means of central planning."[36] The compound's other buildings radiated around these, including separate dormitories for brothers and sisters, and in larger hospitals multiple chapels staffed by different chaplains. These compounds were in turn surrounded by workshops of artisans, such as bakers and masons, who provided goods and services to residents. Running water was recognized as de rigueur for maintaining health, and records of water management survive for St. Bartholomew's and St. Mark's. In 1297, St. Bartholomew's was allowed to cover with wood and stone a foul-smelling watercourse running through the hospital; St. Mark's received piped water from springs outside of Bristol.[37] Along with St. Mary's Abbey, St. Leonard's, York, was the only local institution to have its drain fully encased in stone.[38]

English medieval hospitals were founded in rural, urban, and suburban locations. Many of the earliest foundations were rural, yet urban hospitals also emerged relatively early, between 1170 and 1250.[39] Watson sees
the consolidation of towns and the foundation of urban hospitals as linked
developments in this period, whereby "the locating of new hospitals in
prominent sites proclaimed the emerging town and simultaneously laid
claim to responsibility for its well-being."[40] Cities produced a need for hospitals, since urban areas attracted migrants requiring social assistance and
travelers searching for lodging. Higher rates of urban mortality in turn produced poor widows and orphans. At the same time, cities generated wealth
and were homes to benefactors who could afford to establish hospitals and
give charity.[41] Baronial hospitals tended to be located just outside town walls
(hence technically suburban), welcoming travelers and drawing attention
to the lord from whom the town held its liberty; burgess hospitals were
often sited just inside town gates, announcing governmental independence
and concern for the town's internal population.[42] Hospital residents, sometimes socially marginal people, remained visible to city dwellers as they
circulated within their neighborhoods, sometimes supporting themselves
by begging for alms.[43] Of the three hospitals that I consider, St. Leonard's,
York, was located inside the city walls; St. Bartholomew's, London, and
St. Mark's, Bristol, were sited in the surrounding suburbs of Smithfield
and Billeswick, respectively. Throughout their histories, each hospital remained in constant, sometimes tense contact with the city's spaces, regulations, and people.

## DIVERSE COMMUNITIES

The constant interrelation of hospital residents and larger city is visible in
the makeup of hospital populations. The dynamism of my three chosen institutions as literary communities stems from their heterogeneous natures
as places that drew in people of different ages, genders, religious and class
statuses.[44] J. C. Dickinson makes "diversity" a key term for his analysis of the
regular canons, who often supervised late medieval hospitals. The Augustinian Rule resists uniformity within the community, noting that not every
brother needs the same amount of food or quality of clothing. In its longer
version, the Rule's third chapter reads,

Sed non dicatis aliquid proprium, sed sint uobis omnia communia, et distribuatur unicuique vestrum a praeposito uestro uictum et tegumentum, non aequaliter omnibus, quia non aequaliter ualetis omnes, sed potius unicuique sicut cuique opus fuerit. Sic enim legitis in Actibus Apostolorum, qui erant illis omnia communia et distribuebatur unicuique sicut cuique opus erat.

---

Call nothing your own, but let everything be yours in common. Food and clothing shall be distributed to each of you by your superior, not equally to all, for all do not enjoy equal health, but rather according to each one's need. For so you read in the Acts of the Apostles that they had all things in common and distribution was made to each one according to each one's need.[45]

In most cases, Dickinson notes, "within the order and indeed within the convent diversity was often the order of the day."[46] The three hospitals that I consider were by circa 1350 home to clerical leaders, lay brothers, a range of patients, and other residents of varying ages, sometimes including retirees, families, and orphans.

The late medieval English hospital master, whether a secular or a regular cleric, or occasionally a well-connected layman, oversaw the running of the institution, particularly its financial operations. Depending on his profession and inclinations, he might serve as a spiritual leader to his brothers and other residents. Hospital masters might include royally appointed churchmen, as at St. Leonard's in the early fourteenth century, or longtime brothers who achieved the mastership after years serving the house, as with Master John Colman of St. Mark's in the early sixteenth century.[47] Documents occasionally give insight into a master's authority: for example, these "provisiones et praecepta" issued by Walter de Langton, master of St. Leonard's in 1295, mandating that if any hospital brother "fuerit incontinens, vel inobediens, vel proprietarius, quod nullus possit eum absolvere nisi solus magister, nisi tantum in periculo mortis" (should be intemperate, or disobedient, or property-holding, nobody may absolve him except the master, unless he is in danger of death).[48] If a hospital was staffed by vowed religious, these tended to be canons, usually thirteen, the apostolic number, but this too might vary. Secular chaplains often formed part of the clerical staff, attested at all three hospitals I study. By the mid-fourteenth century, St. Leonard's housed thirteen chaplain brothers living under the Rule of Augustine, along with four secular chaplains. At both houses the secular chaplains are documented as having regular contact with the ill patients, offering them confessions and counsel; chaplains appear frequently in residents' wills as trusted advisors.[49]

The presence of secular chaplains indicates that hospitals frequently employed members of the "clerical proletariat"—a diverse group of highly educated but underemployed clergy that burgeoned between the early fourteenth and mid-fifteenth century.[50] Kathryn Kerby-Fulton's important recent study argues for the centrality of this group to Middle English literary production, highlighting the vocational crises represented by authors such as Langland and Hoccleve and attributing anonymous works such as the York *Second Trial before Pilate* to proletarian authors. The characteristic qualities and institutional commitments of hospitals dovetail in some respects with the priorities that Kerby-Fulton discerns in such literature (including a blurring of religious and secular concerns, a strong concern for the poor, an effort to counsel women, and a notably multilingual culture).[51] Given my focus on hospitals as sites for the convergence of various vowed, secular clerical, and lay interests, Kerby-Fulton's larger conclusions, and in some cases her comments about specific figures, add complementary and suggestive dimensions to my study of hospitals and literary practice.[52]

Whereas hospitals' secular clerics attended to confessions and counsel, the nurses (professed sisters) and the lay brothers, in some cases, cared for the sick poor. Even when both regular brothers and nurses were professed to the Rule of Augustine, the brothers' job tended to religious matters and the nurses cared for the sick.[53] Martha Carlin highlights the injunctions sent to the Southwark Hospital of St. Thomas in 1387 that exhort the brothers to study and pray and the sisters to supervise the patients. We do not generally find detailed statutes for nurses in English hospitals, as in some French examples such as Paris's Hôtel-Dieu or Florence's Santa Maria Nuova, but we do find evidence from St. Leonard's that nurses were enjoined to take vows of poverty, chastity, and obedience.[54] The 1364 episcopal visitation requires the same vows from the "sorores regulares" (nurses) and "fratres conversi" (lay brothers): both must promise "obedienciam, castitatem, et abdicacionem proprietatis" (obedience, chastity, and the renunciation of property).[55] Although the nurses are summarily advised in this same document to "promittendo se necessitatibus infirmorum labore proprio subvenire" (promise to attend to the needs of the sick with their own labor),[56] Cullum argues that experienced nurses probably developed more than basic skills:

Their skills were probably based on a traditional herbal medicine, perhaps modified by access to books in the hospital's library, and quite probably including minor surgery. Evidence that they were indeed in demand as skilled healers outside the hospital is given by the 1364 Visitation which stated that they were not to do work for money but were to concern themselves only with the poor (*non faciant sorores aliquas operaciones venales set tantum pauperum necessitatibus sint intente*), which suggests that they were indeed doing work for money.[57]

Sisters were lower on the spiritual hierarchy than the professed brothers, and their more rudimentary living conditions often reflected their inferior status.[58] Nevertheless, occasional bequests in residents' wills show that patients appreciated the sisters' efforts to care for them.[59] Lay brothers, even lower in status, assisted the sisters in caring for the sick by doing heavy manual labor and fetching food for patients in consultation with the house's cellarer.[60]

In hospitals that treated the sick poor, the types of lay patients could vary considerably, but some hospitals defined their patient populations strictly. Residents might suffer from many different afflictions. The five most common causes were cited in a petition of the House of Commons from 1414, which noted that English hospitals were funded to sustain "veigles hommes & femmes, lazers hommes & femmes, hors le lour senne & memoir, poveres femmes enseintez, & pur hommes q'ount perduz lour biens & ont cheiez en grande meschief" (old men and women, lepers, men and women who have lost sense and memory, poor pregnant women, and poor men who have lost their goods or fallen upon hard times).[61] Leper hospitals were a separate (though varied) category and were sometimes repurposed for more general use after leprosy became less prevalent after 1350.[62] Poor pregnant women were admitted to many hospitals, but among the three that I study here, only St. Bartholomew's is recorded as welcoming pregnant women to give birth there. Some hospitals explicitly rejected pregnant women for fear they would distract brothers from religious practice or bring shame upon the house. The Hospital of St. John in Cambridge enjoins brothers as follows: "infirmi et debiles admittantur benigne et misericorditer, exceptis mulieribus pregnantibus, leprosis, vulneratis, contractis et insanis" (the infirm and the weak should be admitted kindly and with mercy, except for pregnant women, lepers, the paralyzed and the insane).[63] Such rules bespeak a generalized anxiety about contact between the sexes at hospitals. At St. Leonard's, York, in-house ordinances mandate the separation of brothers and sisters within the hospital, ordering sisters to congregate in a "locus honestus" (respectable place) in the lower part of the church, away from the brothers at all times.[64] The mixing of men and women comes up periodically in episcopal visitations of both St. Leonard's and St. Bartholomew's, which note inappropriate relationships between brothers and sisters, or masters and sisters.

Despite prohibitions on the mingling of brothers and sisters, the larger lay communities that congregated at hospitals tended to be of mixed genders and ages. Corrodians (older residents who paid fees to retire at hospitals, or who received free places if they were royal favorites) became prominent, and in some cases they created significant financial drains on larger institutions, such as St. Leonard's.[65] Many retirees were married couples, but sometimes widows gathered at hospitals for the congenial spiritual and social life and perhaps also for the safety that their compounds afforded.[66] Other lay residents at the larger hospitals included retirees renting tenements, as in the close of St. Bartholomew's, sometimes including families with children. At St. Bartholomew's, younger residents might include orphans plucked from the streets or infants whose mothers had died in childbirth at the hospital. Some of these children may have become students at the hospital's grammar school. In a good example of the hospital's multiple functions converging, in 1447 one John Stafford endowed a chantry at the hospital's altar of St. Nicholas and also left money for the master to arrange "for instructing boys in grammar and singing." Stafford's bequest supported both his own commemoration and the poor children who were educated free of charge at the hospital.[67] Such glimpses of multigenerational community allow us to see hospitals as dynamic places that brought young and old, clerical and lay into a range of relationships.

## THE AUGUSTINIAN CANONS AS HOSPITAL LEADERS

Despite the variations found among late medieval English hospitals, one striking point of commonality is the prominence of the regular (Augustinian) canons as their clerical leaders. Dickinson notes the "well-known flexibility of the order," and it has become a commonplace in English hospital scholarship that this flexibility made the Augustinians ideally suited to manage the varied requirements of hospital administration.[68] Yet each hospital had its own complex history, and the Rule of Augustine was not a default or a foregone conclusion. Many hospitals came under Augustinian rule long after their foundations, as was the case with St. Leonard's and St. Mark's.[69] Although the Augustinian Order encompassed not only canons but also hermits and friars, it would seem that the order's overall outlook (characterized by a commitment to *caritas* and teaching) was conducive to hospital work.[70] The Rule's opening words proclaim the dual commitment to love God and neighbor that defines Augustinian observance: "Ante omnia, fratres carissimi, diligatur deus, deinde proximus, quia ista sunt praecepta principaliter nobis data" (Before all else, dear brothers, love God and then your neighbor, because these are the chief commandments given to us).[71] Dickinson stresses "the maintenance of a full common life," in accordance with the apostolic commandment, as the most essential aspect of canonical practice preceding the adoption of the Rule, which was a gradual process over the eleventh and twelfth centuries.[72] Monastic observance often militated against contact with the world, and mendicant observance theoretically precluded ministry in a single established place, but canons sought out both a regular liturgical life and steady pastoral commitments, which became central features of many hospitals.[73]

The details of English Augustinian observances are often difficult to track, yet scholars of Augustinian culture as a wider European phenomenon have made arguments that may help us to understand the connection between canons and hospital settings in later medieval England.[74] As Eric Saak has shown, the twelfth-century canon Philip of Harvengt was an early definer of St. Augustine's meaning for the medieval order, presenting the saint's mixed life of action and contemplation as a model for canons.[75] Although Saak focuses on the hermits, who made more extensive contributions to theology, many fundamental assumptions were shared by hermits and canons, despite their later battles for primacy as the true "sons of Augustine." Saak argues that in the later Middle Ages, "theology as affective knowledge, a knowledge of the heart, rather than of the mind, became a hall-mark of Augustinian theology."[76] Love was paramount within the Augustinian Order: "Acts of mercy, the giving of alms, were love made concrete and real."[77] This emphasis seems very suggestive for the connection between the Augustinians and hospitals.

Caroline Walker Bynum has argued that twelfth-century regular canons, though they might look and act much like monks, developed a distinctive emphasis in their nonpolemical spiritual writings on "the canon's sense of a responsibility to edify his fellow men both by what he says and by what he does."[78] The canons' devotion to teaching, the assumption that they should offer "pattern (*forma*) and example (*exemplum*) to those who encounter them" is manifest in their original writings and in their use of sources, in which they highlight or "add a concern for the educational responsibility of the individual brother."[79] Bynum points to works such as the *Expositio in regulam beati Augustini*, a long commentary that had become by the thirteenth century a standard adjunct to the Augustinian Rule, as exemplifying this concern for brothers as teachers.[80] In chapter 4, I show how John Colman of St. Mark's Hospital combined texts, including the Rule and *Expositio*, into clusters that highlight the responsibilities of canons and lay readers for teaching each other within the Augustinian hospital.

Jean-Pascal Pouzet's characterization of the English Augustinians further enhances our understanding of how the order's priorities might have influenced hospital literary practices. He notes an Augustinian focus on the New Testament and pastoral work, the practices of humility and sobriety, and "perhaps above all, a taste for study."[81] All houses of canons under the governance of the General Chapter were enjoined to have a master to teach novices the Rule and the Statutes of the order.[82] Although most hospitals, including the ones that I study, were under episcopal governance, not subject to the General Chapter, we nevertheless see substantial testimony to the "expectation that canons should be educated" through the evidence of surviving books.[83] Some hospital canons are recorded as having attended university to study theology.[84] Dedication to the collection and copying of books was another established Augustinian value,[85] and Pouzet draws attention to Augustinian hospitals as particularly conducive to the *otium* required to develop scribal expertise.[86] We can detect in the manuscripts associated with hospital scribes a strong devotion to teaching "verbo et exemplo," inflected by the particular settings, functions, and reading populations of St. Bartholomew's and St. Mark's. The teaching of children in grammar schools was a related facet of hospital practice, and such schools are documented via the wills of schoolmasters and benefactors at St. Leonard's, York, and St. Bartholomew's, London, for the fifteenth century.[87]

Augustinian contributions to wider late medieval catechetical trends were important for English pastoral and devotional practice, and hence for hospitals as spaces of spiritual advice and reading. As Saak shows, the

Augustinians contributed extensively to pastoral literature of the late fourteenth century, offering "model sermon collections, treatises on the Ten Commandments, expositions of the Lord's Prayer, treatises on the virtues and vices, on the Ave Maria, and on the articles of faith."[88] They were also instrumental to integrating Passion devotion within the larger matrix of religious practice.[89] All of these genres were well represented among the literary practices of the hospitals in question.

## THE THREE HOSPITALS: EARLY HISTORIES

The three hospitals I feature in this study show important variations, yet they all share connections to major cities and to the Augustinian Order. They are all marked by rich literary histories and extant archives. I introduce them here in the chronological order of their foundations. St. Leonard's originated as an appendage of York Minster and gradually developed its own identity. By the fourteenth century, the hospital was a large, complex institution that combined liturgical functions with the care of patients, housing religious and secular personnel and residents of both sexes, including the ill, the poor, aged priests, and retired laypeople.

It is difficult to pinpoint an exact foundation date for St. Leonard's. According to a dubious *Historia fundacionis* surviving in the hospital's cartulary, the Petercorn or "thraves" (twenty-four sheaves of corn from every working plow in the diocese, one of the house's main sources of income) was granted in 936 by King Athelstan to the church's canons "sustinere pauperes confluentes hospitalitatem tenere et exercere alia opera pietatis" (to give hospitality to the poor gathering there and to exercise the other works of mercy).[90] A more solid piece of early evidence for the hospital lies in the gift of land in front of York Minster to the cathedral canons, circa 1089–95. The Rawlinson Cartulary's editor, David Carpenter, notes that Nigel d'Aubigny's gift of land "for the sustenance of the poor brethren next to that church" indicates that a hostel or hospital existed next to the minster circa 1109–14. D'Aubigny also makes a reference to "the hostel (*hospitio*) of poor brethren of the said church."[91] The earliest hospital charters date from the 1130s throughout the reign of King Stephen. An inquisition of 1280 found that William II had founded the chapel of St. Peter, endowing it with the thraves. Stephen was responsible for the church of St. Leonard and had changed the name of the hospital to St. Leonard's.[92] Although it is uncertain when the hospital priests adopted the Augustinian Rule, Cullum speculates that Archbishop Thurstan (1114–40) may have imposed the Rule, having founded several other Augustinian houses during his tenure.[93]

Although some places at St. Leonard's Hospital were endowed or purchased, the majority of hospital beds were free to the "weak, infirm, poor people" who were the institution's main concern.[94] St. Leonard's was unusual among large hospitals in admitting not only the chronically ill but also those with hope of recovery, who were encouraged to leave as soon as they could work again.[95] The only Yorkshire hospital to provide for children, by 1287 St. Leonard's maintained an orphanage for approximately eighteen boys and girls.[96] The house also supported a separate grammar school, which by 1289 had thirteen scholars and two boys sent by the queen. By the mid-fourteenth century, the 1364 visitations reveal, the house was the largest hospital in the north, caring for about two hundred patients. It was staffed by thirteen Augustinian brothers who performed the liturgical offices, four secular chaplains, eight professed sisters, and various lay brothers and lay servants who helped minister to the residents' spiritual and physical needs.[97]

And even though it remained administratively independent from the city and had historically derived significant revenue from landholdings and other investments, St. Leonard's was deeply enmeshed in York's social fabric and depended for its survival upon the generosity of local people. From close to its foundation, St. Leonard's had occupied its own liberty outside the city's jurisdiction; the house had resisted the city's thirteenth-century attempt to gain its patronage, a move that may have alienated some possible civic supporters.[98] As I show in chapter 1, St. Leonard's has the most paradoxical history of the three: it had the most venerable and grandest foundation but also suffered the most precipitous economic decline over its history and now has the poorest surviving textual record. Yet it was the source of one of our most famous late Middle English texts: a pageant of the York Play. I suggest that sponsorship of drama, building upon existing performance traditions, may have helped the house to gain attention within the broader York community, functioning to promote the hospital's mission and distinguish it from other local charitable institutions.

Like St. Leonard's, initially attached to York Minster, St. Bartholomew's Hospital was founded in 1123 as a dependent house. Unlike St. Leonard's,

St. Bartholomew's was home to an Augustinian community from the start.[99] The hospital was founded jointly and under the supervision of an Augustinian priory, a twinned relationship that soon proved fractious. Ultimately St. Bartholomew's Hospital would become administratively separate, outlasting the priory after the sixteenth-century Dissolution. It is the only hospital of the three that still functions today as a medical institution, having been "refounded" by Henry VIII as a secular institution that nevertheless retained many of its original spiritual commitments in a reformed setting.

Founded by Rahere, one of Henry I's royal clerks, St. Leonard's soon received a royal charter.[100] The first charter, from Henry I in 1133, jointly gave the priory and hospital absolute tax exemption and protection of clergy to all members.[101] Equipped to care for about two hundred patients, the hospital was staffed by an unspecified number of Augustinian brothers, and also by secular chaplains, nurses, and lay brothers. The hospital's documents tell a story of friction with and increasing independence from the adjacent priory. Even though the hospital remained linked to the priory church, in 1147 the priory named a new hospital master, a layman named Adam the Merchant. The prior's charge grants him "potestas in pauperes orphanos pueros projectos vicinos pauperes infirmos quoslibet et sine hospicio vagantes quantum ei deus inspiraverit, misericordie visceribus habundante" (the power [to care for] poor, homeless orphans, neighboring paupers, and the sick wandering outside the hospital as much as God shall inspire him, from the mercy abounding in his heart).[102] The hospital's privileges increased with the grant of papal protection in 1183, which permitted the hospital its own burying ground and freedom from interdiction, but in continuing controversy with the priory, the burial ground was rescinded in 1224 by the bishop of London. After receiving exemption from the Statute of Mortmain in 1281, a change that enabled the hospital to hold property, over the next hundred years St. Bartholomew's developed endowments of land and established chantries within its chapels, expanding relationships with Londoners and benefactors farther afield.[103] Injunctions of 1316 offer a detailed picture of practices and requirements of the house, mandating that the house have only seven brethren, four sisters, and no more. They are all to attend the sick poor and not to quarrel.[104] Although some irregularities of daily worship and diet were criticized in 1318, the hospital continued to expand and by 1373 received from Bishop Simon Sudbury a new set of ordinances enshrining the rights to appoint its own master and control its own burial ground.[105]

A copy of these ordinances receives pride of place in the hospital's cartulary, the house's most precious book, which was partially copied by John Cok, a fifteenth-century brother who documented the institution's expansion under Master John Wakering. This is the period whose books and readers will occupy chapters 3 and 4.

St. Mark's Hospital, Bristol, locally known as the Gaunts, was first conceived as an almonry by a layman, Maurice de Gaunt, a Bristol magnate, who made arrangements with St. Augustine's Abbey between 1216 and 1230 to endow a "daily dinner for 100 poor in the almonry which Maurice had constructed for them, and to maintain a chaplain there to pray for the souls of Maurice and his ancestors."[106] None of Maurice's early charters survive, but these agreements were formalized and expanded by his nephew Robert de Gournay within two years of Maurice's death. Robert made provisions for more chaplains and removed the priests from the abbey's control, placing them under an independent master.[107] By 1259 the house seems to have come under the Augustinian Rule, even though the bishop's charter written in this year, which imposed the customs of the nearby Augustinian hospital at Lechlade, does not explicitly mention the rule.[108] At this time the house was allotted staff, including a master, three chaplains, three clerks in holy orders, and five lay brethren, numbers that fluctuated over the years and declined during the fourteenth century.[109] By 1269 the hospital was in fraternity with an Augustinian priory, and there is a reference to the brothers as canons by 1300.[110]

In contrast to St. Leonard's, York, and St. Bartholomew's, London, St Mark's, Bristol was a small institution. It was less prominent in the civic realm than Bristol's other hospitals of St. Leonard or St. John. Yet after gaining independence from St. Augustine's Abbey, St. Mark's became deeply connected on its own terms to local religious and charitable networks.[111] The house did not originally have resident ill or poor people but was required by the terms of its early charter to feed twenty-seven poor daily.[112] In addition to delineating the clerical staff and lay brethren, the bishop's charter of 1259 made the institution responsible for the housing and care of twelve poor scholars. The "duodecim scolares" were to serve "in choro tantum ministrantes pro disposicione Cantoris" (in the choir . . . under the direction of the precentor).[113] "Although we hear nothing more specifically of the scholars, we can perhaps see here the beginning of a gradual transition from a system of daily doles for the poor at the gate to the provision of board and lodging for a much smaller number of resident almsmen," says Ross.[114] Despite a paucity of documentary evidence for teaching, an educational tradition evidently persisted throughout the hospital's history. Thomas Tiler, master at the turn of the sixteenth century, testified in 1496 to having been "brought furth in the said place of Gauntes from yowth,"[115] and at the hospital's suppression in 1539, several resident children and choristers are recorded.[116]

With fewer external functions, a small contingent of brothers and a powerful master, the house assumed a more traditionally monastic character than the hospitals of St. Leonard's, York, or St. Bartholomew's, London. Yet like these two others, the Augustinian community of St. Mark's developed relationships of control and patronage with the larger community. The house maintained close ties with prominent lay benefactors, extended control over its own parish and chantries, and welcomed a small contingent of retirees, clergy, and laity to live and worship within its precincts. St. Mark's' manuscripts include a copy of the Augustinian Rule, giving us important clues about the house's observances and literary culture, as I show in chapter 4. My study of devotional reading at St. Mark's will be concerned with how its small Augustinian brotherhood used books to construct canonical spirituality and to advise lay community members.

In framing this study with the dates 1350 to 1550 I take a cue from Orme and Webster, who note that the years between the great plague of 1348–49 and the Reformation of the 1530s have been seen as especially "distinctive" and eventful for English hospitals.[117] I do not attempt to narrate the histories of these three foundations in detail, nor do I judge their successes or failures as charitable, liturgical, or medical institutions during this long period. Historians have made varied arguments about how different hospitals changed, declined, or reinvented themselves in the face of social changes, such as the plague, consequent population reduction, and rising wages.[118] Taking up texts that served important educational, medical, devotional or political functions within these three hospitals from the late fourteenth to the mid-sixteenth century, I show how literary practices shaped and narrated the lives of the varied people residing in or adjacent to these institutions. I also investigate how texts intervened into the larger urban world to shape wider understandings of the hospitals' charitable and civic roles, which were always subject to negotiation during these fraught years. In considering the evolutions of various English hospitals, Rawcliffe observes the "increasing use of ritual and ceremony in the country's older urban hospitals," including St. Leonard's, York, and St. Mark's, Bristol, which developed elaborate liturgies requiring ever-more choristers and altar boys.[119] For St. Leonard's, this requirement dovetailed with its longtime function as a grammar school and an orphanage whose children probably attended the school.[120] The combination of functions evokes the diversity of people, practices, and texts that we find in these three hospitals as dynamic spaces of charity, liturgy, and literature.

My first two chapters uncover women's central but understudied roles in the literary lives of English hospitals. In chapter 1, "St. Leonard's Hospital, Civic Drama, and Women's Devotion," I begin with the earliest foundation in the study and ask why York's great Hospital of St. Leonard sponsored a dramatic pageant representing the Purification of the Virgin as part of the city's annual Corpus Christi play cycle. Sponsorship by a religious house was unusual within a civic dramatic event produced mainly by artisan groups, and this practice suggests the hospital's desire to promote its mission within the urban sphere. In this chapter, I use hospital and civic records together with the extant play text to reconstruct the Purification pageant's early form. Connecting the pageant's early fifteenth-century form to the hospital's distinct devotional culture and economic concerns, I show how St. Leonard's used the woman-centered episode of Mary's purification to appeal to the experiences of female audiences and donors. The hospital channeled its well-established devotion to the Virgin Mary into a moving public spectacle of her purification, placing her miraculous maternity in the context of female spiritual community. By exploiting links between Mary's purification and the churching of ordinary women, and by giving unique prominence to the widowed prophetess Anna, St. Leonard's advertised itself as a worthy recipient of charity from York's townspeople, particularly women, and as an appealing institutional home for older women interested in donating or retiring to its precincts. Offering a new understanding of the *Purification* as a drama linked to the hospital's female patrons and populations, I show how St. Leonard's used performance to position itself strategically within the charitable economy of York at an economically challenging early fifteenth-century moment.

Chapter 2, "Corruption and Purification at St. Bartholomew's Hospital, London: *The Book of the Foundation* and John Mirfield's Compilations," initiates a sequence of two chapters on literary practice at this richly documented hospital. Unlike St. Leonard's in York, St. Bartholomew's of London admitted unmarried pregnant women and housed them through childbirth until their ritual purification forty days later. It is therefore notable that several major texts written in the hospital's orbit manifest concern for women's well-being at all stages of their life cycles. The dialectic of contamination and purification that attended the hospital, in its disreputable Smithfield location, was most urgently embodied by women, with their presumed physical and moral weaknesses. This chapter considers constructions of women in three late fourteenth-century works: a Middle English religious narrative (*The Book of the Foundation of St. Bartholomew's Church*) and two Latin compendia (John Mirfield's *Florarium Bartholomei* and *Breviarium Bartholomei*). Whereas the priory's foundation narrative writes anxiety about women's sexuality into the early history of priory and hospital, Mirfield's *Breviarium* implies a more nuanced, socially situated view of the sexual lives and requirements of urban single women. In keeping with the hospital's outward-looking focus, one fifteenth-century afterlife for Mirfield's gynecology shows that the remedies he compiled for a particular set of patients were later seen as valuable treatments for sexually active women beyond the specialized setting of the hospital. The therapeutic commitments of the *Breviarium* are thrown into relief by Mirfield's *Florarium*, a theological compilation for priory brothers that presents women as dangerous agents of temptation and impediments to well-regulated spiritual or medical practice.

Chapter 3, "Lay Reading Community in St. Bartholomew's Close: John Shirley's Final Anthology," keeps the focus on St. Bartholomew's, moving into the fifteenth century. I reconstruct lay reading practices adjacent to the hospital through the translations and manuscripts made by the London bibliophile John Shirley during his retirement in the hospital close. London historians Caroline Barron and Euan Roger have suggested that the group of educated, well-off lay Londoners, including Shirley, who lived in the hospital's orbit at midcentury, may have formed a textual community.[121] Building upon their groundbreaking work, I take a fresh look at the texts Shirley translated, copied, and compiled in the hospital close in an effort to understand the particular reading practices that its environment fostered. As a microcosm of urban society with links traveling in many directions, via ecclesiastical channels, social networks, and patronage relationships, St. Bartholomew's became in the fifteenth century a unique site for book production and reading. I consider the evidence that wills provide of shared devotional and literary concerns among this cultivated network of residents. Then I turn to Shirley's late literary productions, particularly his final Middle English anthology, Bodleian Ashmole MS 59, to argue that we can best understand its unique combination of didactic texts within the hospital's cultural framework. The Ashmole collection combines formative lessons for the hospital's multigendered, multigenerational reading context, creating a unique configuration of works for mature men, matrons, and children. Key texts for this investigation include a fragmentary translation of *Secretum Secretorum*, Chaucer's "Chronicle of Ladies," and several Lydgate works, notably the "Complaint" for the Duchess of Gloucester, the "Epistle to Sybil," and "Stans puer ad mensam."

Chapter 4, "Collaborative Devotional Reading at St. Bartholomew's and St. Mark's," turns to the interface of lay and priestly agents through the medium of books. This chapter engages with devotional manuscripts copied by priestly scribes living in the hospitals of St. Bartholomew and St. Mark. John Cok, a fifteenth-century canon of St. Bartholomew's and John Colman, master of St. Mark's from 1517 to 1539, copied Latin, vernacular, and bilingual collections expressly for hospital residents: clerical and lay, male and female. These custom-designed books structure devout practice within the two hospitals, developing modes of instruction and friendship that linked clerical and lay readers within Augustinian devotional frameworks.

I focus first upon Cok, a brother of St. Bartholomew's by 1421, seeking to understand how his religious books figured in his communal life and in his relationship with John Shirley. Cok and Shirley knew each other well, for Shirley named Cok as an executor in his will. One of Cok's smaller books is a varied collection of Latin religious texts (British Library MS Additional 10392), dated 1432; he also copied a volume including Middle English versions of Richard Rolle's *Form of Living* and *Emendatio vitae* (Cambridge, Gonville and Caius MS 669/*646), which was ultimately owned and annotated by Shirley. In the Latin collection, Cok visualized and performed the care of souls, extending penitential imperatives into programs of prayer and meditation to be shared with clerical and lay readers alike. In the next section of the chapter, on Colman's Bodleian MS Lyell 38, which features the Latin *Emendatio*, I consider how Colman annotated *Emendatio* to guide fellow Augustinian readers. In the final section of chapter 4, I consider two multilingual anthologies from St. Mark's, copied by Colman and his Augustinian brother William Haulle. I show that these two kindred pastoral collections combine Latin and vernacular texts in an Augustinian mode, guiding clerical and lay readers in the hospital who followed different religious routines alongside and in constant contact with each other.

Chapters 5 and 6 treat the tumultuous late fifteenth century, the Dissolution years, and the two decades following, in which all three institutions were obliged to "adapt or perish," in Rubin's terms. Here I bring together little-studied sixteenth-century polemics, poems, and records to consider how the three hospitals endured critique and dissolution, and, in some cases, reconstituted themselves in a reformed religious world after 1539. Chapter 5, "Poverty, Charity, and Poetry: Critique and Reform before the Dissolution," shows how linked concerns about religious practice, endowment, and poverty coalesced in critiques of English hospitals from the late fourteenth through the mid-sixteenth century. Early critiques articulate positions (both lollard-reformist and establishment-bureaucratic) that adumbrated the dissolution of the religious houses under Henry VIII and Edward VI and in some cases also anticipated reformed visions of the hospital. Having considered this range of critique, and changes in hospital foundation over the course of the fifteenth century, I turn to Robert Copland's *Hye Way to the Spyttell Hous* (ca. 1536). I understand this overlooked poem as central to the debate over hospitals in the early sixteenth century as the fear of "rogues" and "vagabonds" intensified in London. Copland expresses a complex understanding of the hospital's historical role and contemporary predicament in a poem that is central to a literary history of St. Bartholomew's Hospital. In a satirical vein that nevertheless actively searches for answers, Copland asks how St. Bartholomew's might fit as a charitable institution into the increasingly poor, overrun, and religiously reformed world of London.

Building on chapter 5's discussion of representation and critique, chapter 6, "Dissolution, Disappearance, and Refoundation: Textual Strategies of Reconstitution," considers how the hospitals' own textual responses enabled them (in some cases) to survive the dissolutions forced upon them. St. Leonard's Hospital remained visible and viable in York even after the loss of its signature Corpus Christi pageant, contributing to public religious ceremonial and the "worship of the city" up to its surrender in 1539. A unique set of political circumstances conspired to prevent St. Leonard's from reconstitution, but the refoundation and reformation of St. Bartholomew's and St. Mark's into new civic forms depended upon textual means—civic letters, hospital orders, regulations, and new liturgical forms. I juxtapose St. Bartholomew's 1552 *Ordre of the Hospital*, which expresses a fear of "slander" and textualizes the house's officers, procedures, and prayers, with the house's contemporary records, the product of this new system. Despite the seemingly clear-cut categories and exclusions that the *Ordre* creates to forestall sexual scandal, the hospital's records suggest that St. Bartholomew's remained flexible enough to superintend a range of charitable care for women in the neighborhood.

In my epilogue, I speculate about the changed meanings of St. Mark's, Bristol, after its refoundation as a civic chapel in 1540. Repurposing the chapel as a civic institution under mayoral control removed the hospital from the nexus of charity and poor relief into which St. Bartholomew's had been reinserted, yet it returned St. Mark's to visible participation within a reformed religious system, with a former hospital brother as its curate. I suggest that rites for the dead, even if performed according to the radically changed English prayer services, might have retained some of the complex associations with purgatory and intercession that the medieval institution had cultivated. Even as these two hospitals took on significantly changed forms and functions, their historic and textual connections to commemoration, charity, and care persisted well into the early modern period.

# ONE

# St. Leonard's Hospital, Civic Drama, and Women's Devotion

From the late fourteenth century until 1569, the York Corpus Christi cycle's forty-plus episodes dramatized providential history from the *Fall of the Angels* to *Doomsday*. Students of this well-known body of texts are familiar with the pageants as preserved in their late fifteenth-century forms, each associated with an artisan or mercantile sponsor. In this chapter, I recover an earlier form and cultural meaning for the *Purification of the Virgin*, which was originally produced by York's Hospital of St. Leonard. By restoring the link between hospital and pageant, I offer new insights into performance as a means of expressing institutional identity, and I shed fresh light on the Hospital of St. Leonard as a site for cultural production. Theresa Coletti has characterized the late medieval hospital as "a place where performative aspects of religious expression found a venue in a more broadly conceptualized late medieval theater of devotion."[1] I build on this astute observation to show how St. Leonard's intervened in civic life with its own "theater of devotion." A large, venerable foundation, St. Leonard's gathered many social groups into proximity, including regular and secular clerics, the poor and the infirm, widows, and children. The hospital's liturgical life and performance customs gave rise to a pageant that expressed Marian devotion to foreground feminine concerns and rituals within the civic space, demonstrating women's devotions as integral to the hospital's life and worthy of public celebration alongside masculine artisan and mercantile interests. Like the craft and trading companies that sponsored most of the York pageants, this proudly independent religious house developed a biblical drama that reflected and promoted its own interests.[2]

The *Purification* has two important textual witnesses. The first is a cast list (but not a play text) from the 1415 York *Ordo paginarum*. Listed as cast members are the Virgin Mary with Jesus, Joseph, Anna, the midwife with doves, Simeon and his two sons. The second textual witness to this drama consists of a play text, labeled *Purification of the Virgin*, not entered into the York Register until 1567, and differing in some respects from the play suggested in the 1415 cast list. The pageant's early form, judging from the 1415 text, seems to have given particular prominence to female characters: the Virgin Mary, her midwife, and the widowed prophetess Anna. The unique features of the extant 1567 pageant include its conflation of Mary's purification with the churching of women (the new mother's return to church forty days after childbirth) and its emphasis on Anna as a spiritually empowered widow. These features allow us to glimpse a performance that once foregrounded the Virgin Mary and highlighted the importance, to the hospital and the wider urban community, of women's devotional rituals and implicit economic power. This emphasis on women's religious lives as part of York's civic structure had largely disappeared by the later fifteenth century, as the cycle came fully under the control of masculine urban regimes and artisan sponsors.

Looking beneath textual accretions and behind changes of sponsorship, this chapter seeks to understand the relation between the hospital and dramatic performance during the York cycle's early days. Some scholars speculate that local craftspeople developed dramatic pageants as a "devotional enterprise" that was gradually co-opted by civic leaders. Others contend that the organization of the cycle went hand in hand with the city government's organization of craft work in the 1370s, with the corporation creating craft specializations pursuant to the 1363 Statute of Laborers, then assigning thematically appropriate pageants to each artisan guild.[3] Whether one holds to a gradual theory of evolution or subscribes to a "big bang" theory, documents show that the early period of the cycle (1370s through 1460s) featured a greater variety of sponsors and perhaps more extensive participation for women, while the later period (1460s through 1569) saw increasing control by civic authorities together with local artisan and mercantile companies. Not only did St. Leonard's Hospital originate the *Purification*, but the *Coronation of the Virgin* was first sponsored by York's mayor, with both pageants coming under artisan control in the later fifteenth century.[4] By uncovering the prominence of female roles and concerns with the early text, I reconnect the pageant to its hospital context and expand our understanding of women's importance within the early play cycle.[5]

## THE HOSPITAL'S PAGEANT: EARLY DOCUMENTS

The vicissitudes of history have nearly erased the link between the Hospital of St. Leonard and its *Purification* pageant. The earliest reference to the hospital as a pageant sponsor appears in the York *Ordo paginarum*, a civic document of 1415, without identifying the pageant. A second pageant list in the same volume, copied a few years later, assigns St. Leonard's the *Presentation of Christ in the Temple* (*presentacio christi in templo*). Frustratingly, there are no references to a pageant in the hospital's own extant records.[6] In 1477, York's mayor reassigned the *Purification of the Virgin* pageant (*pagina pureficacionis beate Mariae virginis*), presumably after a period of nonperformance, to the artisan groups of Masons and Laborers, yet made no mention of St. Leonard's as its original sponsor.[7] To complicate matters further, the extant pageant text is a very late copy, not entered into the York Register until 1567.[8] Thus no airtight evidence exists to prove either that St. Leonard's produced a *Purification* or that the late text has any relation to the hospital's pageant as performed over sixty years earlier. Yet these are precisely the connections that I shall draw, arguing that the later fifteenth-century play text preserves significant material from the hospital's pageant as it may have looked in its early days. My argument relies upon close scrutiny and new interpretation of the pageant text in comparison with other vernacular *Purification* pageants, together with deduction from relevant civic and hospital documents.

The key civic document, which for my purposes establishes the hospital's early pageant as a depiction of Mary's purification, is the *Ordo paginarum*, the "order of pageants" included at the back of York's A/Y Memorandum Book, dated 1415. This difficult text, much revised during the fifteenth century, later damaged by flood and vandals, was compiled by York's common clerk. Meg Twycross has argued that "the second and third decades of the fifteenth century were a time of drastic change in the organization and content of the Corpus Christi Play. . . . The very existence of the *Ordo* suggests that it had reached a stage where some kind of increased control was felt necessary."[9] The *Ordo* contains a list of pageants together with guild sponsors, apparently designed to serve as a "working checklist" of plays for the city's use.[10] Updated over the years as some pageants were merged, eliminated, or changed sponsors, the *Ordo*'s descriptions offer "a cast list" for each pageant.[11] Twycross notes that it is "an historical document which more than most reflects the processes of *change* in the event it records."[12] Among other changes are many disparities between the contents of these lists and the pageants as they survive today. One such disparity will be central to my argument for how the *Purification* pageant evolved away from its original form as a Mary-focused hospital drama into a Christ-focused artisan drama.

My discussion picks up on Sue Niebrzydowski's tantalizing specula-tion that a freestanding play celebrating the Virgin's purification "may lie behind the entry in the York *Ordo Paginarum* of 1415."[13] The *Ordo* descrip-tion provides the only firm evidence for how the hospital's pageant looked in 1415. Featuring the Virgin Mary, her midwife, and the widow Anna, this early version makes women visible as mother, caregiver, and widow. The de-scription reads, "Maria cum puero Iosep Anna obstetrix cum pullis colum-barum, Symeon recipiens puerum in vlnas suas & duo filij Symeonis" (Mary with the boy, Joseph, Anna, the midwife with the young doves, Simeon re-ceiving the child into his arms, and the two sons of Simeon).[14] Noting the "static quality" of the descriptions, Twycross suggests that the pageants might at this point have occupied "a sort of halfway house between tableau and play."[15] Given the various references to speeches throughout the *Ordo* and the definite reference to "materia loquelarum" (pageant speeches) in a document of 1422, my reconstruction of the 1415 pageant will follow this line of argument, positing speeches that perhaps punctuated an otherwise largely "static" tableau.[16]

As Twycross's detective work has shown, Mary's prominence in the St. Leonard's description is reflected elsewhere in the *Ordo*, where a slightly later hand (probably that of city clerk Roger Burton) has moved "Maria" to the head of the description for the mayor's pageant (the *Coronation of the Virgin*), "displacing respectively 'Angelus' (Gabriel), 'Iosep,' and 'Ihesus.'"[17] This alteration suggests that Burton wished to establish Mary as the "focal point" of the mayor's pageant, consistent with her prominence in the St. Leonard's pageant description.[18] Although the *Ordo* description clearly de-lineates the hospital as pageant producer (later crossed out and replaced

with "iam Masons" (formerly masons), presumably after the 1477 reassignment, the *Ordo* gives the pageant no name. Pageant identifications appear in
a second, slightly later list of the pageants, copied onto fol. 255r. This brief
list, written by Burton some time before 1421/22, attributes to St. Leonard's
the episode of *Presentacio christi in templo*.[19] Mary's purification and Christ's
presentation at the Temple were intertwined events celebrated on the same
day; it is therefore not surprising that Burton used "presentacio" to name
the pageant described in the *Ordo*. Though he tinkered with the *Coronation*
description, Burton seems not to have altered the *Ordo* description of
St. Leonard's pageant, preserving its intentional foregrounding of Mary,
her midwife, and the widow Anna.

## PURIFICATION AND PRESENTATION:
## ORIGINS AND REPRESENTATIONS

In order to place the *Ordo* and the extant pageant into a precise relation to
each other, we need to understand what is meant by the terms "purification
of the Virgin" and "presentation of Christ" and how these rituals were commemorated in English liturgical and dramatic practices. Mary's purification and Christ's presentation are overlapping events in Luke's Gospel,
both deriving from the demands of Mosaic law. These two events provide
the narrative backbone for the dramatic representations that later developed. Leviticus 12:6–8 requires the postpartum woman to wait seven days
after childbirth to resume sexual intercourse, then another thirty-three for
a boy child or sixty-six for a girl before coming to the Temple with an offering for the priest:

> And when the days of her purification are expired, for a son, or for a
> daughter, she shall bring to the door of the tabernacle of the testimony,
> a lamb of a year old for a holocaust, and a young pigeon or a turtle for
> sin, and shall deliver them to the priest: Who shall offer them before the
> Lord, and shall pray for her, and so she shall be cleansed from the issue
> of her blood. . . . And if her hand find not sufficiency, and she is not able
> to offer a lamb, she shall take two turtles, or two young pigeons, one for
> a holocaust, and another for sin: and the priest shall pray for her, and so
> she shall be cleansed.[20]

Luke's Gospel describes Mary's appearance at the Temple forty days after Christ's birth for her purification ritual and for the presentation of Jesus. Luke represents Mary's purification as coinciding with the ritual presentation of the firstborn at the Temple, but strictly speaking these two rituals should have occurred ten days apart. Exodus 13:2 requires, "Sanctify unto me every firstborn that openeth the womb among the children of Israel, as well of men as of beasts." Numbers 18:15–16 specifies, "Only for the first-born of man thou shalt take a price, and every beast that is unclean thou shalt cause to be redeemed. And the redemption of it shall be *after one month*, for five sicles of silver" (emphasis added). Dorothy C. Schorr notes, "St. Luke's account, which describes the two ceremonies as occurring at the same time, does not correspond to the practice as laid down by the Mosaic law" (Luke 2:22–28).[21] Although Mary's virginal conception technically rendered her purification unnecessary, she dutifully follows the law and appears at the temple:

> And after the days of her purification, according to the law of Moses, were accomplished, they carried him to Jerusalem, to present him to the Lord. As it is written in the law of the Lord: Every male opening the womb shall be called holy in the Lord. And to offer a sacrifice, according as it is written in the law of the Lord, a pair of turtledoves, or two young pigeons. And behold there was a man in Jerusalem named Simeon, and this man was just and devout, waiting for the consolation of Israel; and the Holy Ghost was in him. And he had received an answer from the Holy Ghost, that he should not see death, before he had seen the Christ of the Lord. . . . And when his parents brought in the child Jesus, to do for him according to the custom of the Law, he [Simeon] also took him into his arms, and blessed God.

In the Gospel narrative, Mary's purification and Christ's presentation overlap, with the offering of turtledoves serving for both Mary and Jesus. After Christ is handed to Simeon for a blessing, the widow Anna appears: "And there was one Anna, a prophetess, the daughter of Phanuel, of the tribe of Aser; she was far advanced in years, and had lived with her husband seven years from her virginity. And she was a widow until fourscore and four years; who departed not from the temple, by fastings and prayers serving night and day. Now she, at the same hour, coming in, confessed to the Lord: and spoke of him to all that looked for the redemption of Israel" (Luke 2:36–38). Here we have an outline of the cast of characters and a sense of how these two sacred events intertwined.

As Luke's vision of this composite event came to be commemorated in liturgy, the Western Church developed a feast celebrating both the Presentation and the Purification. By the seventh century, an early February Roman feast of purification had been replaced with a Christian festival and candle procession in honor of the Virgin, heralding the English term "Candlemas."[22] Blessing of the candles held in the procession was incorporated into the liturgy in the eleventh century, at which point the feast came to be denoted simply the Purification.[23] Yet as Schorr demonstrates, the Western iconographic tradition chiefly focused on Mary's handing of Christ to Simeon, who came to be garbed as a priest. Karl Young contends of the Purification that "in the Western church it assumed the character of a feast of Christ rather than of his Mother."[24]

Although the feast was known as the Purification, medieval English liturgies tend to privilege Christ over Mary, even as they show significant reverence toward the mother of God. In the York *Purificatio Beatae Mariae* Mass, the presentation of Christ is mentioned first, with Simeon's embrace of the child recalled repeatedly during the service. Mary is invoked as Christ's bearer and later addressed with antiphons at her own altar. She receives sequences lauding her virginity and showering her with epithets, such as "decus mundi, regina caeli" (glory of the world, queen of heaven).[25] Son and mother receive veneration in descending degrees: Christ appears as the "light unto the gentiles," recalling Simeon's words, while Mary remains the vessel who "bears the king of glory."[26]

Though Christ received precedence in the York liturgy, Mary sometimes took a starring role in extraliturgical performance. A procession mounted by Beverley's Candlemas Guild of St. Mary, described in a guild certificate of 1388–89, included "omnes fratres et sorores gilde" (all the brothers and sisters of the guild) led by "quidam de gilda qui ad hoc aptior inuenietur, nobilissime et decentur vestitus et ornatus vt Regina Virgo instar gloriose Virginis Marie, habens quasi Filium in vlnis suis" (one of the guild who shall be found most fitting, dressed nobly and beautifully as the Virgin Queen, like to the glorious Virgin Mary, having what may seem a son in her arms).[27] Here, in a religious guild production, the Virgin in glory occupies the primary position, while Jesus, "what may seem a son," though necessary to the tableau, goes unnamed, functioning primarily as a prop, an adjunct to her stunning presence.[28]

Perhaps owing to the popularity of the Purification feast and related local devotions, Mary's purification came to feature prominently in the English vernacular drama as well. Although not every known dramatic cycle featured a Purification, the episode appears in the extant dramatic texts of York, Towneley, Coventry, Chester, and N-Town.[29] A freestanding example also survives in the "Candlemes Day and the Kyllyng of þe Children of Israelle" from the East Anglian Digby manuscript (Oxford, Bodleian MS Digby 133). We cannot be certain of the auspices for all these plays, yet we can discern a latent tension between the Purification and the Presentation played out in the thematic differences among them. Religious groups, whether monastic foundations or devotional guilds, tend to cast Mary as a heavenly queen with numinous power, reinforcing connections to Candlemas. In contrast, *Purification* plays associated with artisan production tend to highlight the encounter between Christ and Simeon, privileging masculine spiritual experience and knowledge.

The thematic emphases of these pageants are consistent with the concerns of their larger compilations or cycles, which were produced by varying groups with disparate interests. As Gail McMurray Gibson has shown, the plays of the N-Town compilation, once thought to have a monastic origin, and more recently associated with a religious guild, place the life of Mary at their center, privileging female relationships and rendering "the Virgin Mary—perhaps even more than Christ himself—the very emblem of Christian mystery."[30] The Digby Candlemas play is also linked to religious auspices, perhaps produced by Bury St. Edmunds's prominent Alderman's or Candlemas Guild, a religious fraternity that "probably exhibited a commitment to ceremonial practices, especially on festive occasions associated with its dedication to the Virgin Mary's Purification."[31] In contrast, the northern cycles associated with artisan production (York, Chester, and Coventry) channel their expressions of devotion differently, foregrounding the concerns of the master craftsmen who produced them: company membership, localism, and distinctions between master craftsmen and others, particularly apprentices and women.[32] What makes the York *Purification* unique (and uniquely problematic) is its movement from religious to artisan auspices, a transition that I argue is detectable in the palimpsestic text that remains.

Purification pageants organized by religious groups evince a striking interest in venerating Mary. The East Anglian Digby Candlemas pageant opens by praising Mary as "this glorious maiden doughter vnto Anna, / . . . And by resemblaunce likenyd vnto manna, / . . . Chosyn for to bere mankyndes Savyoure, / With a prerogative aboue each creature!"[33] From the start, Mary's glory, beauty, and native rights eclipse those of all others, except Christ. In the *Purification* pageant from the N-Town compilation, Simeon and Anna hail Mary just after they greet Jesus: "All heyl also, Mary bryght! / All heyl, salver of seknes! / All heyl, lanterne of lyght! / All heyl, thu modyr of mekenes!" Though carefully placing Mary second to Christ ("also"), the Temple-dwellers credit Mary with healing power and draw attention to the "lyght" associated with Candlemas.[34] Later Joseph explicitly enfolds the presentation of Christ within the iconography of Candlemas: "Take here these candelys thre— / Mary, Symeon, and Anne— / And I shal take the fowrte to me / To offre oure childe up, thanne" (163–66). Thus even in acknowledging Christ as savior, both pageants cast Mary as their brightest star.

In contrast, within the artisan-sponsored cycles that dramatize biblical episodes, *Purification* pageants tend to downplay Mary's power and highlight bonds among men. Along with York, Coventry and Chester are the two cycles firmly associated with craft sponsorship.[35] Brandon Alakas shows how the Coventry Weavers' pageant, which combines the Purification/Presentation with Christ and the Doctors, locates these episodes within the contexts of "the craft fellowship, the household, and the civic council," working to contain threats to the "hierarchy of authority" on each front.[36] Mary and Joseph appear as a couple reminiscent of fabliau, with Mary nagging Joseph to go find the "turtyll dowis" for their ritual offering, while Joseph draws upon misogynist stereotypes to rally other men in sympathy for his plight. He complains,

> How sey ye all this cumpany
> Thatt be weddid asse well ass I?
> I wene þat ye suffur moche woo;
> For he thatt weddyth a yonge thyng
> Must fulfyll all hir byddyng,
> Or els ma he his handis wryng.
> (461–66)[37]

Even as it sets Mary and Joseph at odds, the Weavers' pageant emphasizes the search for harmony between masters and apprentices, framing the action with a senior and a junior prophet speaking to each other as master to apprentice.[38]

York is the only English town where we can trace a single pageant's transition from religious to artisan auspices.[39] The thematic differences between religious- and artisan-sponsored *Purification* pageants are encapsulated in miniature in the changes from the hospital's early Marian pageant, commemorating her purification, to the later form the pageant took when reassigned to artisan groups. These changes may have come about during the effort around 1476 to consolidate the Corpus Christi play into a civic event expressing a thoroughly masculine, commercial orientation.[40] In 1476–77, the mayor and civic authorities were, in Richard Beadle's words, "paying special attention to the organization and indeed the integrity of the Play."[41] The mayor issued a decree requiring auditions for actors, and two Marian pageants were revived and reassigned: the *Purification of the Virgin* and the *Funeral of the Virgin*.[42] The *Purification* was to be sponsored by York's Masons and Laborers and the *Funeral* by the Linenweavers. Beadle speculates that at a moment when the city was cultivating its relationship with Richard of Gloucester, the "good lord" influential in installing both Mayor Thomas Wrangwish and the Common Clerk Nicholas Lancaster, the play was "not only to be spruced up, but it was to be relaunched with its entire repertoire fully functioning."[43] The Marian plays were required to complete the cycle's "entire repertoire," yet their feminine devotional emphases may have fit awkwardly within a cycle emphasizing masculine control and patronage. The *Purification* required some revision, as I will suggest in the next section. As I have argued elsewhere, the York pageants in their late fifteenth-century forms consistently perform male artisan concerns about mastership, knowledge, and local belonging.[44] After considering what remains in the extant text, I work to recover what has been lost: the links among the hospital, the text, and the female communities that the pageant once celebrated.

## THE LATER PAGEANT: ARTISAN REVISIONS

The surviving pageant text looks very different from what is suggested by the *Ordo* description of 1415. Mary's midwife has disappeared, as have the sons of Simeon. A Temple priest and an angel have appeared in the pageant, both with significant speaking parts. The pageant's sequence of events conforms roughly to Luke's narrative, except that whereas the prophetess Anna appeared after the Presentation in the Gospel, in the pageant Anna appears and speaks before Simeon. The priest opens the play with a lengthy speech detailing ritual purification requirements that are later repeated by Joseph. After Anna speaks, introducing herself and prophesying Christ's birth, Simeon offers a very long speech, first bemoaning his physical weakness, then anticipating the Messiah's arrival. Mary and Joseph appear, discussing her purification, and then ritually present Christ to the priest, who proceeds to praise the "blyssyd babb" at length. These praises are followed by thanksgiving from Anna and Simeon, who, after a brief conversation between Mary and Joseph, concludes the pageant with a long benediction.

The extant text presents numerous challenges to an archaeological reading that might reveal older strata and newer areas of revision. As Beadle has noted, its stanzaic forms are more varied than those of any other York pageant: these include quatrains, octaves, tail-rhyme stanzas, and a complex nine-line stanza.[45] Stanzaic forms often vary even within a single character's speech, and the meanings of these variations are hard to interpret. Since the Temple priest did not appear in the *Ordo* cast list, I assume that his speeches were added to this later version. I speculate that the same is true for the angel, who has two similar speeches at intervals (lines 165–74 and 340–44), both addressing "Olde Symeon," in which he urges the elderly man to enter the Temple and welcome Christ. These deductions help to narrow the scope of the pageant slightly, but it is impossible to associate particular stanzaic forms with older or more recent strata of the text, because one finds the same forms used both by original (for example, Simeon) and added characters (for example, the Temple priest).

In addition to noting speeches that probably did not appear in the 1415 version of the pageant, attending to duplicated material and internal thematic variations may also help us to detect which sections were revised to reflect the reassignment of the *Purification* to the Masons and Laborers in 1477. Beadle suggests that the text performed by the Masons and Laborers replaced "the lost or superseded version formerly brought forth by St Leonard's."[46] I suggest that what survives today is not a wholly new text, but a palimpsest or composite, a work revised for artisan sponsorship but still bearing some traces of its earlier form as hospital drama. Rather than commissioning a wholly new play script, the Masons and Laborers could have

obtained an existing text from the hospital when they received their play as-
signment and then subsequently revised the text. This scenario becomes
plausible in view of the close connections between local masons and the
hospital during this period. As Sheila Christie points out, like York Minster,
St. Leonard's was a large complex of stone buildings needing frequent re-
pair, and it hosted an on-site masons' lodge.[47] Masons were thus an integral
part of the hospital community. Offering an alternative possibility for the
Masons' history of dramatic production, Christie has even speculated that
perhaps from 1477 "the pageant remained the responsibility of St Leonard's,
but became specifically associated with the masons whose lodge served the
hospital."[48] Although the lack of documentary evidence makes this theory
impossible to prove, Christie's argument posits a relation of cooperation between hospital and Masons that would have facilitated the transfer of materials associated with the pageant. Whether or not the Masons and Laborers
produced the pageant independently of the hospital, it is logical to suppose
that they built upon the hospital's existing text to fashion their own artisan-
inflected performance.

Although it is impossible to know exactly how the pageant's speeches
looked in 1415, we can be fairly sure, given that the priest and angel do not
appear in the *Ordo paginarum*, that these characters' speeches were not
originally included. In keeping with the change from religious to craft
sponsorship, the male artisans who took over the York *Purification* probably revised the pageant to heighten the emphasis on the male encounter
with divinity that is found in other artisan *Purification* pageants. Pamela
King contends that the York pageant's emphasis on the encounter between
Simeon and Christ (the *hypapante* in the Eastern Church), with its Eucharistic resonances, was "probably always" present in the York *Purification*, but I suggest that the 1477 change in sponsorship led to a significant
alteration in dramatic representation.[49] We cannot know what changes
might have been made between 1477 and 1567, but we can see that the
extant York *Purification* highlights artisan identity in particular ways. The
most salient, for it comes early on, is the emphasis within Simeon's opening speech on his aging masculine body in relation to productivity and
livelihood.

Simeon's first speech has the main purpose of expressing his longing to
see the Messiah before he dies. About midway through his speech, Simeon
expresses the pain associated with this long wait:

A lorde God, I thynke may I endure,
Trowe we that babb shall fynde me here;
Nowe certys, with aige I ame so power
That ever it abaites my chere.
(141–44)[50]

He grows increasingly desperate:

A, trowes thowe these ij eyes shall see
That blyssed babb or they be owte?
Ye, I pray God so myght it be—
Then were I putt all owte of dowte.
(161–64)

Whereas the biblical account simply references Simeon's hope to see the Messiah before he dies, the drama enables Simeon to voice his increasing anxiety as he waits.

His speech proves to be so long (seventy-seven lines, far longer than similar comments in any other *Purification* pageant) that one can imagine it straining an audience's attention.[51] This speech would function perfectly well as a set piece of lament were it to begin with "A lorde God" and finish with "owte of dowte," the lines cited above. Yet at the very outset of his speech, even before the lines just quoted, Simeon has spent two stanzas bemoaning the ravages of age upon his body, in lines that are not strictly necessary to convey his age or his eagerness to see the Messiah, but that would be particularly poignant in an artisan drama. He laments,

For I am wayke and all vnwelde,
My welth ay wayns and passeth away,
Whereso I fayre in fyrth or feylde,
I fall ay downe for febyll, in fay.
(91–94)

This emphasis on male physical weakness in connection with economic loss is also salient in the Chester and Coventry pageants, the other *Purification* dramas securely associated with artisan production.[52] The Chester *Purification*, produced by the town's Smiths, presents Simeon (more traditionally) as a priest but also emphasizes the toll taken by waning masculinity:

> Mightie God, have mynd on me,
> That most art in majestee.
> For many a winter have I bee
> preist in Jerusalem.
> Myche teene and incommoditie
> followeth age, full well I see,
> and nowe that fytt may I not flee,
> thinke me never so swem.
>                                   (1–8)

Here Simeon speaks more metaphorically, yet his language still evokes work and the market, deploring the physical pain ("teene") and economic losses ("incommoditie") that "follow" old age.[53] In the Coventry Weavers' pageant, which begins by juxtaposing older and younger prophets, Simeon is portrayed as a priest, but one for whom old age brings with it pain and "decrepitude," as he begs,

> Yett, Lorde, þi grace to me now extende:
> Suffur me rathur yett to lyve in peyne
> Then to dy or [before] thatt I thatt solam syght haue seyne.
>                    (Weaver's pageant, lines 214–16)[54]

Given these close parallels between the two artisan versions, which both present old age as a painful and (implicitly) economically draining loss of physical powers, this particular line of emphasis in York would seem to derive from the revision for artisan production. With the addition of a Temple priest in the later version, Simeon's lay status becomes more evident by contrast: he clearly adumbrates a worker, one whose ailing body will, he hopes, be revived by the infant Christ.

The Laborers and Masons were newcomers to this pageant in 1477 and may have revised the text to highlight the role of their crafts in a version of salvation history that, like other artisan productions, emphasizes Christ's importance over Mary's. Their cosponsorship of a pageant in 1477 represented a new level of organization on the part of both crafts, the Laborers in particular. Yet the pageant looked different in its earlier fifteenth-century form, lacking the Temple priest, the angel, and probably parts of Simeon's speech. How might this early version have sounded and signified as a hospital drama, before it became an artisan drama? If we attempt to reconstruct this earlier version using the 1415 *Ordo* description, hospital records, and the extant pageant minus the sections almost certainly added later, then a different kind of performance begins to emerge. Emphasizing links between the early pageant and two key life stages for late medieval English women—churching after childbirth and pious widowhood—in what follows I connect this early version to the hospital's fifteenth-century culture and practices.

ST. LEONARD'S HOSPITAL AND
THE DRAMA OF PURIFICATION

The Purification of the Virgin was clearly an event ripe for dramatic performance, but the link between St. Leonard's and the episode has not been well understood or fully investigated. "How a religious house rather than a craft came to be associated with it is a matter for speculation," notes Beadle.[55] I contend that this particular performance emerged from the institution's devotion to the Virgin Mary and St. Leonard, promoting the hospital's devotional and charitable functions, in which women featured prominently, as integral to civic life. As Christie argues of the Masons' involvement in the Corpus Christi play, drama might function as a means of civic participation by those outside craft or franchise membership, expressing "a conception of civic identity that could expand beyond the jurisdictional limits of the franchise to encompass the social community of the city as a whole."[56] This capacious conception of civic identity may help us to recover the origins and function of St. Leonard's *Purification* pageant.

As I noted in the introduction, St. Leonard's Hospital was a large, complex institution that combined liturgical functions with the care of patients. It housed religious and secular personnel and residents of both sexes, including the ill, the poor, aged priests, retired laypeople, and children. Although the hospital was well known for sheltering orphans, we do not find any references to the care of pregnant women in its surviving records. One grant of a church income specified that the money was to support the hospital in "ministering to the poor and sick, and to infants exposed there," indicating that these infants were foundlings, not born at the hospital.[57] Building upon its existing religious performance traditions, sponsorship of a pageant in the cycle may have helped the house to gain attention within the broader York community, functioning to promote the hospital's mission and distinguish it from other local charitable institutions.

St. Leonard's participated visibly in York's annual civic celebration of Corpus Christi, perhaps before adopting a pageant in the annual play. The hospital played a major role in the annual Corpus Christi procession, an event attested from the late fourteenth century and originally taking place on Corpus Christi Day, before the play began.[58] In the procession, representatives of the church, city government, and guilds followed the consecrated Host through the city with lighted torches. The procession ended at St. Leonard's, where the Host was deposited. Beadle plausibly suggests that "this association with the procession may have led the hospital to identify itself with the civic celebrations of Corpus Christi to the extent of adopting one of the pageants."[59]

Complementing its association with the Corpus Christi procession, St. Leonard's had a tradition of in-house performance for major feasts. The hospital's fragmentary records indicate festive performances occurring from at least 1370. In that year, the hospital paid "various men" to perform an "interlude" at Christmas, throughout the 1370s minstrels were hired to celebrate the Feast of St. Leonard, and in 1385 two minstrels performed on the occasion of the Virgin Mary's purification.[60] The Feast of the Purification was one of the great Marian feasts, privileged at other hospitals as well. For example, Florence's Hospital of Santa Maria Nuova celebrated the Purification as one of its three main feasts.[61] At St. Leonard's, an existing tradition of performance for the Purification suggests a basis for an official pageant in the annual civic play, a performance that would both consolidate and publicize the hospital's civic identity. One can imagine that the hospital, with its numerous personnel and choirboys to play the dramatic roles and sing, with its ecclesiastical vestments for costumes, would only have had to pay for construction and decoration of a pageant wagon in order to mount an impressive production.

Who performed in the hospital's early pageant? If we make an analogy to other York cycle pageants, in which roles were largely played by company members, with occasional extraguild artisans, priests, and singers, it seems likely that male hospital personnel acted in the pageant. Pamela King has speculated that the role of Simeon was played by a cleric in the early version.[62] We have scattered evidence of women performing in the urban cycles, most famously in the lost Chester Wives' *Assumption* play, and also under religious auspices, in convent and parish dramas.[63] It is thus plausible that sisters or laywomen residents played female roles in the York *Purification*, during a period when, James Stokes argues, "women participated (as actors, producers, and patrons) in every performative aspect of local culture."[64] The character of the early *Purification*, the production of a mixed-gender religious institution within the civic space, recalls the aforementioned male and female Purification procession of Beverley. In that procession, the "one most fitting, dressed nobly and beautifully as the Virgin Queen" would almost certainly have been a woman performer.[65]

Although the connection between St. Leonard's and the *Purification* has puzzled some scholars, this conjunction is a logical one, for the pageant seems to have emerged from the hospital's devotion to the Virgin and St. Leonard.[66] As Carole Rawcliffe has noted, devotion to the Virgin was pervasive in medieval English hospitals: Mary was "a ubiquitous presence in the wall paintings, statuary and altar-pieces of hospital chapels and infirmaries throughout Christendom."[67] St. Leonard's evidently viewed the Purification as a feast day worthy of performance, and on a daily basis, the Virgin Mary featured prominently in the hospital's liturgical practice. The foundation's 1294 ordinances, attributed to Master Walter de Langton, require liturgical veneration of Mary to punctuate the day. The ordinances direct that after matins and the Mass every day, at least four brothers "intersint missae Virginis gloriosae, a principio usque ad finem" (shall take part in the Mass of the glorious Virgin, from beginning to end).[68] Considering that by this period the Mass of the Virgin had become an elaborate polyphonic affair in many churches, this requirement indicates the resources that the hospital devoted to Marian worship.[69] After dinner, hymns and antiphons were to be sung to Mary at an altar dedicated to her; the hospital church also featured a "porticus beatae Virginis" (porch of the Virgin).[70] In requiring the brothers to say the "Salve Regina, vel aliquam aliam Antiphonum Virginis gloriosae solempnem coram altari ejusdem Virginis" (Salve Regina, or some other solemn antiphon of the glorious Virgin before the altar of that same Virgin), the statutes assume a repertoire of Marian music.[71] Such a repertoire, and a standing choir, would come in handy for the performance of a pageant containing significant liturgical music. We see evidence of devotion to the hospital's Lady altar: John de Stokeslay, a priest and recluse associated with the hospital, made a personal bequest in 1400 to the altar of the Virgin.[72]

In view of St. Leonard's tradition of Marian devotion, one can readily see how producing a *Purification* pageant might broadcast the house's customs of honoring "the glorious Virgin" into the civic realm.[73] The dedication to St. Leonard is also related to the subject of the Purification and complementary with the institution's Marian devotion. In the realm of religious practice and popular belief, the Virgin and St. Leonard were both renowned protectors of pregnant women. Prayer scrolls, girdles, and amulets frequently invoked the Virgin's aid for an easy delivery, and St. Leonard too had a connection to childbirth.[74] Numerous hospitals across medieval England were dedicated to St. Leonard, a sixth-century French hermit, nephew of Emperor Clovis.[75] His patronage of pregnant women derives from an episode in which his prayers brought Clovis's wife to a safe delivery. In the *vita*, Leonard shows a pronounced devotion to the Virgin Mary. After being rewarded by Clovis with a forest in which to build a monastery, Leonard founds an oratory in the Virgin's honor.[76] This gesture suggests an enduring link between St. Leonard and devotion to the Virgin such as we see in the hospital's liturgical life.[77] The hospital's own customs explicitly linked devotion to St. Leonard and the Virgin Mary. When lay brothers joined the house, their profession included a vow to serve God, the Virgin, and St. Leonard, and to serve the poor to the best of their ability; the sisters made a similar profession.[78] A connection between Leonard and childbirth is evident elsewhere in medieval England. Katherine French notes that after childbirth, women in Newbury, Berkshire, made offerings in "a hospital chapel dedicated to St. Leonard."[79] Given the hospital's devotion to St. Leonard and Mary, the relation between these two saints, and their traditional appeal to women, it was fitting for St. Leonard's to adopt the *Purification* as a means to project its devotional identity into the civic sphere and appeal to devout citizens, perhaps women in particular.

Mounting the *Purification* pageant in the Corpus Christi play might also have helped St. Leonard's to maintain its visibility in York during the financially challenging late fourteenth century. During this period, the need to compete in the charitable marketplace became acute. Isolated records show local individuals' continued support for St. Leonard's during the last decades of the fourteenth century,[80] but masters of the 1390s mismanaged the house's finances at the very moment when the larger York economy was beginning to improve and local citizens starting to have more money to donate. During the 1390s, the hospital began selling large numbers of corrodies (support packages for older individuals), many of which proved more costly than expected. By 1399, the hospital owed the resident poor almost £100 in arrears of money and food,[81] and Master William Waltham petitioned the king for permission to stop all payments except to the house's resident hermits and paupers.[82]

During this difficult turn-of-the-century period, when St. Leonard's most needed support, the city saw a boom in new private charitable foundations that began to siphon off benefactions to older foundations like St. Leonard's.[83] A particularly popular new type of foundation was the maison-dieu, a house or part of a property endowed to support a small number of poor, infirm, or otherwise vulnerable people. It became common in the later years of the fourteenth century for citizens to give small bequests in their wills to each of the city's maisons-dieu.[84] Women were newly prominent in the foundation of maisons-dieu, which were cheaper to endow and maintain, sometimes located simply in an individual's house or garden.[85] Probate evidence shows that not only were women more generous than men with their bequests, even when they had fewer means, but they particularly tended to support institutions with primarily female inhabitants.[86] Female residents often populated maisons-dieu, some of which were reserved for vulnerable women, sometimes widows in particular.[87] Moreover, after 1380, the local hospital of St. Nicholas began to accept women residents only and may thus have become a more appealing target than St. Leonard's for local women's donations.[88] Cullum speculates that around the turn of the century, more people wanted to found or donate to newer institutions, while older institutions suffered a "neglect bred by familiarity."[89] Would-be donors may have looked elsewhere because they disapproved of the practices at St. Leonard's, which was increasingly selling its beds rather than giving places freely to the poor.

The form that the early *Purification* performance took, featuring Mary with her midwife and placing the widow Anna in a prominent position, indeed first to appear in the pageant, highlighted the hospital's function in the community and its physical and spiritual care of women. To present Mary as a mother with her midwife is to connect her with the familiar women's ritual of churching, a representational choice that promotes identification from female audience members, most of whom would have personally experienced this ritual. (In suggesting that the pageant created a visual link between Mary's purification and ordinary women's churching, I am not, however, arguing that St. Leonard's was advertising itself as a site for churching, a closely guarded parochial privilege because of the income involved.[90]) To present Anna explicitly, as no other extant *Purification* pageant does, as a widow living in religious retirement, linked this figure to contemporary widows who lived in and around the hospital—highlighting the hospital as a place of holy retirement and celebrating such women's devotions within the civic sphere.

## MARY'S PURIFICATION AND THE CHURCHING OF WOMEN

In my effort to excavate the hospital's original *Purification* pageant, I assume that the work drew to some degree upon the institution's liturgical and festive traditions that I have outlined thus far. Although the authorship of the plays remains unknown, Alexandra Johnston's speculation about the influence of York's Augustinian friars over the texts is suggestive for understanding how the pageant might have emerged from the hospital setting. Johnson discerns a certain theological and literary consistency in the cycle's texts, even over their many years of revision and change, finding "a remarkable theological and philosophical sophistication on the part of the playwright, or playwrights, steeped in the learning of the Fathers (particularly Augustine) for both its theoretical framework and specific theological insights."[91] Johnston speculates that this continuity may indicate participation by York's Austin friars in the composition and revision of pageant texts. The friars, whose house was located just across the street from the hospital, possessed a late medieval library of nearly 500 volumes, the largest recorded for York. Of the later Marian pageants, Johnson notes that "the Friary possessed the major patristic writings on the Virgin Mary that embellish her story with the details dramatised in the plays of the *Death*, *Assumption* and *Coronation of the Virgin*."[92] Numerous contents among the library volumes could have also provided material and inspiration for the *Purification*, including texts and commentaries on the relevant biblical sections (Leviticus and Luke) and material on the Virgin Mary, including Hugh of St. Victor's treatise "de virginitate beate Marie" and Anselm's "de laude virginis Marie."[93] The library's books also included material on women's life stages, including Augustine's "de bono coniugali" and "de bono viduitatis" in one volume.[94] Such texts might have helped to give language for the *Purification* as it simultaneously evoked the Virgin Mary's life and the customs of secular women, as I show in the remainder of this chapter.

Together with St. Leonard's liturgical traditions, the 1415 *Ordo* description, with its inclusion of a midwife, strongly suggests that the hospital's early pageant blended liturgical devotion to the Virgin with the trappings of a late medieval churching, a celebration forty days after childbirth, in which mothers received a purification echoing the Virgin's. In the *Ordo* description, the term *obstetrix* creates a link between Mary's purification and the postpartum ritual familiar to late medieval women. The churching ceremony has been subject to varied modern interpretations, some emphasizing the aspect of ritual purification imposed by men upon women, others stressing the ceremony's complex social function and appeal for women.[95] Becky Lee argues of medieval English churching that the ceremony combined "themes of transition or integration, purification, and thanksgiving."[96] Late medieval people were probably unconcerned to disentangle these intertwined threads. The aspect of celebratory thanksgiving was prominent in the service, which commenced after the new mother had processed to her parish church with her midwife and female friends. The women were met at the church door by the priest, who took the new mother's hand and welcomed her inside. The short liturgy, performed in conjunction with a Mass, might vary in its content but always included Psalm 120, beginning, "I have lifted up my eyes to the mountains, from which help shall come to me."[97]

The churching ceremony, the mother's first church visit since childbirth, without her baby, was generally a festive occasion for the women involved.[98] Gibson notes that churching was "the only liturgical ceremony in the medieval church provided by the clergy for women only," one in which "men remained literally marginal, on the outskirts of the ceremony and its meaning."[99] Churching sacralized the motherhood of ordinary women, and the shared ritual of processing with candles worked, in Gibson's terms, to connect "the purity of Mary's body" with "the ritual purification of the individual female body."[100] Such links were made explicit in the churching ceremony, which often culminated with the mother placing her lighted candle on her church's Lady altar.[101]

Given the familiarity and frequency of the churching ritual, the inclusion of an *obstetrix* in the *Purification* pageant as of 1415 seems to be intentional, not merely a scribal idiosyncrasy, as Beadle implies. He suggests that the term "midwife (*obstetrix*) was evidently the compiler's way of describing the maidservant who is sometimes shown accompanying the holy family in late medieval pictorial representations of the episode."[102] But why write *obstetrix* if *ancilla* was intended? The *Ordo paginarum* scribe recognized the figure as a midwife, central to the episode. No midwives are mentioned in Luke's account of Christ's birth, but the apocryphal "infancy gospels" told the Nativity story featuring two midwives, who found their way into medieval visual art and drama, including Latin religious plays.[103] We find midwives in the N-Town and Chester *Nativity* pageants: Denise Ryan shows that both pageants dramatize the midwife's role as one who authenticated the virgin birth and in her professional capacity "stamped the occasion with propriety."[104] The midwives of the Chester *Nativity* serve a combined devotional and civic function: in testing and testifying to Mary's virginity, they serve as "guardians of the civic honour in relation to the rites of childbirth."[105]

It was not an eccentric choice to feature a midwife at the events surrounding Mary's childbirth, but an intentional means of connecting Mary's maternity with the devotional concerns and life cycles of contemporary women. Elsewhere in the York cycle, whereas the extant York Tilers' *Nativity* pageant contains no midwives, the 1415 *Ordo paginarum* description of that pageant features an *obstetrix* who, like the *Purification* pageant's midwife, subsequently disappeared.[106] And thus we can only guess at what these midwives might have said. Their presences in the early *Nativity* and *Purification* pageants suggest a purposeful connection between Mary's childbirth history and the ritual experiences of ordinary women in York. In turn, their disappearance marks the elision of women's devotional practices and traditions from the texture of the York cycle.

There is an intriguing parallel between the loss of the midwives in these two York pageants and the post-Reformation disciplining of Chester's midwives, both actual and impersonated. In 1539–40, reforming mayor Henry Gee issued a decree against excessive food and drink after churchings and limited postchurching visitors to the midwife only, perhaps out of a mistrust for all-female gatherings without male supervision, Ryan speculates.[107] Several decades later, in response to Puritan critiques, Chester's Late Banns acknowledged the nonscriptural status of the *Nativity*'s midwives, among other popish elements in the plays.[108] The revisions in York and Chester have different motives, but in both cases they seem to stem from a desire to place civic drama and festivity under masculine control, rendering female experience marginal to these performances and to civic identity.

York's fourteenth-century iconographic traditions also support the idea that a midwife attended Mary's purification. In the York Minster Lady Chapel clerestory, a stained glass window depicting the Purification fea-

tures a wimpled woman behind Mary and Joseph, carrying a candle and a
basket that may originally have contained the two doves (see fig. 1.1).[109] Although Beadle speculates that this figure is a maidservant, this visibly wimpled (and thus probably married) woman accompanying Mary is more
likely her midwife, in an image that, like the early pageant, blends purification with churching iconography.[110] Art historian Richard Marks considers
the presence of the midwife to be an iconographic norm in English medieval images of the Purification. Of the winter Candlemas holiday, Marks
notes that the procession of parishioners with lighted candles "is reflected
in the tapers carried by Joseph and the midwife in manuscript illuminations of the Presentation."[111]

Other recent research into contemporary purification imagery reveals
similar scenes. Beyond England, Paula Rieder notes that from the fourteenth
century onward, French devotional manuscript images of the Purification included a woman carrying either the basket of doves or a candle, and
some began to feature larger groups of women with Mary in the center surrounded by female attendants and spectators. Rieder argues that such images emphasize the Virgin's association with "the community of ordinary
women," connecting her visually and imaginatively to the "custom of other
women."[112] St. Leonard's original pageant of the *Purification*, much like the
surviving *Purification* from the East Anglian N-Town cycle, placed Mary
within this female community, emphasizing not only her singular purity
but also her connection to "ordinary women." Niebrzydowski has emphasized the appeal of Marian drama to secular female audiences, arguing that
"Mary's perpetual virginity was no real bar to the many correspondences
felt by real women between their life-cycle and that of Mary."[113] Having suggested that St. Leonard's *Purification* may have originated in a freestanding
Candlemas play, Niebrzydowski observes that the original characters, including the midwife and the sons of Simeon, imply a connection between
Mary's purification and the churching of ordinary women.[114]

The early pageant's tableau of Mary with Joseph and the midwife,
along with Simeon and his sons, offers a striking representation of family:
a dramatic vision that sacralizes parental bonds while evoking the ritual of
churching. The obscure figures of Simeon's sons, mentioned in Matthew
27:52 as among those who rose from the dead at Christ's resurrection, also
witnessed the harrowing of hell and offered an account of their own baptism,
according to apocryphal sources.[115] They would have been adults, perhaps

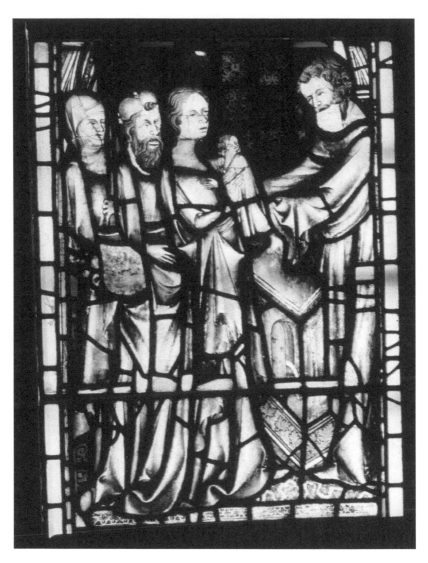

FIGURE 1.1. Purification of the Virgin. York Minster, Lady Chapel, clerestory, south window. © Crown Copyright. Historic England Archive. Reproduced with permission.

wearing the white robes they describe having received for baptism. Though, as Beadle contends, their function here was largely "prefigurative"—looking ahead to Christ's future resurrection—the tableau of mother, fathers, and sons would have suggested links between the spiritual family of the hospital, which included religious brothers and sisters, lay brothers, children and students, and the ordinary families watching the play from the streets of York.[116]

If we turn again to the extant pageant text, the presence of redundant material in the extant *Purification* text may indicate zones of accretion and revision. For example, the content of the priest's opening speech detailing ritual requirements is almost entirely duplicated in the conversation between Mary and Joseph, when they arrive onstage discussing her intention to be purified and to present Jesus to the priest. It is therefore likely that their conversation represents an older stratum of the text. Within this conversation appear elements unique to this play, which lack equivalents in the other Middle English Purification dramas that I have considered. These elements afford glimpses of the pageant's prehistory as hospital drama: a production mounted to extend the hospital's Marian devotion into the civic realm. If we assume speaking parts for the characters who appear in both the early and the revised versions (Mary, Joseph, Simeon, Anna), we can begin to consider how these characters' existing speeches might have emerged from a differently configured pageant, one that emphasized women's communities and familial connections rather than masculine bodies and knowledge.

Not only does the original pageant's cast evoke a churching ritual, but in the extant text itself, Mary's construction of her purification strongly associates the Temple visit with the churching of women. At the outset the York text, more explicitly than any other *Purification* drama, even the Digby Candlemas play, produced by a St. Anne guild, casts Mary's purification as parallel to that of "other women," to recall Rieder's phrase. When Mary announces her intention to go to the Temple to present Christ, she is clearly adhering to the forty-day tradition of churching and following a time-honored, festive custom:

Ful xl days is comme and went
Sens that my babb Jesu was borne,
Therefore I wolde he were present
As Moyses lawes sais hus beforne,

Here in this temple, before Goddes sight,
As other women doith in feer;
So methynke good skyll and right
The same to do nowe with good chere,
After Goddes sawe.

(191–99)

This gesture by Mary, together with the mention of the forty days, appears in some form in most *Purification* pageants, but Mary's opening conflation of her visit with the custom of "other women" and her description of churching as the "right" thing to do, a practice undertaken "with good chere," or festivity, are unique to the York pageant.[117] By characterizing the occasion in this way, Mary evokes the celebratory context of contemporary churching that "other women" in the audience would surely recognize, since the churching ritual was typically a joyful occasion followed by a banquet full of "good chere."[118] A kindred evocation of churching festivity appears at the end of the Digby Candlemas play. After the presentation of Christ, a group of virgins processes with candles, singing the *Nunc dimittis* hymn, and to end the play the expositor figure Poeta invokes minstrels: "Also, ye menestralles, doth your diligens; / Afore oure departyng, geve vs a daunce!" This gesture strongly associates churching, feasting, and minstrels.[119] In this section of the Digby play, the "virgynes, as many as a man wylle," were probably played by local girls.[120] The first virgin has a substantial speech. Coletti has argued that this section of the Candlemas drama "foregrounds ordered female ritual and the private, domestic realm of the family."[121] The York pageant's emphasis on women's ritual and churching festivity does not seem particularly well suited to a masculine artisan context. However, under hospital sponsorship, such a discourse, in connection with Marian devotion, evoked the centrality of women to the hospital's life and, by building the action around the churching ritual, made women's devotional lives integral to the larger civic cycle.

Mary's initiative appears in some form in every *Purification* pageant, yet equally striking in the York version is Joseph's interest in why "other women" require purification. Following upon the previous passage, this interest may reflect a desire to appeal to the devotional impulses of local women. We have no evidence that the hospital admitted pregnant women who would require churching forty days after childbirth, and it does not seem that the hospital itself was a site for churching. Yet the pageant's evocation of this ritual fosters recognition in female onlookers, a recognition that might lead community members to appreciate the hospital's Marian devotion as a valuable element of civic identity. Joseph goes on to reassure Mary:

> Mary, my spowse and madyn clene,
> This matter that thowe moves to me
> Is for all these women, bedene,
> That hais conceyved with syn fleshely
> To bere a chylde.
> The lawe is ledgyd for theme right playn,
> That they muste be puryfied agayne,
> For in mans pleasoure, for certayn,
> Before were they fylyd.
>
> But Mary, byrde, thowe neyd not soo
> For this cause to be puryfiede, loo,
> In Goddes temple.
> For certys thowe arte a clene vyrgyn
> For any thoght thy harte within,
> Nor never wroght no flesly synne,
> Nor never yll.
>                                          (200–215)

By way of explaining Mary's exemption from the ritual requirement ("thowe art a clene vyrgyn"), Joseph dwells extensively on the duties of "these women" who "must be puryfied agayne," having been "fylyd" by sexuality. Such a detailed explanation is unparalleled in other contemporary English dramatic representations. Whereas in the N-Town pageant Mary never explicitly mentions her purification, in the Chester pageant Joseph says merely,

> Yea Marye, though yt be no neede—
> syth thou art cleane in thought and deede—
> yett yt is good to do as God bade
> and worke after his sawe.
>                                          (127–30)

Joseph's lengthy speech in the York pageant has more in common with contemporary English homiletic explications arguing that since Mary did not conceive after "having received seed," then she did not technically require purification. Mary's virginity sets her apart from other women, but her eagerness to undergo the ritual as they do exemplifies her humility, which should be exemplary for other women. The Midland Augustinian homilist John Mirk introduces the feast as

> þe puryfycacyon of oure Lady, þat ys in Englys, þe clansyng of oure Lady—for no nede þat heo hadde þerto, for heo was clansed so wyth þe wyrchyng of þe Holy Gost in þe conseyuyng of hure Sone þat þer was laft in hure no mater of synne ne of non oþur fulþe, but for þat day was þe fortyþe day fro þe burth of hure Sone and was kalled in þe Iewes lawe þe day of purgacyon, not onlyche for oure Lady but for *alle oþur wymen* of þat lawe.[122]

Deploying a familiar discourse that distinguishes pollution from purity, sin from innocence, Mirk emphasizes that, although Mary had no need to undergo "purgacyon," she voluntarily submitted to the custom of "alle oþur wymen," a phrase similar to the one Mary uses in her speech. Mary's obedience not only connects her to other Jewish women, but it also offers a pattern to contemporary Christian women, as Mirk makes clear a bit later. Explaining to parishioners Mary's reasons ("skyles") for going to Temple, he notes that the fourth "was for ensampul to alle crysten wymmen þat þey schulden come to chyrche aftur here burth and þonke God þat hadde saued ham fro perel of deth in hure trauaylyng of hure chyld."[123] Mirk's description of Mary's voluntary Temple visit explains and reinforces what "other women" must do, here in an explicitly didactic mode. Placing the York pageant and Mirk side by side helps to highlight the homiletic quality of Joseph's lines: he is not only instructing the much younger Mary, but also preaching to the pageant's audience.

Joseph's speech draws attention to the need of "other women" to be purified "agayne," repeatedly, with each successive child. This conversation between Mary and Joseph creates a link between Mary's churching and their own, fostering identification with the life cycle event that nearly every female "spowse" experienced multiple times.[124] Ultimately in explaining why "other women" must undergo purification, Joseph's speech promotes Marian devotion by emphasizing what is special about Mary: her virginity.

The speech insists on the difference between the sexuality of "other women" and the perpetual virginity that makes Mary, who "never wroght no flesly synne," worthy of special veneration. She manages to be "spowse and madyn clene": a paradoxical spectacle inviting identification and devotion from ordinary women.[125]

## PROPHETESS ANNA AND THE APPEAL TO WIDOWS

In addition to appealing to women of childbearing age populating the pageant's audience, the hospital's *Purification* pageant also highlighted the institution's connection to older women and widows. By the late fourteenth century, the hospital had a sizeable community of female residents, including caregivers, patients, and corrodians. As Cullum shows, the hospital sisters provided most of the medical care at the house. Their efforts were sometimes rewarded with recognition in bequests dedicated to them rather than to the hospital brothers.[126] Caregivers were outnumbered by the hospital's laywomen, who fell into several categories. These included ill and poor women patients; women who had purchased beds in the hospital, known as liveries; and finally those who had bought corrodies, or retirement packages, either together with their husbands or as independent widows.[127] Such women would live in the hospital precinct, either in the infirmary or in separate dwellings, about which little information survives.[128] During the period 1392–1409, two women, probably widows, purchased an allowance that financed a servant for the price of a "habitum sororis." These women might have been living as vowesses, in a quasi-religious state of regular prayer and religious observance.[129] In late medieval York, widows were quite visible as providers and recipients of charity. To sponsor a drama that emphasized voluntary submission to religious law—not only mother Mary's, but also widow Anna's—would have highlighted the hospital's community of devout laywomen and perhaps appealed to mature women contemplating where to donate and how to live out their own final years. Widows were prominent donors and (along with young women on the verge of marriage) were the most likely to receive charity from other women.[130]

A promising source of information about fifteenth-century widows at St. Leonard's survives in a manuscript register of wills proved in the hospital's peculiar jurisdiction.[131] Among these diverse wills, which include those of hospital porters, servants, and others residing in the precinct, we find several made by widows. Most of these date from the mid-fifteenth century, when the hospital maintained its association with the *Purification* pageant. Although one must treat wills circumspectly, given that a minority of York residents made them and in view of their formulaic nature, these documents may afford some insight into the devotional priorities and communal ties of widows nearing the ends of their lives.[132] All these widows lived within the precinct, two of them naming themselves "Margareta Usburn vidua infra hospitalem Sancti Leonardi" (Margaret Usburn widow within the hospital of St. Leonard) and "Matilda Wighton de hospitali Sancti Leonardi" (Matilda Wighton of the hospital of St. Leonard), designations that suggest residence within the hospital.[133] Like many of the testators, most (though not all) of the widows included in the register requested burial within the hospital's church, indicating ties to this location as a spiritual home and final resting place.[134] Some specify funerary observances for hospital personnel to perform after their deaths. In 1445, Katherine Aslaby, the widow of former hospital porter John Aslaby, detailed payments toward tolling the church bell, for wax for candles to be burned around her body during funeral services, and for a hospital brother to perform Mass on her burial day.[135] This particular widow seems to have understood herself as part of the extended hospital family, having probably resided there for many years.

Even if they had not lived in the hospital for a long time, it seems notable, given their self-appellations as widows "of" and "within" the hospital, that Margareta Usburn and Matilda Wighton offer detailed lists of bequests to the broader hospital community: not only to the brothers and chaplains, but also to the sisters and the poor. In addition to leaving money to priestly brothers participating in her funeral services, Usburn also makes bequests "cuilibet sorori in habitu dicti hospitalis" (to each sister in the habit of the said hospital) who takes part in her funeral services, and for a provision of bread "cuilibet pauperi in infirmarium" (to each pauper in the infirmary).[136] Wighton, though she chose her former parish church over the hospital as a burial place, includes bequests to brothers who participate in her funeral services and "cuilibet sorori habitum habenti et portanti" (to each sister having and wearing the habit of the house).[137] She also leaves a bequest "cuilibet pauperi homini et mulieri moram trahenti in Sent Lennardis garth" (to each pauper, man and woman, residing in St. Leonard's garth).[138] Although we cannot assume too much from wills, Usburn's and Wighton's detailed bequests evoke the strong connections that these widows felt to the hospital's complex, mixed-gender community.

One can only speculate as to why these widows had moved to the hospital. Although evidently Wighton had belonged with her late husband to the parish of St. John the Evangelist, she had settled at St. Leonard's in her retirement. Euan Roger suggests of widows recorded in the rental roll of St. Bartholomew's Hospital, London, at mid-fifteenth century, "These women may have sought out the hospital precinct for the perceived security of its walls, or even for the care and devotional environment that the community offered to those of mature years."[139] Hospitals became places of spiritual retirement for many widows across England. Mary Erler has documented the lives and devotional reading habits of several later medieval widows living at St. Mark's Hospital in Bristol. These women were supervised by the hospital master, who copied works concerned with women's spiritual development. Erler views the hospital setting as a "suitable staging-ground" for widows "seeking to progress spiritually, reading and studying, connecting with female friends, carrying out family obligations, advocating for members of one's circle, choosing particular charities to support."[140] Evidently the hospital offered an agreeable site for older women seeking to perform a religious life, a phenomenon that brings us back to the *Purification* pageant and how it might have evolved from or reflected life at St. Leonard's Hospital.

Given the evidence for widows living on-site or in the hospital precinct, and the appeal of hospitals as sites for devout retirement, there are several remarkable features in the York *Purification*'s depiction of the widow Anna. She is described in Luke's account as "a widow until fourscore and four years; who departed not from the temple, by fastings and prayers serving night and day" (Luke 2:37). In the late medieval English context, Anna's closest analogue might be a vowess or a devout older woman attracted to retirement at a hospital, or a pious woman living in a churchyard.[141] In the context of the dramatic performance, an actual widowed resident might well have relished the chance to inhabit this plum role, which reflected her own life choice and advertised the hospital as a refuge for kindred spirits.

If we remove the opening speech of the Temple priest, which I have argued is a later addition to the pageant, the first character to appear onstage is the widow Anna. She thus occupies a more prominent position in the York *Purification* than in any other dramatic rendition of this episode. Appearing onstage before Simeon, Anna takes on a spiritually powerful, prophetic role that also represents a major departure from Luke's account, which introduces her well after the action of the Presentation.

Anna explicitly defines her status and describes her life in terms that imply a kind of profession. This is the only English *Purification* drama in which Anna identifies herself as a religious widow or speaks in detail about herself:

> Here in this holy playce, I say,
> Is my full purpose to abyde,
> To serve my God bothe nyght and day
> With prayer and fastynge in ever-ylk a tyde.
>
> For I have beyn a wyddo this threscore yere,
> And foure yere to, the truthe to tell,
> And here I haue terryed with full good chere
> For the redempcyon of Israell.
>
> And so for my holy conversacion
> Grete grace to me hais nowe God sent,
> To tell by profecy for mans redempcion,
> What shall befall by Goddes intent.
>
> (57–68)

Anna paraphrases but expands upon her description in Luke, articulating that she is a widow and expressing an intention to stay indefinitely in the "holy playce," enjoying a religious form of retirement. Her phrase "my full purpose to abyde" bespeaks an intent to stay forever, as might an older woman who had committed financially and emotionally to spending her old age at a hospital. Particularly striking is Anna's term "holy conversacion," defined in the *Middle English Dictionary* as "a life dedicated to the ideals of Christianity."[142] This rich term might encompass a wide array of conduct and practices: not necessarily the vowess's formal pledge, but a commitment to a way of life involving "prayer and fastynge in ever-ylk a tyde," and perhaps other good works, such as participation in the caring activities of the house: tending the sick or distributing alms. Its elasticity seems well suited to expansions and changes that might occur within the religious life of a woman retired to a hospital. A widow's "holy conversacion" might

include living devoutly as a liveried resident or tenant in the hospital precinct, or becoming an active member of the religious community.[143] By
placing Anna up front in the pageant, the drama appeals to women directly,
suggesting that widows are integral to the institution's spirituality.

Not only does the York pageant render Anna uniquely prominent as an
object of identification and perhaps charity, the drama also casts her as a
powerful prophetess. In the other *Purification* pageants that I have considered, regardless of auspices, Anna always appears after Simeon, sometimes
long after. In N-Town, with the consistently strong feminine focus that Gibson has noted, Anna has the greatest visibility, seconding Simeon's prediction
of Christ's passion and resurrection and later collaborating with Simeon to
hail the infant Christ. In the Digby Candlemas pageant, she is called "Anna
Prophetissa" but does not appear until the end of the play, and even then
she utters no prophecy.[144]

In contrast to her role as Simeon's subordinate in these other pageants,
in York Anna confidently speaks before him:

> I tell you all here in this place,
> By Godes vertue in prophecy,
> That one is borne to oure solace,
> Here to be present securely
> Within short space,
> Of his owen mother, a madyn free,
> Of all vyrgens moost chaist, suthly,
> The well of mekenes, blyssed myght she be,
> Moost full of grace.
>
> (69–77)

Anna conveys in this compact speech "the redemption of Israel" that her
biblical description promises, describing Christ's coming in terms of imminent comfort and consolation ("solace," "within short space"). Yet her
speech is also striking in its divergence from strictly biblical content. N-
Town, the only other *Purification* pageant in which Anna prophecies, pre-
dicts Christ's passion and resurrection "*For redempcyon of all mankende,* /
That blysse for to restore, / Whiche hath be lost fro oute of mende" (91–94;
emphasis added). York's Anna, who has already addressed "mans redemp-
cion" (67), now describes the relation between Christ and Mary in a sequence

that shows Christ's holiness arising from Mary's. This speech may borrow phrases from the York Purification liturgy, in which we find the antiphon beginning "Ave Maria gratia plena. Dei genitrix, virgo; ex te enim ortus est sol justitiae illuminans quae in tenebris sunt" (Hail, Mary, full of grace. Mother of God, virgin, out of you the sun of justice is risen, illuminating those who are in shadows).[145] In the antiphon, Jesus's light rises out of Mary's perfect purity in a movement similar to that of the dramatic stanza, which suggests that Christ has risen from Mary "*Of his owen mother*, a may-den free, / *Of all vyrgens* moost chaist, suthly" (emphasis added). Here the anaphora reinforces Mary as the source, the "well of mekenes" and "grace" from which Christ draws these qualities. In this singular dramatic rendition of Anna, this prophetic widow announces Christ while praising Mary, inviting audience members to do the same.

Thus the early hospital-sponsored drama stages the veneration of Mary as an expression of holy widowhood. Anna has another remarkable speech, which in the extant *Purification* appears after a much longer speech by the Temple priest. If we were to strip away the priest's speech as we did his opening discourse, Anna's speech would gain prominence, and the praise of Mary at this point would precede the praise of Jesus. The priest speaks the following:

> A, blyssyd babb, welcome thowe be,
> Borne of a madyn in chaistety,
> Thowe are our beylde, babb, our gamme and our glee
> Ever sothly.
> Welcome, oure wytt and our wysdome,
> Welcome our joy, all and somme,
> Welcomme *redemptour omnium*
> Tyll hus hartely.
>
> (316–23)

Here we find Christ the "blyssyd babb" exuberantly welcomed by the priest; Anna and Simeon later use the same phrase (lines 332 and 354).[146] And as I have argued elsewhere, the key term "beylde," meaning "comfort," with its aural similarity to "bilden" (to construct), contains within it an argument for artisan community.[147] Yet if we were to omit the priest's speech, we would move straight from Joseph's lines offering the infant Christ to Anna's speech, which begins by hailing not Jesus, but *Mary*:

Welcome, blyssed Mary and madyn ay,
Welcome, mooste meke in thyne array;
Welcome, bright starne that shyneth bright as day,
All for our blys.
Welcome, the blyssed beam so bryght,
Welcome, the leym of all oure light,
Welcome, that all pleasour hais plight
To man, iwysse.

(324–31)

Beadle connects Anna's lines, with their repetition of "Welcome," to the "formulae used in levation prayers uttered quietly to themselves by the faithful at the elevation of the Host during Mass."[148] This liturgical echo is certainly present, but to stop with a comparison to Eucharistic worship assumes that Anna is praising only Christ, who as an infant upon the altar prefigures the Eucharist. Yet Anna explicitly names Mary here before Christ. Mary is welcomed first as the "bright starne that shyneth bright as day" (328), the light upon whom Christ depends for his existence. If we regard these lines from a Marian perspective, we see that even as Anna's speech shades into praising Christ (the "blyssyd beam" and "leym of all oure light," who has already received the epithet "lemer of light" in the York *Nativity* pageant), her speech has decidedly begun with Mary.[149] Here Christ's light emerges from Mary's brightness, similar to Anna's earlier prophetic speech, where Christ arose from Mary's "well of mekenes." The Feast of the Purification makes that dependence upon Mary visible, even if at various points throughout both the liturgy and the drama Mary is celebrated primarily as the carrier, the "wombe" redeemed by the privilege of bearing Christ.[150]

Like Anna's previous speech, this later speech of praise may draw inspiration from the most sustained praise of Mary to appear in the York Purification Mass, whose final sequence hails Mary as "star of the sea" and "glory of the world, queen of heaven," emphasizing her brightness, beseeching her to recognize her suppliants: "Virgo, decus mundi, regina caeli, praeelecta ut sol, pulchra lunaris ut fulgor, agnosce omnes te diligentes" (Virgin, glory of the universe, queen of heaven, first chosen as the sun, in radiance beautiful as the moon, acknowledge all those who love you).[151] Thus Anna's final speech to Mary—devout widow speaking to virgin mother—may offer us another trace of Mary's capital importance in the original pageant.

This earlier pageant may have more closely resembled other *Purification* dramas in which Mary shines with particular brightness: the N-Town *Purification*, for example, echoes the Sarum Candlemas liturgy.[152] As Gibson has argued, the epithets used to hail Mary in N-Town ("salver of sekenes" and "lantern of lyght") emphasize her numinous status and evoke this liturgy, casting Mary as "mystical queen who is celebrated in a high lyric style derived from the Latin sacred lyric."[153] Anna's final speech opens onto a version of the York *Purification* that more strongly emphasizes Mary's role as the source of light that Christ will cast over the world.

York's Hospital of St. Leonard, devoted to Mary and St. Leonard, used drama to position itself publicly as a spiritual resource, a potential home, and a worthy site for patronage. By foregrounding the experiences of Mary, her midwife, and Anna, the hospital's early pageant reflected the importance of women's devotion to the hospital and the civic realm in which the institution was embedded. The hospital may have ceased to perform its pageant in the years leading up to 1477, when the drama was reassigned. It is also possible that the hospital's original aims had come to compete with the agenda of the Corpus Christi play as it developed into a more uniformly civic production, tightly linked to artisanal and mercantile interests. As the hospital's Marian pageant became subsumed into a larger civic performance of artisan identity, it came to focus, like Chester's and Coventry's versions of the Purification, on masculine spiritual experience and the man-to-man transmission of knowledge. A mixed-gender institution such as the hospital, with its particular interest in and appeal to women, no longer fit the masculine civic and artisanal vision of the cycle. But if we view the extant text as a palimpsest, the unique features of the *Purification* still testify to Mary's centrality in the late medieval hospital's history and to women's prominence in the devotional and social life of the larger city.

# Corruption and Purification at St. Bartholomew's Hospital, London

## The Book of the Foundation
### *and John Mirfield's Compilations*

### WOMEN AT ST. BARTHOLOMEW'S HOSPITAL

The image of the newly delivered Virgin Mary seeking purification in the Temple was central to the devotional life and public presentation of St. Leonard's Hospital, York. Yet we have no evidence that the hospital admitted pregnant or laboring women. St. Leonard's dramatized the Virgin's miraculous maternity amid a female community that included wives, widows, and sisters, but possibly no new mothers. We know, however, that poor, unmarried pregnant women were commonly admitted to English hospitals, forming one of the five main categories of patients: the "poveres femmes enseintez" cited in the House of Commons petition of 1414. Some hospitals even catered to pregnant women, among other patients, particularly in London, where the proliferation of servants, widespread poverty, and prostitution led to many lonely, unsupported pregnancies.[1] Along with the suburban London hospitals St. Mary without Bishopsgate and St. Thomas in Southwark, St. Bartholomew's of Smithfield admitted pregnant women seeking a safe place to give birth and rest until their own purification forty days later.[2] Pregnant women are referenced as objects of the hospital's care in a 1352 decree by Edward III and in a declaration of Henry VI in 1437.[3]

These late medieval women left few textual traces, but they drew the concern of male clerics writing at the intersection of priory and hospital, institutions that were linked from their 1123 founding until the late fourteenth century. In this chapter, I begin to show how the late medieval literary history of St. Bartholomew's Hospital centers around the treatment of women. A dialectic of contamination and purification attended the hospital from its foundation in seedy suburban Smithfield, infamous for its fair, criminals, and prostitutes. Women, with their presumed physical and mental debilities, were strongly associated with this dialectic. I consider women's treatments in three works written around the turn of the fifteenth century: a Middle English foundation and miracle narrative (*The Book of the Foundation of St. Bartholomew's Church*) and two Latin compendia (John Mirfield's *Breviarium Bartholomei*, a medical encyclopedia, and his *Florarium Bartholomei*, a theological compendium).

The treatments of women in these three texts give us insights into the hospital's function as a haven for marginal women in a notorious part of London. *The Book of the Foundation*, written at the priory, writes anxiety about female sexuality, especially prostitution, into the twinned founding and early history of priory and hospital. In contrast, Mirfield's *Breviarium*, compiled for use in the hospital, reveals a pragmatic, nonjudgmental view of single women's sexual requirements. The *Breviarium* treats virginity as a physical state and an ongoing performance within a larger therapeutic system that includes contraception. The therapeutic commitments of the *Breviarium* are thrown into relief by Mirfield's *Florarium*, a theological compilation for priory brothers that presents women as agents of temptation and impediments to well-regulated spiritual or medical practice. By triangulating these texts, I show how their varying perspectives present an ambivalent vision of the hospital in which its function of care for women could be variously seen as socially threatening or recuperative, with implications for the institution's role within the wider city. Whereas the *Book* and *Florarium* tend to link sexual purification to a retreat from the city and from sexuality itself, the *Breviarium* facilitates the "corrupted" woman's return to the city and, perhaps, to sexual respectability. In keeping with the hospital's outward-looking focus, one fifteenth-century manuscript afterlife for Mirfield's gynecology shows that the remedies he compiled for the hospital's single women were later seen as valuable for sexually active married women far beyond the hospital setting.

BOOK OF THE FOUNDATION:
FROM CONTAMINATION TO PURIFICATION

As its title suggests, the *Book of the Foundation of St. Bartholomew's Church* tells the story of the hospital's and priory's simultaneous founding and relates many of the early miracles wrought there by St. Bartholomew. The *Book* was translated circa 1400–1425 from the Latin *Liber fundacionis ecclesie Sancti Bartholomei Londoniarum pertinentis prioratui eiusdem in Weste Smythfelde.*[4] Latin and English texts appear together in a single manuscript, British Library MS Cotton Vespasian B ix.[5] It is not clear why the translator made an English version; the dating suggests that it was prepared around the time when the hospital became administratively independent of the priory.[6] Laura Varnam has argued that the translation's timing corresponds to a moment when the priory church was itself undergoing a "Great Restoration."[7] In its narration of foundation and miracles, the *Book* creates an early, persistent connection between women and corruption, casting the hospital and priory as places of purification, both physical and spiritual. Although the miracles narrated in the *Book* do not exclusively depict women, female subjects are particularly useful for promoting St. Bartholomew's healing powers. The *Book* features virgins, matrons, and prostitutes—women of every sexual status except widow—and shows the saint restoring proper conduct and hierarchies within these roles or enabling women to be healed and thus occupy them properly. The roles of virgin, wife, and prostitute inform Mirfield's *Breviarium* as well. Though all medieval women were defined by their sexual roles and behavior, prostitutes were "entirely defined by their sexuality," and they become key figures, sometimes implicitly, in the literature of the hospital.[8]

The *Book* has the primary aim of glorifying the priory church, where the saint's relics were housed and most of his miracles took place. Yet the simultaneous foundations of hospital and priory were closely connected during the time period that the *Book* depicts, when the priory controlled the hospital in a tense relationship marked by controversies over funding and ritual, until the hospital gained independence by the late fourteenth century.[9] Norman Moore terms hospital and priory "twin works of piety, the one in accordance with the vow which he [the founder, Rahere] had made, the other as had been enjoined him by the apostolic command."[10] The *Book* acknowledges the hospital's priority in Rahere's intention, yet it depicts the priory church as the main site of Bartholomew's miracle cures and the hospital as something of an appendage. As Nellie Kerling observes, working between circa 1174 and circa 1189, a period of tension between priory and hospital, the author's "aim was to show that the Priory was the more important of the two and that the Hospital . . . should not take a line of development of its own."[11] The *Book* author does not always make a distinction between the priory and hospital, except when necessary to emphasize the priory as his location or its church as the site of a cure. Sometimes he mentions the hospital as the site for a miraculous intervention, as in the case of the mad prostitute, which I consider at the end of this section.

The *Book* draws attention to the foundation of hospital and priory as a continual effort to transform corruption into purity. This effort begins with the spiritual conversion of its founder, Rahere, and continues with the institution's foundation in the polluted borough of Smithfield. The work's opening moments detail Rahere's youthful errancy, conversion, and vow to found the institution. Although Rahere, "Funder of owere hoely places," is initially praised as having "prouyd puryte of soule / bryght maners, with honest probyte / experte diligence yn dyuyne seruyce / prudent besynes yn temperalle mynystracyun," the description of his preconversion life links sensuality and depravity, implicating corruption into the foundation story.[12] A low-born Anglo-Norman youth, Rahere spends his days entertaining noblemen and princes, first coming into view at the "housholdys of noble men and the palicis of prynces / where, vndir euery elbowe of them / he sprede her coshynys, delectably anoyntynge her eerys / by this maner to draw to hym ther frendschippis." His efforts to win friends seem homosocial yet seductive, as he "inforsid hymself with iolite and carnale suauyte / by the whiche he myght drawe to hym the hertys of many oone" (3). This extreme sycophancy is given a more pointedly gendered meaning when Rahere is suddenly plucked by God from his idle way of life:

> This manere of leuynge he chose yn his begynnyge / and yn this exercisid his yough: but the inwarde-seer and mercyfull God of all / the whiche oute of Mary Magdalene cast oute vii feendys / the whiche to the Fysshere ʒaue þe keyes of heuyne / mercyfully conuertid this man fro the erroure of hys way / and addid to hym, so conuerted, many ʒiftys of vertu / for why they that are fonnysch and febill in the worldys reputacioun / oure Lorde chesith, to / confounde the myghte of the worlde. (3)

The author makes a striking choice of Mary Magdalene and the apostle Peter ("the Fysshere") as exemplary recipients of Christ's mercy. These figures offer two different gendered analogues for Rahere: the demoniac woman whose composite biography mirrors the "anoyntynge" and seduction of Rahere's preconversion life, and the priestly figure who becomes Christ's second in command, protector of heaven's sacred space.[13] Rahere will leave behind the first model, with her problematic femininity, to emulate Peter, the most celebrated early Christian cleric.

By citing Mary Magdalene's exorcism as the paradigmatic female conversion, the author makes this reputedly sexual sinner a reference point not only for Rahere but for all who are "fonnysch and febill in the worldys reputacioun." This phrase translates "stulta et infirma sunt mundi" from the Latin text.[14] Although the *Book*'s use of "fonnysh" is glossed in the *Middle English Dictionary* as "foolish or innocent," I suggest that given the association with Mary Magdalene the term also encompasses the sense of "sinful," another listed definition.[15] Although the hospital has not yet entered Rahere's mind, the very moment of his conversion connects him imaginatively both to Mary Magdalen and the sexually compromised women that the hospital will shelter in the future.

The hospital's care of unmarried pregnant women was well known in late medieval London. In a detailed list of London city churches included in the fifteenth-century miscellany BL MS Egerton 1995, this description of St. Bartholomew's Hospital appears:

> Bartholomewe ys spetylle; hyt ys a place of grete comforte to pore men as for hyr loggyng and yn specyalle vnto yong wymmen that haue mysse done that ben wythe chylde; there they ben delyueryde, and vnto the tyme of Puryfycacyon they haue mete and drynke of the placys coste and fulle honestely gyded and kepte. And in ys moche worschyppe as the place maye, they kepe hyr conselle and hyr worschyppe. God graunte that they doo so hyr owne worschippe that haue a fendyde. Amen.[16]

The author draws attention to pregnancy as a result of women's sexual failings ("wymmen that haue mysse done that ben wythe chylde"). The care that these fallen women receive includes not only sustenance but secrecy ("they kepe hyr conselle and hyr worschyppe"). And although the passage implies that these unmarried young mothers deserve care during the vulnerable period from childbirth to purification, the author also blames them for their lapses: "God graunte that they doo so hyr owne worschippe that haue a fendyde." The repeated term "worschippe" signifies chaste reputation.[17] The hospital is involved in safeguarding these women's reputations while they remain there, but this duty reverts to the women themselves after they are "delyueryde" and purified. Alert to the danger that pregnancies posed to young women's futures, this description suggests that with the hospital's help, their "worschippe" may be preserved. Within the *Book* and the wider public imagination of Londoners, women's sexual offense is always a subtext for St. Bartholomew's, wrapped up with the very founding and purpose of the institution.

The Smithfield site that St. Bartholomew himself selects as the church's location must first be purged of filth before the salutary institution may be founded. This scene too is replete with gendered meanings. St. Bartholomew appears to Rahere in a vision, announcing that he has "chosyn a place yn the Subbarbis of Londone, at Smythfeld ; where yn myn name thou shalte founde A Chirche / And it shalbe the house of God / there shalbe the tabernacle of the lambe / the temple of the Holy Gost. . . . Trewely euery soule conuertid / penytent of his synne / And in this place prayng / yn heuyn graciously shall be herde" (5). St. Bartholomew envisions the new church in terms of holy enclosed spaces ("house of God," "tabernacle," "temple," with a direct link from "euery soule conuertid" to "heuyn"), spaces whose purity and masculinity ("penytent of *hys synne*") link them to Peter, keeper of heaven and the masculine model for Christ's mercy. However, the location of Smithfield, a large open site in northwest London, was notorious for contamination and death, home to a raucous fair, public executions, and prostitution. "Smithfield had a symbolic resonance in the English consciousness," notes Andrew Taylor. "It offered a space for large public gatherings on the very edge of the metropolis and had long been associated with trickery, haggling, louche diversions, and punishment."[18] Before any "conuertid" or "penytent" supplicants may enter, the site must be cleansed, in a section bearing the title "de loci emendacione" in the Latin version.[19] This "clensynge" is framed in penitential terms that also seem markedly gendered:

> Truly thys place aforne his clensynge / pretendid noone hope of goodnesse / right uncleene it was / and as a maryce dunge and fenny with water almost euerytyme habowndynge / And that / that was emynente,

a-boue the water drye . was deputid and ordeyned to the Iubeit or gal-
owys of thevys / and to the tormente of othir that were dampnyd by
Iudicialle auctoryte. (12)

With its "uncleene" swamp overflowing with moisture, topped by a "drye"
gallows affording punishment to "thevys," this cursed space manifests the
worst of feminine qualities: a dangerously moist environment enabling illness and sin to proliferate, culminating in death on the gallows.[20] Not only
is the area unclean, with the muddy fens creating an unhealthy miasma
whose vapors were understood to spread disease, but before its "purgacion"
it is rife with feminine associations.[21] Building on Joan Cadden's work on
the humors and gender, Nancy Caciola has shown that women were considered cool and moist in their complexions. Whereas "coolness was a pre-
dictive sign for moral instability, moistness begets a changeable, incon-
stant, and highly impressionable nature, like mud retaining a footprint."[22]
This metaphorical mud of femininity is tangible in the Smithfield swamp.
A royal manor outside the city of London, Smithfield was administratively
independent, subject to the lord's jurisdiction. Like Southwark, Westmin-
ster, and Walworth, Smithfield was a location in which prostitutes and
bawds were frequently brought to court and fined.[23] The earlier mention of
Mary Magdalen, usually viewed as a penitent harlot, highlights this association, making prostitution an implicit context for the work. Even as Rahere
purges the site of its uncleanness, the unsavory atmosphere of Smithfield
persists, and fallen women, descendants of Mary Magdalen, populate the
area as potential hospital patients.

The Smithfield Decretals (BL MS Royal 10. E. IV), an early fourteenth-
century canon law collection owned by the priory and decorated with extensive marginal illustrations during the 1340s, offers another intriguing
portal into the priory's literary treatment of women. This volume speaks
obliquely to the figure of Mary Magdalen and to the context of prostitution
that subtended Smithfield literary productions. The translator of the *Book
of the Foundation* may well have been familiar with the lavish Decretals
manuscript and its striking illuminations. Taylor reads the Decretals manuscript, whose legal content is surrounded with extensive pictorial marginalia, including bawdy and comic scenes, in relation to this liminal location,
noting that in contrast to its learned content, the volume's marginal illustrations "represent the vigor of alternative and more popular traditions."[24]

In another reading that stresses the Augustinian setting, Alixe Bovey notes the prominence of the Eucharist and related miracles within the visual narratives, including saints' lives and Marian miracles, that are illustrated in the manuscript's *bas-de-page* illuminations.[25] She suggests that as a production of an Augustinian priory, the images may reflect the order's characteristic focus on educating the laity about the sacraments.[26]

One of the manuscript's most striking features is the inclusion of images representing penitent prostitutes: St. Thaïs and St. Mary of Egypt.[27] The illustrations emphasize in both cases the importance of the sacrament and Christian burial of the saints, rituals that enfold the women into "Christian community despite their years of deliberate isolation from it."[28] The *bas-de-page* image of Mary of Egypt receiving Communion is a prime example (see fig. 2.1). These images might complement the *Book of the Foundation,* which explicitly evokes the dangers of the Smithfield location in the allusion to Mary Magdalen and offers the hope of spiritual healing and "delivery" to the fallen women of its narratives via St. Bartholomew's interventions.

Returning to the *Book*'s narrative, we see that the purgation of the filthy site has not yet been accomplished. Under Rahere's charismatic leadership, which includes gaining the "felischipe of children and seruantis" who secretly help him gather materials to build his church, he manages to purge the site and frame the church in short order: "Of this almen grettly were astonyd / boeth of the nouelte of the areysid frame / and of the wonder of this newe werke / Whoe wolde trowe this place with so sodyan a clensynge to be purgid / and ther to be sette vp the tokenys of [the] crosse! And God there to be worshippid / where sumtyme stoid the horrible hangynge of thevys" (13–14). The dangerously gendered place has been miraculously purified: the swampy place "purgid" of its fetid miasma, the threateningly "emynente" gallows replaced by Christ's glorious cross. This first purgation sets up the gendered nature of the miracles that follow, in which women's vulnerably liquid bodies become entry points for corruption.

The *Book*'s miracles of purification from sexual sin inscribe the possibility for women to move from "fonnysh and febill reputation" toward purity.[29] The *Book* includes a wide range of women, conventionally defined by their sexual status as maids, mothers, single women, or matrons. And even though not all of the miracles involving women relate to illness of body or spirit (in one story, a faithful matron wards off a house fire by invoking the saint), the majority of the *Book*'s women appear afflicted in some way,

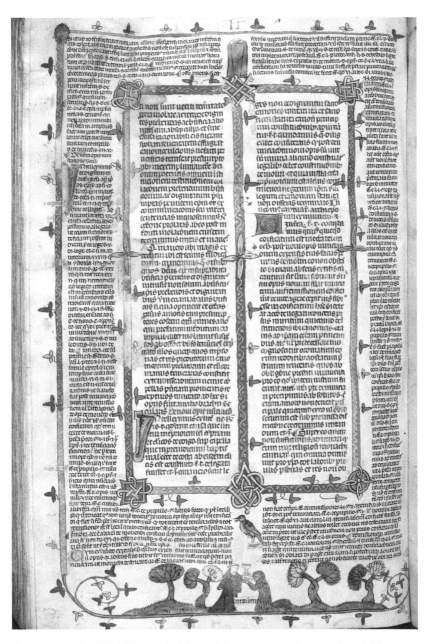

Figure 2.1. Smithfield Decretals: Mary of Egypt receives Communion. © The British Library Board, MS Royal 10. E. IV, fol. 286v. Reproduced with permission.

sometimes by minor ailments, such as a swollen tongue.[30] Although it is not obviously sexual, even this sickness is gendered, given the pervasive cultural association between women and excessive speech. This particular woman's tongue "so gretly was swolle that she myght nat schete here mowth" (20).

As in the earlier description of the "uncleene" Smithfield site before its purgation, women's corruption is always tied to their physicality: consistent with the earlier image, the first miracle story in the collection describes divine mercy as "that welle of pyte / that was and is opyne to the menstruat womane and synful man" (18). As in the image of the corrupt site, women's physical processes make them objects of pity, with menstruation the paradigmatic female infirmity.[31] An attention to the sexualized female body is striking within the *Book*, notably in connection to bodies at the limits of sexual experience: virgins, pregnant women, and prostitutes.[32] I focus on the last category in order to show how prostitution forms a constitutive subtext for the hospital and its literature. The *Book* tends to privilege the priory church as the site of St. Bartholomew's miracles, but in this story the hospital is specifically mentioned as the site of his intervention.[33]

The *Book*'s story of a young prostitute, who is brought to the hospital after losing her virginity and going mad, highlights the hospital as a place where St. Bartholomew's power can mitigate even the worst effects of sexual corruption. This story emphasizes a young girl's unwitting entry into urban prostitution. This "certayne yonge woman" starts out innocently enough as a "hyryd seruant / wounte to serue many men" but enters into sexuality once she is "by a bawde bigilid from the profite of her iust laboure / to voluptuousnes of vncleyne synne . . . robbid of yncomperable tresure" (57).[34] The fact that she starts out serving "many men" offers an early warning of her fate as a prostitute. As Karras argues, the medieval prostitute was defined by her public association with multiple men: "Medieval society attempted to control such women by treating them as though they belonged to men in common (though they were not legally property)."[35] This subject is a young woman lacking resources or protection, already occupying a circumscribed status, since single women had no choice other than entering into service.[36]

It is also revealing that the "bawd" [Latin *leno*] is blamed for turning the girl toward sin. Although the term *leno* could refer to a male or female, female bawds feature more prominently in prostitution narratives. It was often not the male client but the female facilitator who was blamed for the girl's loss of virginity: "In the church courts both parties to the sex act as well as the procurer might be accused, but in the secular courts it was usually only the procurer."[37] Such figures were typically female: thus the *Book* implies a moral failure on the part of women for corrupting other women.[38]

As a reward for her accidental entry into prostitution instead of continuing in the "iust laboure" of service, the unfortunate girl goes mad and becomes united with the devil: "Ne it was nat longe / but Loo, the reward of syne folowid / and where her hole body and fleysse she made sugget to synne uttirly she lost her hole mynde / and that membris that were armoure of wykkidnes / be turned to armur of woodness. the herte that is pryncipall of man / with oppressioun of the feende the whiche was onyd to hym / was derkid" (57). Here possession is depicted as the "reward of syne," demonic corruption the "baleful result of sinful behavior."[39] Having carried her into "wykkidnes," her body becomes the vehicle for "woodness" as she is overcome by madness. In Caciola's terms, "Sin alters the composition of the body, opening up the flesh so as to allow the demon to enter in."[40] Thus in addition to being corrupt of body and mind, she also becomes blasphemous and must be physically restrained: "these bondys with her woodnys myght lightly y-broke . othir were addid therto / thus she was browght to the hospitale of the seyid chirche / and yn short tyme folowid contraxioun of all membris . that yn no wyse myght she vse them frely" (57). After being brought to the hospital for treatment of her combined promiscuity and madness, she experiences a "contraction" (unexplained sudden paralysis) that is common in the *Book*'s other miracle stories.[41] Yet, while still in the hospital, this woman too receives "mercy" from St. Bartholomew: "And in so grete a wrechidnes / was presente the mercy of the blessid Apostle / the whiche the madde woman losid of her woodnes mercyfully / and erectid the contracte myghtly / and fulhole went home to her owne" (57). In her extremity, St. Bartholomew's mercy reaches the woman to relieve madness and paralysis, though unfortunately without restoring the "yncomperable tresure" of her virginity. The prostitute is sent "home to her owne," taken out of circulation and presumably off the marriage market.

The story depicts exorcism as a process that responds to the "exemplary illness" of female possession and requires an escape from sexuality and from the city simultaneously.[42] John Mirfield, a rough contemporary of the *Book*'s translator, will invoke some of these same misogynist ideas in his spiritual encyclopedia, yet his medical compendium, which treats virginity as both a process and a practice, suggests that a wider spectrum of women may be able to return to urban society rather than being removed from circulation or permanently stigmatized.

## John Mirfield's *Breviarium*:
## Constrictives and Contraceptives
## for Smithfield Single Women

*The Book of the Foundation* inscribes tension between corruption and purification into the twinned founding and early years of the hospital and priory. In its account, women appear primarily as victims, subject to miraculous cures if they are lucky. Turning to two late fourteenth-century Latin
texts written at the intersection of priory and hospital, we continue to see a
complex understanding of women in relation to physical and spiritual health,
corruption, and purification. The *Breviarium Bartholomei* and *Florarium
Bartholomei* compendia are both attributed to John Mirfield (d. 1407), a
cleric ambiguously linked with priory and hospital.[43] Mirfield's split literary personality illuminates the hospital's complexity as a multigendered
spiritual, social, and medical community that may have struggled to balance these many functions. By considering the treatment of women in Mirfield's *Breviarium* and *Florarium*, I discern an implicit tension between hospital and priory and between their views of sexually active single women.
In this section, I focus on Mirfield's *Breviarium* and its fifteenth-century
afterlife. I show how the *Breviarium* suppresses the antifeminism of its
own medical sources to provide pragmatic recipes for sexually active single
women, giving them strategies for preserving their bodies and reemerging
into civic life. The practical afterlife of the *Breviarium* in Oxford, Bodleian
Library, MS Bodley 682 suggests that one of Mirfield's literary legacies was
to bring the work's hospital-inspired gynecology into the wider world of
medical treatment.

Although Mirfield's name appears in documents including ordination records and a will, his exact relationship to the priory and hospital
remains unclear. He refers to himself as "capellanus" in his will, and in
several London ordination records he derives his clerical title from the
Hospital of St. Bartholomew. Documentary evidence indicates that in
1362, Mirfield was granted an annual pension by the priory and the right
to rent a room on the priory's south side.[44] We might consider Mirfield as
a member of London's large clerical proletariat who managed to establish
relatively stable employment in connection with the hospital and priory.
Editors Hartley and Aldridge conclude, "He may perhaps have acted as an
amateur physician in the Priory until his ordination, and then have be-

come a chaplain in the Hospital. All that can safely be postulated is that, though not a Canon of the Augustinian Order, he resided within the walls of the Priory."[45] Mirfield lived, ministered, and wrote at the intersection of the two institutions, which by the late fourteenth century had become quite distinct communities.

The *Breviarium Bartholomei* and *Florarium Bartholomei* are very different works, but the *Florarium* features one chapter, "De medicis et eorum medicinis" (on physicians and their medicines), whose discussion of the regimen of health overlaps with the *Breviarium*'s final book.[46] Faye M. Getz notes, "*Florarium Bartholomei*, or *Flowergarden of Bartholomew*, concerns the well-being of the spirit while the *Breviarium* concerns the health of the body."[47] Getz argues persuasively for the *Breviarium* as a work composed in and for the hospital. My discussion builds upon her work and that of Monica Green, who has noted the *Breviarium*'s responsiveness to the particular needs of single women. Getz argues that the contexts of priory and hospital shaped Mirfield's emphasis in the two works:

> The *Florarium* was prepared for a community of friars, men who lived a well-regulated religious life. Good health lay in moderation, and the truest health was that of the spirit. The *Breviarium* was prepared for a population that was poor, secular, often transient, and sometimes women or children. . . . For these people, Mirfeld prepared a huge encyclopedia of recipes, devoid of the moralizing and antifeminism of the *Florarium*. . . . Prayers and charms were also incorporated, as Mirfield sought out anything that could mitigate the suffering of the hospital's poor.[48]

Getz's point about divergences in audiences, attitudes, and functions for the two texts is crucial. In the *Breviarium*, Mirfield's mission to "mitigate the suffering of the hospital's poor" is linked with a concern for the sexual circumstances of hospital patients, many of them pregnant or newly delivered single women. Working against the larger trend in medical writing toward detailing the "secrets of women" in order to theorize conception and birth, Mirfield's gynecology works pragmatically within the hospital context to "restore" virginity and prevent conception, reclaiming secrecy as a form of discreet care that shields women from social shame.[49]

From the start, Mirfield's *Breviarium* emphasizes pragmatic healing for a range of readers:

quasdam notabilitates medicinales quas in diuersis locis textuum et glossarum artis medicine necnon et in opusculis plurimorum de ista sciencia subtiliter et copiose tractancium inueni et collegi quas nunc tenet labilis memoria mea hortatu quorundam amicorum meorum iusta ingenii mei modulum sub quodam compendio collocare disposui.

_____

I have found and gathered together certain noteworthy matters of a medical nature, culled from various sources, such as texts and glosses of the Art of Medicine, as well as the works of many writers who have treated of this science skilfully and fully; and since now I merely retain these things in my mind, from whence they are prone to slip away, I have endeavoured, at the instigation of certain of my friends, and according to my own ability, to collect them together and set them down in an abridged form.[50]

Mirfield insists upon the ignorance of medical matters that he shares with his intended readers. He protests that his reason for compiling his "rudam . . . collectam" (clumsy compilation) "plus fuit ex desiderio simplicioribus mihi similibus proficiendi quam ex cupiditate alicuius inanis iactancie procurande" (was more the desire of assisting simpletons such as myself, than any passion to indulge in empty-headed ostentation).[51] Mirfield proposes a brief, useful work, striving to

remedia collecta velut in vno breuiario vt predictum et conscriberem. Vt quocunque venirem huiusmodi impostores vitare possem et vt mihimet ipsi et Christi pauperibus scirem mederi si in languoribus curabilibus et lenibus incidere oporteret.

_____

write down within one breviary the various remedies applicable to each disease; so that, wherever I might come, I might by this means be able to escape the impostors of this kind, and might be able to relieve, not only myself, but all the other poor followers of Christ, who should happen to be afflicted by those diseases which are not serious but curable.[52]

Having perused many medical compendia, Mirfield was aware of the division within medical culture between the empirical and the theoretical, a pronounced rift by the end of the fourteenth century.[53] Even as he draws from a range of learned works, Mirfield emphasizes practical remedies over etiological or humoral explanations. John Riddle defines practice as "the execution of health regimen, generally by drug and diet therapy. In pharmacy, practice was a constant tradition of unstructured testing of the relationships between drugs and ailments (a form of experimental controls), a mode of transmission of recipes, and a commitment to drug therapy."[54] In delineating his reasons for occasionally including multiple remedies for the same ailment, Mirfield claims a pragmatic rather than a theoretical rationale: "Quoniam de proprietate medicaminum est quod iuuabunt vno tempore et non alio. Et hoc est mirabile" (For it is a peculiarity of medicaments that at one time they are beneficial, and at another time they are not—a fact which is a matter for wonder!).[55] Mirfield's approach contrasts with contemporary pharmacological works in which theory sometimes took precedence over practice: such copying would manifest the kind of "empty-headed ostentation" that he deplores.[56] In the realm of gynecology, my focus in this section, Mirfield resists the tendency toward "natural-philosophical speculation" that had begun to seep into gynecological texts since the thirteenth century, as Green has shown. Mirfield prefers "medical practicality" (Green's phrase) in line with his stated intent to relieve those "afflicted by those diseases which are not serious but curable."

Mirfield's *Breviarium* is hardly brief: the text fills more than 200 folios in Oxford, Pembroke College MS 2. Yet the work's organization, previewed at the end of the Proemium, seems designed for ease of reference. In the Pembroke manuscript, the text is followed by an index that allows readers to locate sections quickly. Mirfield organizes his work in the head-to-toe scheme familiar from other contemporary medical compendia: first treating fevers (1), then "de morbis aliis vniuersalibus occupantibus totum corpus" (general diseases that attack the whole body) (2), dividing the body from the head down in the subsequent sections, moving from head and upper chest (3) to lower and inner chest (4), the mid-body, chest to genitals (5), genitals (6), "ab ano vsque ad extremam partem pedis" (from the anus downward to the extremities of both feet) (7). The remaining sections treat abscesses (8), wounds (9), fractures (10), dislocations (11), simple drugs (12), compound medicines (13), laxatives and purgatives (14), and blood-letting and health regimen (15).[57] Mirfield's discussion of surgery in the ninth book has been singled out for its extensive and largely reliable advice on treating wounds.[58] Robert Gottfried highlights the relatively unusual inclusion of a surgical manual within a medical treatise as well as Mirfield's statements on the importance of harmonizing the two pursuits. Mirfield's effort to integrate medicine and surgery speaks to his pragmatic emphasis in a book that strives to include all necessary information within one "promptuarium" (repository).

For whom did Mirfield compile his *Breviarium*, other than himself? In his Proemium, Mirfield claims to have compiled the work for his own use, "ad labilitatem mee memorie supportandam" (to provide a support for my unreliable memory).[59] He envisions the book helping a reader "si rudis sit lector sicut et ego" (if the reader be as ignorant as I am) and "simplicioribus mihi similibus proficiendi" (assisting simpletons such as myself). Even as Mirfield obviously employs a humility topos, he also seems to be projecting the work's utility for those without formal medical training. There are few records of physicians presiding at St. Bartholomew's until the sixteenth century, except for a 1479 bequest by London mercer John Don to pay a surgeon to cure "poure, sore and seke peple" at St. Bartholomew's and two other London hospitals.[60] As at other English hospitals, St. Bartholomew's patients received most of their care from nurses or servants. A *Breviarium* reader would have to be Latinate, which would preclude most of the nursing sisters at St. Bartholomew's: Rawcliffe argues that Mirfield's Latin text would have had "limited use" for nurses.[61] Yet channels existed for nurses to learn these recipes, perhaps by hearing them read and translated. Monica Green and Linne Mooney speculate in their edition of the Middle English *Sickness of Women* that obstetrical recipes may commonly have been read aloud to midwives "or communicated to them through other indirect means."[62] The hospital's Augustinian canons probably had little contact with postpartum women or nurses, but St. Bartholomew's chaplains seem a more likely group of available Latin readers. They circulated among the poor and ill, as chaplains did at St. Leonard's Hospital, ministering and hearing confessions. One may perhaps imagine chaplains reading and translating Mirfield's recipes for women caregivers such as nurses or visiting midwives.

The care of postpartum women did not necessarily stop with their departures from the hospital. The information contained in Mirfield's recipes could have been transmitted orally within a network of neighborhood women who cared for other women, perhaps including those discharged after purification. As Montserrat Cabré has shown, late medieval women's acts of health care took place primarily in the "domestic sphere, normally

left outside the histories of the art of maintaining health and alleviating illness."[63] The hospital's post-Reformation records document neighborhood
women caring for those rejected from the hospital, as I show in chapter 6.
Such care, spanning arrangements from "the ordinary to the occupational,
from gratuitous therapeutic attention to paid acts of health care," surely
took place during the fourteenth and fifteenth centuries also.[64] Mirfield issues an invitation to the "prudent reader" to correct the book as needed.
And though this gesture invokes a familiar literary topos, it also conveys a
hope that a relatively broad range of readers or hearers might use and
modify its information in their own practice of caring for patients in the
hospital and perhaps beyond.[65]

Only two copies of the full *Breviarium* survive, along with several
copies of sections or extracts.[66] Given Mirfield's stated emphasis on practicality, it is worth pausing over the two full manuscript witnesses to consider what their functions might have been. What we can determine about
their original provenance and later owners suggests that the texts were copied as medical reference works. The better copy, Oxford, Pembroke College
MS 2, is a large, clearly written book that originated at Abingdon Abbey in
Berkshire, for it bears the abbey's arms on the frontispiece. This is not a
well-thumbed physician's manual but a large, fairly ornate volume. Yet it
may have been copied for a practical purpose rather close to Mirfield's conception of the work as a compendium for hospital use. By the early twelfth
century, Abingdon Abbey had a hospital that operated until the mid-fifteenth century, when it was converted into an almshouse. The hospital's
buildings included rooms for the brothers and sisters, a chapel, and "either
one or two dormitories for the sick and infirm poor living there."[67] This
setup sounds similar to that of St. Bartholomew's, and although smaller
than the London hospital, the abbey's hospital may have catered to a similarly mixed population. Surprisingly, the Pembroke manuscript lacks chapter 15, the *Regimen sanitatis*. This omission may indicate that the abbey already had other such books in its library.

The practicality of this manuscript is enhanced by two appended reference texts: the *Sinonoma Bartholomei*, evidently Mirfield's own glossary,
which offers English synonyms for certain terms (e.g., *ambrosia* is glossed
as "wilde sauge," *armoniaca* as "selfehele"), and a *Quid pro quo*, a pharmaceutical reference work offering substitutes for ingredients that might not
be readily available.[68] The *Sinonoma* contains alphabetical synonyms for

pharmaceutical ingredients, symptoms, and other difficult terms. The drugs include many of those cited in the constrictive recipes that I consider later in this section, including *mastix* ("gumma est") and *agnus castus* ("frutex est, i. bischopeswort").[69] Such terms link the *Sinonoma* to St. Bartholomew's Hospital, with its range of patients, for it defines symptoms that one might expect from expectant or nursing mothers: for example, *nausea* ("est voluntas evomendi sine effectu"), and body fluids, including new mother's milk, *colostrum* ("lac statim post partum mulsum").[70] The *Quid pro quo* likewise adds practical value to the volume: this sort of reference work was considered de rigueur among late medieval Continental physicians, and such texts were widely used in England.[71] The one copied in this manuscript is extensive, featuring similar entries to other contemporary examples.[72]

Later owners of these *Breviarium* manuscripts seem to have valued their practical information, but we cannot know exactly how they used the books. Pembroke MS 2 was owned in the sixteenth century by the Oxford graduate and physician Richard Bartlett (or Bartlot), a founding fellow of the Royal College of Physicians.[73] Although Bartlett (d. 1556) did not have a known connection to St. Bartholomew's Hospital, he was buried in the erstwhile priory's church of St. Bartholomew the Great.[74] BL Harley MS 3 belonged to another well-known scientist, Dr. John Dee, the mathematician and astrologer.[75] Dee's annotations indicate interest in the work's recipes, Getz notes: he added two more medical recipes, one "Against childrens worms" (fol. 302v) and another "For the Eye syght clearing" (fol. 303r). He may have viewed the volume as a repository for useful medical guidance.

Mirfield's gynecology suggests not only a pragmatic but also a socially perceptive view of the hospital's female patients. Focusing on his discussion of vaginal constrictives and contraceptives, I show how Mirfield responds to his sources by extracting and enhancing therapies while minimizing the moralizing content: actually *removing* misogynist content in an effort to support the hospital's marginalized and suffering female patients. In her history of medieval European women's health care, Green makes a comment that can help us to understand how Mirfield's *Breviarium* fits into the literary and cultural history of St. Bartholomew's. The twelfth-century Salernitan treatises on women's health are critical texts for the development of medieval gynecological works. One of these works, *Treatments for Women*, derived ultimately from the pragmatic knowledge of Trota, a noted twelfth-century female healer. The *Treatments*, together with the "probably" male-authored *Conditions of Women* and the "certainly" male-authored *Women's Cosmetics*, were shaped by successive editors into an ensemble that circulated widely from the late twelfth century.[76] These works were in turn plumbed for information on women's health by later medical encyclopedists, such as Gilbertus Anglicus. Although the *Trotula* ensemble represented an amalgam of different authors' work, Green discerns a distinctive integration, in the Salernitan corpus, of the "physical" with the "social" woman:

> In the Salernitan view, a woman is a body with a uterus that can be displaced or become intemperate, with a vagina that can develop lesions or become overstretched, with breasts that can become turgid with milk or eaten away by cancerous lesions. This physical woman shades imperceptibly into the social woman who induces menstruation in order to become fertile, who is concerned to dye her hair and modify the colour of her face or teeth or gums in order to be attractive to men or maintain her social position, *the woman who endures painful intercourse or fakes virginity or chooses chastity because of current assumptions about female sexuality. This latter woman is a performer, an active agent choosing to use or manipulate her body in specific ways.*[77]

In the gynecological sections of his *Breviarium*, Mirfield enhances this integration of the "physical" with the "social" woman. In the *Breviarium*, virginity is treated as a performance, a process, not an absolute state but one that may be simulated in response to social requirements. Getz argues that Mirfield compiled the *Breviarium* to aid the treatment of vulnerable and poor patients, and women were prominent among these. Such women, like the unfortunate one described above in the *Book of the Foundation*, had lost their "yncomperable tresure" and moreover had become pregnant. Mirfield does not attempt "originality" in his compilation, but he does make meaningful choices to borrow, amplify, or suppress material from his sources, resulting in a collection tailored to the particular context of the hospital. Building on the work of these historians of medicine, I delve in more detail into this process of compilation in order to show how, as Getz argues, the *Breviarium* becomes "devoid of the moralizing and antifeminism of the *Florarium*," and in order to suggest the significance of this new emphasis within the hospital context. Unlike Georg Kraut, the later humanist editor of the *Trotula* material who removed most of the constrictive recipes from his 1544 printed edition, Mirfield added *more* of the remedies that he seems to have judged practical for hospital patients.[78]

In her insightful discussion of Mirfield's *Breviarium*, Green notes the author's recipes for the "restoration" of virginity, which borrow liberally from other authorities, including Gilbertus Anglicus, Robert Frugardi, and Lanfranc of Milan. Mirfield includes all of Gilbertus's and Lanfranc's gynecological sections, and

> Mirfield even included topics like procedures to 'restore' virginity and contraceptives which, one would think, would be quite problematic for a cleric to approve—as in fact they were, for the latter topic appears in cipher in at least one of the extant manuscripts. Obstetrical chapters included aid in difficult birth and means to expel the dead foetus, both of which may have been important at Saint Bartholomew's since, included among the poor and sick whom it took into its walls, there were pregnant singlewomen who had 'done amiss' (and who may have been particularly desirous to 'restore' their virginity).[79]

Mirfield tackles the challenges facing these women and takes seriously the task of making a "corrupta" look like a virgin again, in order to be able to reenter London society. In the above passage, Green notes the presence of "pregnant single women who had 'done amiss,'" referencing the description of St. Bartholomew's hospital that I noted from the list of city churches in BL MS Egerton 1995. A similar phrase appears elsewhere in the list, where the author notes that Mayor Richard Whittington had endowed a room for pregnant single women in Southwark's Hospital of St. Thomas: "And that nobyl marchaunt Rycharde Whytygndon made a new chambyr with viij beddys for yong wemen that hadde done amysse in truste of a good mendement. And he commaundyd that alle the thyngys that ben don in that chambyr shulde be kepte secrete with owte forthe, yn payne of lesynge of hyr levyng; for he wolde not shame no yonge womon in no wyse, for hyt myght be cause of hyr lettyng of her maryage."[80]

If we recall the language seen in the earlier description of St. Bartholomew's concern to "kepe [unmarried mothers'] conselle and hyr worschyppe," it seems that some version of Whittington's rules about secrecy was in place at St. Bartholomew's too.[81] The stern warning to complete secrecy reveals a fear of public "shame," the irreparable damage to reputation, and probable association with prostitution (common to Southwark and Smithfield) that could ruin a young women's marriage prospects. Not only was pregnancy grounds for dismissal from service, making it virtually impossible for women to support themselves licitly outside of marriage, but marriage to a former prostitute (actual or reputed) was generally avoided for the legal complications it might entail.[82]

The concern for secrecy at both hospitals seems particularly notable given the prevalence of prostitution in their neighborhoods, for secrecy was the very privilege denied to prostitutes. Fifteenth-century regulations governing the brothels of Southwark, surrounding St. Thomas's Hospital, mandated that brothel employees work openly, requiring "the wommen that ben at common bordell be seyn every day what they be, an a womman that liveth by hir body to comme and go."[83] Women making unauthorized attempts at secrecy were prohibited, fined, and punished by humiliating exposure: if they attempted to hide in the brothel "and wold be kept privee withynne, and it be not the stewholders wil, thei shal doo the officers for to wite, upon the peine of xl.s.; and the same womman shal be take and made a fyne of xx.s., and be sette thries upon de cokyngestole, and than forswere the lordship."[84] Attempting to hide in a brothel resulted not only in display on the cucking stool, the paradigmatic public punishment for women, but also in banishment from the borough, making future employment impossible.

This predicament must have been one in which some of St. Bartholomew's female patients found themselves. In contrast to the young woman described in the *Book of the Foundation*, whose return home represented a salutary escape from sexuality and the marriage market, women who survived childbirth in the hospital, whatever became of their infants, would have had to resume their lives as single women in London. Some may have decided to leave their children to be cared for at the hospital.[85] Such a prospect would have been daunting in a milieu that made "single woman" synonymous with "prostitute."[86] The ability to represent themselves as virginal, hence marriageable, would have had immense practical value for such women, as Green suggests, perhaps helping them to avoid the reputation or reality of prostitution. Mirfield was as conscious as Whittington of the need to keep the hospital's treatments "secrete" to prevent social shame, and his remedies demonstrate a pragmatic concern to strip away anything that would bring shame to these patients.

As Green notes, the *Breviarium* contains numerous recipes for the "restoration" of virginity, some of unknown provenance. Mirfield subtly reshapes the inherited material, giving it a revised meaning and function for the hospital setting. Here, pregnant women would be cared for after child-birth until their purification, forty days later. Thus we may assume that the hospital in Mirfield's time housed women at various stages of pregnancy and postpartum.[87]

Like the Salernitan writers and Gilbertus in his *Compendium of medicine*, Mirfield defines a separate gynecological section within his compilation, which he labels with the catchall term "De infirmitatibus matricis" (on infirmities of the womb).[88] The section at the end of the sixth book is organized in a logical order that follows Gilbertus's seventh book to some extent: beginning with menstrual complaints of retention or excessive flow, proceeding through the signs and support of pregnancy, help for difficult births, removal of a dead fetus and afterbirth, and postpartum treatment.[89] It is largely limited to practical gynecology, but there are a few sections outside this purview, such as "De sterilitate virorum" and "De signis concepcioni masculi siue femelle." Much of the content is borrowed from Gilbertus, but Gilbertus's section is longer and more varied, containing a chapter "de urinis" and incorporating discussions of generation (such as "De impedimento concepcionis" and "De generationis embrionis"), which Mirfield does not adopt.

The way that Mirfield labels and locates the recipes for vaginal constriction may be telling of their function within the compilation and, thus, perhaps within the hospital's program of care for an unmarried mother. The section on constrictives comes at the end of the gynecological chapters: Mirfield's rubrics for these final two sections read "c. 22: ut corrupta quasi virgo appareat; c. 23: si vis scire an mulier sit corrupta; c. 24: ne mulier concipiat" (how the corrupted woman may appear to be a virgin; how to know if a women has been corrupted; how a woman should avoid conceiving)[90] (see fig. 2.2). He highlights the contents of these sections by setting them apart, at the end of the gynecological section. In contrast, the corresponding section in Gilbertus is located between "De ydropsici matricis" and "De impedimento conceptionis" and is entitled "De sophisticatione uulve" (on the disguise/adulteration of the vagina).[91] In the *Trotula* source from which some of the recipes come, the relevant title that appears before one series of constrictive recipes is "constrictorium bonum" (a good constrictive), within the Salernitan text *On Treatments for Women*, between sections on vaginal prolapse and swelling.[92] These differences in placement and terminology are subtle but may be significant. By separating out these sections

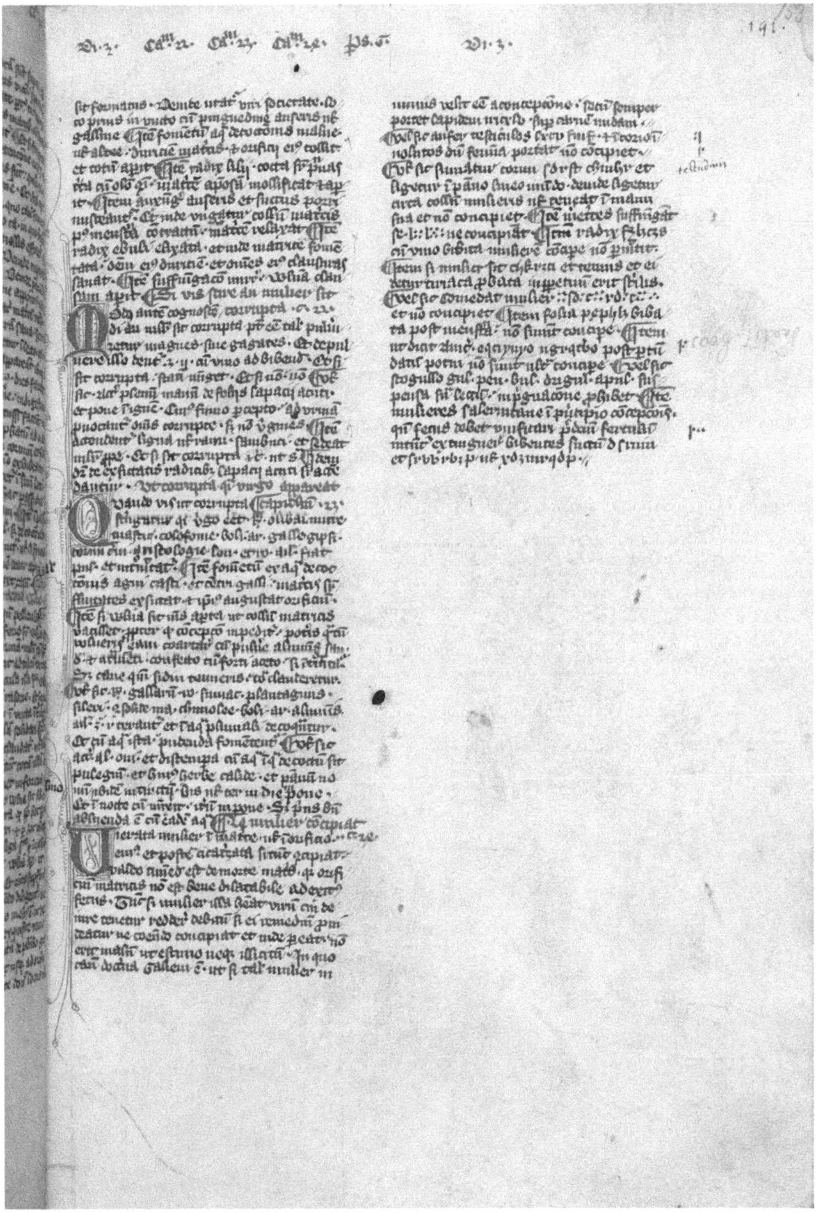

FIGURE 2.2. John Mirfield's gynecological recipes. Oxford, Pembroke College MS 2, fol. 153r. Reproduced with the kind permission of the Master and Fellows of Pembroke College, Oxford.

and titling them clearly, Mirfield makes them easier for readers to locate and to use. He seems to have fashioned this unique bloc of three chapters, related to the detection, performance, and maintenance of virginity, for the particular setting of the hospital and the practical use of women needing guidance in these areas.

Even though the *Trotula* rubric does not carry a judgment, Mirfield and Gilbertus use the terms "corrupta" and "sophisticatione," respectively. Both of these place a negative construction on the loss of virginity. Yet Gilbertus's term "sophisticatio" implies deception, emphasizing the woman's role in falsifying virginity, whereas Mirfield's term "corrupta" in the passive/adjectival sense casts the woman as the victim of sexual contamination. In a single word, Gilbertus's deceiver becomes Mirfield's victim. This shift of terminology is significant in the hospital context, where the female patient might have come, perhaps alone, as a last resort for care. Among such a population, constrictive remedies to simulate virginity might represent one of the few avenues toward regaining respectability in the civic space. As the passage from Gregory's chronicle indicates, what Green has argued for the twelfth-century Mediterranean culture that produced the *Trotula* texts remained true in late fourteenth-century London: "women's honor . . . to a degree that would never have been true for men, was bound up intimately with their sexual purity. If successful, these recipes may well have made the difference for some women between marriage and financial security, on the one hand, and social ostracization and poverty, on the other."[93]

The subtle difference in attitude that the rubrics convey, between suspicion in the earlier sources and sympathetic care befitting the hospital, is reinforced by the content of these sections in the two compendia. The constrictive recipes in Mirfield are borrowed in several cases from Gilbertus and ultimately from the *Trotula* texts in two cases, as Green has shown. Mirfield features several additional recipes, perhaps attempting to add as much useful information as possible on this vital topic. I emphasize not so much the contents of the recipes, which contain fairly standard ingredients, but the suppression of antifeminist commentary and the removal of overtly deceptive recipes that are present, in different forms, in Gilbertus and in the *Trotula* sources.

In keeping with the differences already noted between Gilbertus and Mirfield, Mirfield commences his first recipe, on fol. 153ra, after the rubric "Ut corrupta quasi virgo appareat capitulum 23" (So that a corrupted woman might appear to be a virgin, chapter 23):

Quando vis ut corrupta stringatur quasi virgo esset: Recipe olibani, mirre, masticis, colofonie, boli armenici, galle gipsi, cornu cerui, aristologie longe et rotunde ana. Fiat puluerem et intromittatur. Item fomentum ex aqua decoctionis agni casti, et centri galli: matricis superfluitates exsiccat et ipsius angustat orificium.

——————

When you wish that a corrupted woman should be tightened so that she seems to be a virgin, take some of each of frankincense, myrrh, mastic gum, pitch, Armenian bole, gall, gypsum, stag's horn,[94] round and long birthwort. Make a powder and insert it. Likewise, a fomentation [made] of water of a decoction of chaste tree and clary; this dries out the superfluities of the womb and narrows its orifice.[95]

Thus Mirfield begins, like the *Trotula* source, with a practical directive and then proceeds with the recipe. The ingredients are fairly familiar ones for the period. We find a reference to "cornus cervi" and to oil containing mastic in a fifteenth-century London apothecary's inventory.[96] Most of the ingredients mentioned here are glossed in Mirfield's *Sinonoma Bartholomei*, including mastix, colofonia, galle, cornus cervi, aristologia, agnus castus, and centrum galli.[97]

In contrast to this straightforward presentation, Gilbertus's section on policing and restoring virginity, which shares some recipes with Mirfield (though not this particular one), begins with a long moralizing commentary that at first sympathetically justifies the restoratives but then moves into a condemnation of those who might use them. Green demonstrates that Gilbertus first explains the utility of these remedies within a sexually intolerant system in which "corrumpuntur quandoque virgines, vnde et ianua ampliatur, ita ut corruptela pateat et merito repudium patiuntur et in sempiternum dedecus vel diuortium in vtrisque periculum tam viri quam mulieres sortiuntur" (sometimes virgins are corrupted, whence their 'door' is widened as plainly happens in sexually experienced women ... and they suffer repudiation and perpetual disgrace, or they are fated for divorce, in which there is danger both to men and to women).[98] Green notes that this "unapologetic justification for their presence" does not appear in the *Trotula* sources. Gilbertus's justification is not unsympathetic toward the female subjects, but his discussion veers into antifeminism as he details a method of how "elargatum oportet restringere vitium, et est ipsius mulieris conamine sophisticatum palliare" (to draw tight what sin has enlarged, and to hide what has been disguised by the effort of this same woman).[99] Again we encounter the language of "sophisticatio" and the impulse to "hide" (palliare) the evidence of such tampering. The absence of any such commentary in the *Breviarium* is striking. Mirfield does not explain or justify these remedies or offer judgments of those using them; he transmits them, sometimes amplifying their contents rather than reproducing Gilbertus's rhetoric of anxiety and deceit.

In a similar vein, Gilbertus asserts that virginity may be feigned by "chaste" and "modest" conduct, and thus the only way to tell a virgin from a corrupt woman is through physical testing, examination of urine, or other tests.[100] Mirfield offers several methods of determining whether the subject is virginal, without asserting that women are inclined to deception. One of his recipes, similar to one from Gilbertus, is to make a powder of magnets or jet, then cook it in wine: if the woman, after drinking the mixture, suddenly urinates, then she is not a virgin. If not, then she is a virgin.[101] Mirfield offers no explanation for these methods, nor does he claim that women might be able to falsify virginity through conduct. Yet the recipes that follow acknowledge what must have been the real concern, among hospital patients, for what the loss of virginity meant for a woman's prospects in the city: as a worker, a future wife, or both.

Given the urgency of including recipes for constrictives, it is again notable what Mirfield does not include: any recipes for creating a flow of blood to falsify the loss of virginity. Such a recipe, almost identical in both *Treatments for Women* and Gilbertus, involves putting leeches in the vagina, but not too far (sanguissas ad os vulue caute ne subintret) and then allowing a scab to form, which would break upon penetration.[102] Mirfield suppresses references to such false "adulteration of the vagina," to recall Gilbertus's term. In Mirfield, aids to the simulation of virginity are responsive, but these methods are not explicitly deceptive nor are they associated with immorality. Where Gilbertus used language associating the loss of virginity with sinfulness and its "restoration" with trickery, *Treatments for Women* contains a passage concerning the source of a recipe for simulating virginal blood flow:

> Item quedam sunt immunde et corrupte meretrices que plus quam uirgines cupiunt inuenire, et faciunt constrictorium ad idem, sed inconsulte, quoniam se ipsas reddunt sanguinolentas et uirgam uiri ulcerant. Accipiunt nitrum puluerizatum et uulue imponunt.

---

Likewise, there are some dirty and corrupt prostitutes who desire to seem to be more than virgins, and they make a constrictive for this purpose, but they are ill counseled, for they render themselves bloody and they wound the penis of the man. They take powered natron and place it in the vagina.[103]

This passage did not make it into Gilbertus's compendium, and thus Mirfield may never have seen it; however, I include it because it participates in a similar shaming of the nonvirginal woman that Gilbertus too performs. Despite (or perhaps because of) prostitution as an implicit context for his writing in the Smithfield hospital, Mirfield suppresses such sentiments or mention of prostitutes from his gynecological discussion in the *Breviarium*.

It has been suggested that Mirfield's inclusion of contraceptive recipes at the end of his *Breviarium* may have gotten him in trouble with the Church, or that such recipes might have been "problematic for a cleric to approve."[104] Although some elements of the recipes are obscured by ciphers, many of these recipes, following the constrictives to conclude the gynecological section, are quite legible.[105] The first, most elaborate recipe is derived from the *Trotula* tradition, sharing much of its content with two sections from *Conditions of Women*. Mirfield merges the two sections, the first discussing why women with "uuluas angustas et matrices strictas" (narrow vaginas and constricted wombs) should not engage in intercourse, "ne concipiant et moriantur" (lest they should conceive and die), and the second a set of recipes to prevent conception.[106] In Mirfield the single recipe begins by stating the danger of conception to a woman whose womb and passages are "vierata" (twisted).[107] He continues that conception would result in death for such a woman if the "orificium matricis non est bene dilatabile ad exitum fetus" (the opening of the womb is not expandable enough for the exit of the fetus). Then he offers several recipes, derived from the Salernitan writings, for avoiding conception. The first recipe relies upon the carrying of a stone next to the woman's nude body, and the second calls for carrying a weasel's testicles on her person, wrapped in a linen cloth.[108] The recipes are borrowed, but what seems different is the move that Mirfield makes to combine the two sections, explicitly limiting these recipes to women whose lives would be threatened by childbirth.

A second and related addition is a passage clarifying that the only acceptable sexual intercourse takes place within marriage. This explicit reference to marital sex is not present in the *Trotula* source. Mirfield's work reads, "Tunc si mulier illa habeat virum cum de iure tenetur reddere debitum, si ei remedium prouideatur ne coneundo concipiat et inde pereat, non erit malum ut estimo neque illicitum" (In this case if the woman has sex with the man, as she is required by law to render her debt, and she uses this remedy in order to avoid conceiving so that she does not perish, it will not be sinful, and I don't consider it illicit).[109] This addition is remarkable for two reasons: first, it shows the clerical writer positing a context for contraception that places health, Christian morality, and legality into a proper relationship. Second it seems to presuppose that patients in the hospital will one day be in the position to engage in lawful married sex, envisioning a future of acceptable sexual activity for the women residing temporarily at St. Bartholomew's Hospital.

The combination of virginity tests, constrictives, and contraceptive recipes has a complex meaning in the hospital context. Not only does Mirfield suggest that these three practices might exist in a harmonious and ultimately moral relationship, but he implies that all three may be necessary for the women he envisioned needing his book. For Mirfield, in his capacity as hospital chaplain (if this was indeed his role), there would seem to be no contradiction in the corrupted virgin seeking purification or the wife using contraceptives. Such practices might be necessary at different moments within women's sexual lives, some periods of which may have been spent at the hospital. His practical gynecology does not speculate about motives, nor does it shame women in difficult circumstances. Instead it offers handily organized remedies to help them. One could perhaps describe Mirfield as Richard Whittington was characterized in MS Egerton 1995: "he wolde not shame no yonge women in no wyse."

Mirfield explicitly wrote within and for the hospital, and the Pembroke manuscript's Abingdon Abbey provenance suggests that the abbey recognized the *Breviarium*'s utility soon after its compilation. Yet outside of religious institutional contexts, Mirfield's writings had a wider afterlife in surgery and gynecology, as his work became a source for later compilers, much as he had borrowed from his medical forebears.[110] I turn again to his gynecological remedies to suggest that the poor single women of the hospital may have provided an unexpected inspiration for the care of women more widely in the fifteenth century. The presence of Mirfield's constrictive and contraceptive recipes, with some notable changes, in a later medical anthology, suggests that a fifteenth-century practitioner also found Mirfield's recipes congenial within a health-care regimen. This book, Oxford Bodleian MS Bodley 682, is a large fifteenth-century composite of five parts. Its diversity of contents suggests that the book may have been a physician's personal collection, but we cannot rule out institutional use either.[111] Among other reference works, the volume includes two treatises on urine, a treatise on medical ingredients, a list of synonyms for medical substances, and several recipe collections. One might say that this purpose-made volume approximates the contents of the *Breviarium*, which Mirfield called a "repository" of medical reference material. (This raises the question of whether the compiler was working with a full *Breviarium* or a copy containing only the gynecological section.) As Green has shown, among Bodley MS 682's other medical contents, fols. 172r–196r feature a version of the "standardized" *Trotula* gynecological ensemble, with material added from the *Breviarium* and other authors.[112] Most of the chapters from Mirfield's gynecology are included, albeit often in a different order from the *Breviarium*. However, the three that I examined above (chapters 22–24) do appear in the same sequence as in the *Breviarium*. Although the Bodley 682 compiler places these chapters in the middle rather than at the end of the gynecology, the conservation of Mirfield's sequence suggests that the later compiler considered his section order to have a logic that should not be altered.

Retaining Mirfield's chapter order while making some changes to the content, the fifteenth-century compiler has taken further steps toward rendering the material practical for his or her own purposes. The composite manuscript's comprehensiveness suggests that it may have belonged to a physician with a range of patients and duties, perhaps not limited to a single institutional context. He or she valued the detail and range of Mirfield's collection and was also concerned with determining and simulating virginity. The first recipe under the heading "Si vis scire an mulier sit corrupta an non" (fol. 186r) is virtually identical to Mirfield's as copied in Pembroke MS 2. The second section, with the heading "Vt corrupta quasi virgo appareat," retains two of Mirfield's remedies, including the first one that I examined above calling for "olibani, mirre, masticis, colofonie." MS Bodley 682 then includes an additional *Trotula*-derived constrictive recipe, involving oak apples, roses, sumac, great plantain, comfrey, Armenian bole, alum, and fuller's earth, which is not included in Mirfield.[113]

Most striking is the Bodley 682 compiler's treatment of the final section on contraceptives. Here the recipes have been streamlined and expanded to appear both more legible and more comprehensive. The later compiler retains the expansion that Mirfield made to his source: the passage on marital sex as the proper context for contraceptive use. As in Mirfield, the section is framed as advice to married women, perhaps making it a good fit for some of this later doctor's patients. No user or beneficiary of this volume's recipes need have known the original context for this statement or the marginalized women for whom Mirfield wrote. Retaining this important change by Mirfield, the later compiler has removed the ciphers that made some of Mirfield's recipes illegible and also added content to amplify them, including a variant on the first recipe in the *Liber de Sinthomatibus Mulierum*, not present in Mirfield, advising the woman who does not wish to conceive "ut mulier semper secum portet lapidem que invenitur in matricem capre que nondum fetatur, et non concipiet" (the woman should always carry with her a stone found in the womb of a goat that has not yet given birth, and she will not conceive).[114] Thus the Bodley compilation carries out Mirfield's project of locating contraception within the socially sanctioned context of marriage, while moving the recipes out of the realm of the hospital.

The evidence of MS Bodley 682 shows that for this later compiler, Mirfield's gynecology has become a source for the treatment of patients who may be distant in status and location from the poor women for whom he first wrote. Mirfield's hospital-focused text, which had itself borrowed from the wider women's medical tradition to treat female patients with care and discretion, now conveys practical advice to women in the wider world, who even if not experiencing the marginalized single motherhood of hospital residents, may still have wished to preserve and manipulate their bodies in medically and religiously sanctioned ways.

## Mirfield's *Florarium*: A Return to Misogyny in Theory

I conclude this chapter by framing Mirfield's *Breviarium* and its intriguing fifteenth-century medical legacy with a few passages from his spiritual compendium, the *Florarium Bartholomei*. Mirfield's *Florarium* survives in a comparable number of copies: two full manuscripts and several copies of extracts.[115] It is not clear which work came first, but Mirfield's allusion to his advanced age in the *Florarium* epilogue, noting "modicum illud quod iam restat de vite mee" (the little of life that is left me) suggests that he wrote it quite late in life.[116] This work is a *florilegium* of sententious quotations in alphabetical chapters, beginning with "De abstinencia," ending with "De usura," and including chapters on chastity, the sins, poverty, prayer, and contemplation. The *Florarium* features an unusual chapter entitled "De medicis" (On Physicians), whose section on the regimen of health, derived from the *Secretum Secretorum*, is largely duplicated in the *Breviarium*'s final book.[117]

In some respects Mirfield's *Florarium* looks similar to other fourteenth-century florilegia: clerical compendia that integrate material from various sources under alphabetical headings to aid in the composition of sermons.[118] His choice of "abstinencia" as a first heading, for example, is shared by several other florilegia, but his choice and ordering of authorities is unique.[119] Yet many of Mirfield's topics seem specifically applicable to those in religious orders (e.g., "De monachis et regularibus" or "De vita contemplativa"). And as Christina von Nolcken observes, Mirfield introduces his work not as a preaching aid but as a work for private devotion:[120]

> Autoritates subscripte que ad excitandam legentis mentem ad amorem dei vel timorem seu ad suimet discussionem hic vtique compilate sunt non sunt legende in tumultu sed in quiete nec velociter sed tractatim cum intenta et morosa meditacione.
>
> ———
>
> The authorities given below, since they are compiled for the stimulation of the mind of the reader to love and fear of God, and to the consideration of Him, are not to be read amidst tumults, but in quiet; not speedily but one subject at a time, with intent and thoughtful meditation.[121]

A work intended for private consultation, the *Florarium* marshals its authorities to help clerical readers look inward. The compendium's subject matter and literary purpose differ so much from those of the pragmatic *Breviarium* that it is sometimes hard to believe Mirfield authored both.

Yet in the *Florarium*, the hospital with its pregnant, childbearing women and their children seems to be a ghostly presence. Although he makes no mention of the hospital in the *Florarium*, it seems possible that having compiled the *Breviarium* and faced the challenges of ministering to the hospital's vulnerable, mixed-gender population, Mirfield took the spiritual compendium as an opportunity to assert boundaries between realms that hospital life constantly blurred: spiritual and physical, male and female. Women with their dangerous looks and touches are banished from the spiritual florarium (flower garden), a "locus ubi flores habundant" (a place where flowers abound).[122] Although the *Florarium*'s alphabetical organization precludes an overarching argument, it is notable how Mirfield attempts at various points to prohibit women from the realms of spiritual and physical health. In a book composed for clerical readers, the exclusion of women is not surprising. But by tracing some of the places where Mirfield jarringly contradicts his own statements in the *Breviarium*, we may discern, by contrast, how strongly his medical text advocates for poor, sexually active women. In his discussion of abstinence, in his condemnation of ignorant women practitioners, and in his discussion of women as sexually dangerous, Mirfield voices the misogyny that his *Breviarium* had noticeably extirpated. By putting the two side by side, we can better appreciate the entrenched prejudices and anxieties that the late medieval hospital faced, even from within, in caring for single women patients.

Mirfield proposes abstinence as a way of separating the mind from the body, the physical from the social, rather than integrating them as the *Breviarium* suggested might be possible. In his Proemium, Mirfield claims to have culled these "flowers" of wisdom for an explicitly moral purpose:

> persuadere amatores mundi quatinus relictis immoderatis cupiditatibus suis cum omnibus aliis viciis per sancte pauperitatis et virtutis vias reuerti studeant ad gratiam redemptoris quam fugiunt mundi.
>
> ———
>
> to persuade lovers of this world, that, having left behind them as much as possible their immoderate desires and all other vices, they may, by the paths of holy poverty and virtue, study to return again to the grace of the Redeemer of the world, from which they now flee.[123]

Although his projected readers may once have been "lovers of this world," they are now priests pledged to "holy poverty and virtue," language that would seem to target a professed religious audience.[124] In a work chastising clerical readers to flee the world's allure, abstinence offers a fitting place to begin, not just for its alphabetical primacy but because nullus palmam certaminis spiritualis apprehendet vt ait beatus Gregorius qui non in semetipso prius per afflictam mentis concupiscenciam carnis insentiue deuicerit ideo ad capitulum de abstinencia conueniencius esse videtur inchoandum.

―――――

nobody attains to the palm in the spiritual conflict who does not first, as the Blessed Gregory says, cleanse away the filthy sins of the body by first overcoming the abominable desires of the mind; therefore it would seem most fitting to lay the foundation stone of the work with the chapter on 'Abstinence'.[125]

This is a quality that Mirfield can assume (or at least exhort) from his projected *Florarium* readers, clerics whose role mandates sexual purity. Mirfield presents abstinence as a value with practical and theoretical value for clerical readers, and, crucially, a means to exclude women from their world. It functions as a basis for the avoidance of other sins, beginning as a check upon appetite, which in turn reduces lustfulness:

Et abstinencia libidinem domat et minuat . . . venerabilis Ysidorus: Quia vacuus venter in oracione vigilare facit castitatem quoque gignit abstinencia. Consilium tamen Ysidori est vt qui corpus suum abstinencie dedicat cum feminis habitare non presumat.

―――――

Abstinence moderates and diminishes lust . . . the venerable Isidore says that an empty stomach in prayer creates the chastity by which abstinence develops. Isidore's advice is that he who dedicates his body to abstinence will never presume to live with women.[126]

Not only does abstinence function as a brake on sexual desire, but abstinence may work in a more reflective mode as a remedy for those who have already committed sins. Borrowing from Gregory the Great's *Homily* 35 on Luke, Mirfield writes, "qui se illicita meminit comisisse ab aliquibus et licitis studeat abstinere. . . . Et se reprehendat in minimis qui se meminit in maximis delinquisse" (whoever remembers committing forbidden things should pursue abstinence from those in favor of lawful things. . . . And he should reprove himself lest the smallest memory lead to the greatest delinquency).[127] This first quality expounded in Mirfield's spiritual collection forms a basis for physical and mental asceticism, which preclude either the presence or thought of women.

In his chapter entitled "De medicis et medicinis eorum," Mirfield ponders the relation between spiritual and physical health, transmitting received wisdom, much of it from canon law, on prioritizing the spirit over the body. In keeping with the overall tenor of the *Florarium*, in "De medicis" his borrowings from legal and medical sources assert the paramount importance of spiritual safety in the face of the real dangers involved in medical treatments.[128] Yet before unfolding these issues, Mirfield sounds a strongly misogynist note by showing how women present problems in the medical context as incompetent healers and sources of sexual temptation. He opens the chapter by quoting biblical praise of the physician as an emissary of God and noting the imperative for physicians to be "viri litterati aut quod ab eo qui nouit litteras ad minus artem addiscant" (well educated, or at least that they should learn their profession from a man of literary attainments).[129] Yet this requirement is routinely flouted by women in particular:

> tempore presenti nedum ydiote, verumtamen quod deterius est et horribilius iudicatur, viles femine presumptuose istud officium sibi vsurpant et abutantur eo, que nec artem nec ingenium habent, vnde propter causam sue stoliditatis errores maximos operantur, quibus egri multociens interficiuntur, cum non sapienter nec sub certa radice sed casualiter operantur, et causas et nomina infirmitatum quas asserunt se sanare scire et posse penitus non agnoscunt.

---

> At the present time, ignorant amateurs, to say nothing of—what is worse, and is considered by me more horrible—worthless and presumptuous women, usurp this profession to themselves and abuse it; who, possessing neither natural ability nor professional knowledge, make the greatest possible mistakes (thanks to their stupidity) and very often kill their patients; for they work without wisdom and from no certain foundation, but in a casual fashion, nor are they thoroughly acquainted with the causes or even the names of the maladies which they claim that they are competent to cure.[130]

This diatribe comes from Bruno of Calabria's *Chirurgia Magna* and repeats sentiments found in other contemporary medical writers.[131] Women have no place in the vocational realm of physicians, owing not only to their lack of professional training but also to their natural "lack of ability" and "stupidity," qualities here tied to women's lack of rational capacity and limitation to the bodily realm. Yet these are the very terms that Mirfield uses to describe himself in the *Breviarium*, where he claims to be compiling out of "the desire to assist simpletons such as myself" and to help those "ignorant as I am." Whereas in the passage above he envisions his medical compendium possibly reaching both male or female readers or hearers, here he condemns the ignorant and assumes their (dangerous, even life-threatening) inability to be taught. Notably Mirfield uses very similar terms ("rudis" in *Breviarium*, "ydiote" in *Florarium*) as an opportunity for masculine learning in one case, and as a damning insult to women in the other. Despite writing against the grain in the *Breviarium*, here he reverts to the misogyny that he had avoided in his medical work.

Mirfield picks up the connection between dangers to the spirit and flesh in the chapter "de mulieribus," in which women appear as dangerous, even infectious, to men. My purpose is not to suggest that there is anything original in this pastiche of misogynistic quotations but rather to highlight the contrast between this work and the *Breviarium*, particularly in Mirfield's expression of anxiety about proximity to women.[132] Taking women with all of their dangers as its primary subject, this chapter raises the female threat to clerical purity and rehearses arguments for women's subjection. Mirfield weaves together quotations from biblical and patristic authorities, also including a few choice selections in verse, which make an impact with their formal variation. He frames the chapter with prohibitions on clerical contact with women, beginning with the canonical statement "clerici non debent cohabitare cum mulieribus," then enumerating the only categories of women that might present exceptions (mother, sisters, etc.).[133] Yet as many canonists argued, relying on a chestnut attributed to Augustine, the cleric cannot be too careful, even with female family members: "Augustinus non consentit habitare cum sorore sua, dicens, Que cum sorore mea sunt, sorores meae non sunt" (Augustine did not consent to live with his own sister, saying, Those [women] who are with my sister are not my sisters).[134] Here Augustine is understood to be signaling the danger posed by a female attendant who might accompany his sister.[135] Mirfield sums up this danger with a final framing statement, also attributed to Augustine, fully separating the exercise of holiness from contact with women:

"Amator dei mulieris amore non vincitur" (the lover of God is not defeated by love of a woman).[136] The cleric must struggle constantly between these two forms of love, which in this text at least, can never be reconciled.

Between these two framing statements, Mirfield spends several folios elaborating and rationalizing this struggle in detail. He unfolds the danger that women present through their appearances and touches by embroidering his text at several points with extracts from verse: "Frequens feminarum visus mentem mollificat, sensum hebetat, et sapientem esse non patitur" (the frequent sight of women softens the mind, blunts the understanding, and prevents the wise man from existing).[137] This insight is embellished with lines of verse warning of women's dangers, including, "Est species morbi mulierem tangere [noli], / Si tangis tangit, si tangit, cedere nescit / Est tanti medicina mali fuga si fugis" (It is a kind of illness to touch a woman / If you touch, she touches, if she touches, it is impossible to withdraw. This is a medicine of such evil, that you must flee if you can).[138] This teasing versified play likening the woman to a source of "illness" and to a bad "medicine" that men should avoid echoes the misogynist opening of "De medicis" and recalls but implicitly rejects the mixed-gender, therapeutic world of the hospital. Where the *Breviarium* provided medicine to women, now men are the unfortunate "patients" subject to women's dangerous attentions.

Mirfield's final verse section adapts part of Alexander Neckham's misogynist poem *De vita monachorum* to elaborate on the dangers of women's blandishments. Mirfield splices lines of the poem together in order to emphasize the fearsome strength of women's desires. He creates the following new sequence of lines by transposing the lines of his source: "Femineum fuge colloquium, vir sancte, caveto / Femineas, si vis vincere blandi[ti]as. / Accendit mulier quecumque libidinis ignem / Et sanctis ipsis proxima facta nocet" (I warn you, holy man, flee the conversation of women / If you wish to conquer their flatteries. / Every woman kindles the fire of lust / And an immediate deed destroys even the saints).[139] In a concentrated manner here, Mirfield intensifies the connections suggested earlier between women and danger, both physical and spiritual. Although he does not mention the hospital in the *Florarium*, Mirfield's agitated tone here and in "De medicis" suggests that his involvement with its vulnerable population may have given rise to an impulse near the end of his career to assert order and hierarchy (at least for a clerical audience): the spiritual over the physical, the male over the female. The *Florarium* goes to creative lengths to demote the body, excluding and scorning women from the realm of healing.

Considered together, these three texts, written at the intersection of priory and hospital, reveal deep concerns over the presence of pregnant, laboring, and postpartum single women. At the hospital, poor women seeking cures for their afflictions, a safe place to give birth, and help returning to the civic space populated the hospital and inspired treatment: medical, spiritual, and textual. *The Book of the Foundation* and Mirfield's *Florarium* exclude women's sexualized bodies as dangerous to the priory's ethos. In these works, purification and corruption are seen in absolute terms, and judgment is final. In contrast, without making the picture too rosy, Mirfield's *Breviarium* suggests that in the hospital, marginalized women might have a brief reprieve from judgment, a few weeks of necessary privacy before returning to life in the city. The fifteenth-century movement of Mirfield's gynecology from the hospital into a wider arena of medical practice reveals the enduring utility of his therapies. This movement also shows that the hospital and its literatures could never be cloistered but remained in meaningful conversation with the needs and desires of the wider world.

# THREE

# Lay Reading in St. Bartholomew's Hospital Close

## *John Shirley's Final Anthology*

I turn now to the residential community that encircled St. Bartholomew's Hospital in the mid-fifteenth century and begin to map its literary practices. We can identify the tenants of the hospital close for the years 1456–58, thanks to the survival of hospital brother John Cok's rental list.[1] The close's tenants, many of them retired, included civil and royal servants, lawyers, clerics, city officials and their wives, a few young families, some guildsmen, and numerous widows.[2] Some of the close's widows had come to live there with their husbands; others took up residence alone after their husbands had died.[3] One famously literate resident was the London bibliophile and scribe John Shirley, who continued to copy texts into his eighties, until his death in 1456. Historians of the hospital close have suggested that Shirley and other residents may have formed a "literary community" or "salon."[4] I revisit these suggestions to look with fresh eyes at the texts that Shirley copied and compiled for his neighbors. I argue that Shirley designed his final anthology, now Bodleian MS Ashmole 59, to speak to these residents, who were in many cases his friends: men, women, and children linked to each other and to the wider city through familial and professional bonds, religious loyalties, and personal friendships.

In the first section of this chapter, I argue that even within formal constraints, the wills of hospital close residents testify to their experiences of the close as a site for deep friendships, spiritual expression, and an extended if sometimes fractious family. I then show how Shirley's final anthology may have intervened into this web of relationships with texts promoting particular modes of conduct for the hospital's varied constituencies.

WILLS AS HOSPITAL LITERATURE:
THE HOSPITAL CLOSE AND EXTENDED SPIRITUAL FAMILY

Wills provide textual evidence for the priorities and practices of the hospital close residents who formed Shirley's reading audience. It is impossible to generalize about such a diverse group of people, but I have selected two wills—those of retired lawyer Thomas Gevendale and grocer's widow Beatrice Lurchon—that express some key preoccupations of the elite laymen and prosperous married women who populated the close. Though undeniably formulaic, their wills suggest that these testators understood the hospital community as an extended spiritual family to which they were obligated and upon which they could call for assistance. I also show how the wills of parents, grandparents, and godparents offer evidence for children who lived in the close and formed another of Shirley's potential reading audiences.

Some hospital close residents came from within the institution, including several chaplains and retired brothers, while the close as developed by the charismatic Master Wakeryng also attracted an influx of lay residents from beyond its walls. My focus in this chapter falls primarily upon lay residents who came to the hospital close from various walks of life. By midcentury the close had piped water, multiple chapels, and newly renovated residences. Barron calls the close "a desirable 'gated community': it was secure and attractive, there was a hospital on site and carers (the sisters) on hand and, when the end came, there was a church and a cemetery for burials."[5] But the hospital close was also a "semi-inclusive community," in Geltner's terms, that, rather than separating well-to-do urbanites from undesirables, brought them into productive proximity with the ill, poor, and unfortunate.[6] The hospital represented for its lay residents a site for engagement with friends, with the rhythms of religious life, and with charity in a direct way.

They hailed from different social milieux, but the retired lawyer Thomas Gevendale and the grocer's widow Beatrice Lurchon were acquaintances in the close—Gevendale's 1455 will was witnessed by Beatrice's husband. It is possible that both knew John Shirley in some capacity. From their own vantage points, Gevendale and Lurchon each viewed the hospital as an interdependent community where diverse members might participate, however modestly, in each others' spiritual health. Gevendale's will demonstrates personal piety centered on the hospital and solicitude for the full spectrum of its residents as cooperating to further his salvation. Lurchon's will indicates her active choice of St. Bartholomew's as her spiritual home in life and after death, even though her body's final resting place was elsewhere in London.

Gevendale's will suggests an understanding of the hospital as a community in which lay and clerical, feeble and powerful played evolving roles in each other's care. Like Shirley,[7] Gevendale asks to be buried in the hospital's Lady Chapel. Furthermore, he grants money to support "vni capellano bone et honeste conuersacionis" (a chaplain of good and honest conduct) to celebrate mass and pray for him and other faithful souls for five years after his death.[8] Gathering in a range of members, Gevendale makes a series of gifts to the hospital master, each of the brothers, the sisters, and the suffering patients.[9] Placing the hospital master, brothers, and sisters within one clause (with the sisters receiving more than the brothers) suggests a descending order of power but also a cooperation in prayer by these privileged members "pro salute anime mee" (for the health of my soul). The feeblest members of the community, poor and infirm men and women, are also involved in this effort, each slated to receive three pence. Gevendale also singles out for a gift of three shillings four pence one Mariota Botiller, a woman who had probably been his neighbor in the close.[10] Thus Gevendale evokes the continuum on which the hospital's residents lived, where they might move from financially empowered testators to physically "decrepit" patients. He made further provisions for the poor later, leaving property in St. Martin Ludgate to buy food for the poor and pay a salary for "the chaplain who hears the confessions of the poor lying in the hospital and administering the sacrament to them."[11] If the poor were to pray for the health of his soul, they must also be sustained spiritually.

Within the diverse hospital community, the vulnerable also included poor scholars and destitute girls. Two of Gevendale's bequests create endowments "pro exhibicione trium pauperum scolarum ad scolas in vniversitate Oxoniensi vel Cantebrigiensi disponencium presbiterari" (support for three poor students intending to be ordained for the priesthood in the schools at the university of Oxford or of Cambridge) and dowries for "tribus puellis pauperibus bone et honeste conuersacionis" (three poor maidens of good and honest conduct).[12] Such bequests are not unique, for they participate in a wider effort to support higher education at the hospital.[13]

Yet the categories of poor scholars and girls are distinctive, since the hospital plays a role in supervising their transition from boys to scholars and from girls to wives. Might the young women who came to the hospital to give birth and then returned to the city with their virginity "restored" through John Mirfield's recipes be among the girls eligible for Gevendale's generosity?

Unlike Gevendale, Beatrice Lurchon did not elect burial in St. Bartholomew's hospital: she wished to lie beside her husband, John, in the hospital church of St. Thomas of Acon, located to the east in Cheapside. Yet in contemplating her death, she portrays St. Bartholomew's as her spiritual home, enlisting hospital personnel in a dignified transition from life to death. After requesting to be buried at St. Thomas's church beside her husband, Lurchon adds bequests to St. Bartholomew's fabric, personnel, and poor. She leaves "to the hygh auter of the hospitall of Seynt Bartilmew in Westsmythfeld of London for myn offerynges foryetyn in dischargyng of my sowle vjs viij d."[14] Two of her eight commemorative torches are to be placed at the high altar and in the chapel of St. Michael at St. Bartholomew's. Lurchon recruits a range of hospital members in her transition from spiritual home to final resting place:

> Also I bequeth to the master of the said hospitall iii s, and to euery brother of the same place xij d to th'entent that they shall go with my body to Seynt Thomas of Acres the day of my dyssese. Also I wyll that myn executors distrybute to euery bedred man and woman of the sayd hospitall of Seynt Bartilmew the day of my dyssese iiij d. . . . Also I bequeth to euery chyld of the gramerscole and of the place of the hospytall of Seynt Bartylmew that woll go with my body to Seynt Thomas of Acres and sey de profundis ij d.[15]

Although she asks nothing more than good faith from the bedridden patients, Lurchon makes her charity to the hospital's master, brothers, and children contingent upon their help in the journey to her final resting place. Having resided in the hospital close for nearly twenty years, she seems to view these community members as her trusted spiritual personnel in life and death. (She also enlists members of the "iiij orders of ffreres in London" to accompany her body.) The larger the extended spiritual family accompanying her body to St. Thomas of Acon, the more merit will accumulate to Lurchon, master, brethren, and children alike.

Both Gevendale and Lurchon took pains to include poor university students and grammar school students in their wills. Although we have few records of these children, we know that the hospital housed a school, took in orphans whose mothers had died in childbirth, and was home to the children of younger families residing in the close. Many midcentury lay residents seem to have moved there as retirees, but Lurchon probably raised her two daughters there, perhaps with visits in later years from her grandson Harvey, named in her will.[16] Alice Markby-Shipley-Portaleyn, who came to the close during her first marriage, rented and renovated a large tenement there and raised three sons in the close: her first son by John Shipley, and her second and third sons by Thomas Portaleyn.[17] Alice was a wealthy, capable wife who lived near Shirley in the close and was a friend of his relative Joan Newmarch, who resided nearby. Alice would have known Shirley from the beginning of his time in the hospital.[18]

Elene Joynour, a widow who lived in the close and died in 1430, did not live to make Shirley's acquaintance, but her children grew up in the close under the master's supervision. Joynour's will shows that she had an underage daughter, Margaret, and a son, Richard, who was named a ward of Master Wakeryng in 1436.[19] Looking ahead to her daughter's marriage, Joynour promises Margaret a hefty dowry of cash and household items on the condition that she marry "per assensum et ordinacionem executorum meorum" (by the approval and order of my executors). If Margaret should marry before coming of age (infra etatem), the dowry and other items will instead be donated "in operibus misericordie prout ipsi melius sperent deo placere et salute anime mee et aliarum animarum predictis proficere" (in the works of mercy, by which they may hope to please God better, and for the health of my soul and of the others aforementioned).[20] This stipulation reminds Margaret that she is living in the orbit of a hospital, where commemoration and the works of mercy, in their paramount spiritual importance, could outweigh her own material comforts.

Margaret Joynour and her brother Richard were one audience for Elene's will, and Richard was still Wakeryng's ward in 1443, by this time probably an adolescent and still living in the close.[21] Perhaps he attended the grammar school run by John Reynolds. Richard and other children living in or frequenting the hospital close at midcentury formed a small but important contingent of readers. Later book bequests in parents' wills indicate that these children may have started consuming texts at an early age. Schoolmaster Reynolds (d. 1459) had a son, William, who may have studied at the grammar school alongside resident children. In his will, Reynolds bequeaths William "octo optimos libros meos" (my eight best books).[22] Alice Markby-Shipley-Portaleyn's two younger sons, who might have studied with Master Reynolds, both received book bequests as adults. In her 1479 will, Alice left her youngest son, Thomas, an apprentice mercer, "my boke of praiers with the matens of the Trinite in the same."[23] From Joan Newmarch, Alice's older friend and fellow widow, Alice's son Edmund received a book of matins with services for the dead, featuring an image of the savior's face.[24] Anne Sutton deduces from the will's language, in which Newmarch calls Edmund "Edmundo filio meo et filie Portaleyn" (Edmund my son and Portaleyn's son), that he was her godson.[25] This gift speaks to the close links between the two mothers and the literate piety that they fostered in Alice's sons. Although Joan's children would have been adults by the time she moved to the close in 1440, she may have entertained her grandchildren there and acted as a spiritual mother figure to her younger friend's sons.

Wills tend to emphasize the bonds of friendship and loyalty, but the close community experienced its share of conflicts over the period in question. The generosity of hospital patrons was sometimes obstructed by family members. Although the liberal benefactor John Warner left a large manor to the hospital in 1439, the interference of his daughter and her husband prevented Master Wakeryng from accessing the land and its income until 1446.[26] Not all relations among lay residents were amicable, as seen in a lawsuit brought in 1465 by John Hewek, Thomas Gevendale's cousin, against Beatrice Lurchon, over goods that John had given Beatrice for safekeeping.[27] In another long-simmering family drama, Alice Markby-Shipley-Portaleyn's two younger sons resented her bequest of her entire estate upon her first son, their half brother John Shipley. They eventually brought an unsuccessful suit against him in 1484, five years after her death, to try to recover part of the estate.[28] As I show in the next section, John Shirley's anthology intervened into this multigenerational nexus with edifying texts that often register the difficulties of living generously in community.

## BODLEIAN MS ASHMOLE 59:
### MORAL GUIDANCE FOR MEN, WOMEN, AND CHILDREN

For many of this book's readers, John Shirley will need no introduction. Students of poet John Lydgate know that much of his large literary corpus survives thanks to Shirley's copying.[29] Antiquarian John Stow noted that Shirley "painefully collected the workes of *Geffrey Chaucer, Iohn Lidgate* and other learned writers, which workes hee wrote in sundry volumes to remayne for posterity."[30] Today three of these large autograph volumes survive: BL MS Additional 16165; Trinity College Cambridge MS R. 3. 20; and Bodleian MS Ashmole 59, my chief concern in this chapter. Shirley began his career as a clerk in royal service under Richard II, during which time he briefly held an ecclesiastical benefice but resisted proceeding to the priestly ordination required to maintain it.[31] Thanks to his admiring patron John Norbury, Henry IV's treasurer (1399–1401) and member of the King's Council (1399–1405), Shirley gained favor from the new royal regime and proceeded along a lay clerical track, honing his scribal skills during many years of service to Richard Beauchamp, Earl of Warwick.[32] Shirley was first documented in Warwick's military retinue in 1403 and served in various capacities, including as the earl's secretary from 1421.[33] Having spent the early years of his service in frequent travel with Warwick's retinue, Shirley settled in London by the late 1420s, where he developed contacts within the city's merchant class even as he remained in close contact with the lord's household until Warwick's death in 1439.[34] Reflecting on Shirley's career trajectory, Kerby-Fulton suggestively characterizes Shirley as a "liminal" figure insofar as he "confidently and permanently delayed ordination" in favor of becoming a lay clerk in civil service.[35] This perspective on his career may help illuminate the complex uses Shirley made of his multilingualism and his interest in the hybrid religious/secular institution of the hospital as a home base for his retirement.

As an extension of his scribal work for Warwick, Shirley probably began copying literary texts in the mid-1420s: his earliest collection, now BL Additional MS 16165, is a trilingual anthology including Middle English texts from Chaucer's *Boece* to Lydgate's *Complaint of the Black Knight* and *Temple of Glas*.[36] The volume features a verse prologue that humbly addresses "dere sirs," anticipates that "boþe þe gret and þe comune / May þer on looke and eke hit reede," and asks near the end "þat ye sende þis booke ageyne / Hoome to Shirley þat is right feyne."[37] As Margaret Connolly notes, these features suggest an assumption "that the book would be shared by many people, perhaps passed around Beauchamp's household, but in whatever milieu the manuscript circulated, many different readers would enjoy its contents."[38] Shirley probably compiled his second large literary collection, now Trinity College MS R. 3. 20, in the early 1430s when he was living in London.[39] In this volume, Shirley assembled mainly poetic texts in French, Latin, and English, with a substantial collection of short French verse and numerous Lydgate texts, including most of his performance pieces, such as "The Mumming for the Mercers of London" and "Bycorne and Chychevache."[40] Though it lacks a verse preface, MS R. 3. 20 contains Shirley's bookplate stanza, a rhyme royal verse concluding, "Whane ye þis boke haue ouer redde and seyne / To Johan Shirley restore yee it ageyne."[41] This collection was evidently also shared with various readers: in Veeman's view, perhaps "among Shirley's friends and family . . . members of London's mercantile community, fellow bureaucrats and royal servants, as well as other members of Beauchamp's extended affinity."[42] The volume remained in Shirley's hands during his lifetime, providing him with texts that he would copy into his final autograph collection.[43]

By the time he copied this last volume, now Ashmole 59, in the late 1440s, Shirley was residing in St. Bartholomew's Hospital close. He had been living in the hospital precinct from at least 1444 and perhaps earlier, because by 1438 he is recorded as renting property owned by the hospital.[44] Shirley's attraction to St. Bartholomew's may have stemmed from the fact that his mother was buried in the hospital church's Lady Chapel, where he too would request burial, next to his second wife, Margaret.[45] In Cok's 1456 rental, Shirley is listed as renting a large tenement in the hospital close, including four shops.[46] One may imagine that having once contemplated an ecclesiastical career, he was attracted to life in the orbit of a religious house.[47] Scholars have drawn various connections between Shirley's rental of "shops" and the exact nature of his literary practices. A. I. Doyle, the first modern book historian to consider Shirley's life in detail, suggested that he might have produced books commercially, an idea that Cheryl Greenberg pursued, contending that Shirley's personal networks and the location near St. Paul's would have brought in both customers and book craftsmen as collaborators.[48] In favor of a commercial motive for Shirley's later collections, A. S. G. Edwards suggests that the variation in Lydgate material between MS R. 3. 20 and MS Ashmole 59 creates a "conspicuous element of newness to the poet's appearances," perhaps a marketing strategy.[49] Yet as Connolly has argued, although Shirley's collections influenced other anthologies that circulated during the fifteenth century, there is no direct evidence that he ever sold his books.[50] It seems more likely that Shirley lent this final collection to readers within his immediate community, as he may have circulated the earlier volumes within the noble household, familial, and other personal networks.[51] The "newness" of Ashmole's Lydgate contents would indeed have appealed to Shirley's audience of hospital readers, many of them educated, sophisticated book owners. The Ashmole volume, like MS R. 3. 20, features Shirley's bookplate stanza just before the beginning of the "Epistle to Sibille." Although I do not wholly dismiss the possibility of a commercial motive, I consider the hospital reading community as a primary context for the volume. Shirley compiled Ashmole for a mixed audience of hospital-based readers who might have borrowed, shared, and returned the book to him.[52]

During his residency in the hospital close, Shirley entered into and deepened many friendships, embracing his new community of neighbors as a kind of surrogate household. Upon moving into the close, Shirley drew other prominent residents into his orbit, in 1444 granting all of his English and foreign properties and rents to several friends, including three neighbors (William Baron, gentleman; Robert Danvers, city recorder; and Richard Shipley, gentleman).[53] Euan Roger suggests that Wakeryng, who had renewed the grammar school by poaching John Reynolds from St. Paul's, might have wished to burnish the hospital's intellectual status by cultivating Shirley, with his reputation for book production.[54] Shirley admired Wakeryng: in his 1452 will, he asked the master and several others to assist his wife in carrying out his last wishes.[55]

Shirley compiled Ashmole near the end of his life, in the late 1440s. Connolly notes that the volume is substantively different from his earlier anthologies, including poetry "of a more serious nature" and lacking the verse preface that would signal an appeal to a patron. Although the anthology contains eleven works that Shirley had already copied into MS R. 3. 20, notably secular lyrics such as "Fortune" and the "Complaint of Venus," in Ashmole he presents the texts differently, either with new headings or with textual expansions.[56] Noting the volume's "preponderance of didactic and religious material," Connolly suggests that Shirley's supply of texts might have been influenced by the proximity to neighbors in the close and to the nearby religious communities of St. Bartholomew's priory, Greyfriars, St. Martin-le-Grand, and the London Charterhouse.[57] A close textual connection between Shirley and his neighbors emerges in the fact that three of the later texts in Ashmole 59 are identical to a run of texts copied into a manuscript associated with his pious friend William Baron.[58] Shirley and

Baron, members of the "same bookish environment," evidently had access to some of the same texts.[59]

Ashmole 59, with its strongly didactic focus, contains a unique combination of texts that bear in specific ways upon the needs and experiences of lay life adjacent to St. Bartholomew's Hospital.[60] As with Shirley's earlier manuscripts, the contents of his last collection do not at first seem systematically organized. Yet as Connolly has shown, elements of Ashmole's construction, including catchwords, continuous quire numbers, and consistent ink colors for the main texts and apparatus, demonstrate that Shirley had a plan for the volume.[61] It is true that Ashmole's contents are various, yet Shirley's clustering of material and inclusion of particular texts indicate his awareness of the hospital close reading audience.[62] With its diverse edifying texts and multiple inscribed audiences, Ashmole bears some comparison to the sort of collection that Phillipa Hardman calls a "household library," a multigenre volume designed to serve the needs of varied readers, including adults and children, for "devotional reading, literary entertainment and practical use."[63] The fit is not perfect: such collections tend to contain more elementary religious texts and explicit guidance to readers, and to be associated with a single family.[64] Yet if Shirley viewed his community in the hospital close as a surrogate extended household, the analogy can help us to understand Ashmole as an intentionally compiled volume for a range of readers: men, women, and children.

Shirley's final manuscript offers a range of formative texts to the close's multiple readerships. Some works target elite men as potential readers: notably, the Middle English *Secretum Secretorum*, a popular *speculum principis*, which appears as the first text in Ashmole. A number of the volume's texts, particularly those in a moralizing vein, have particular relevance to women. The wives of the hospital close were important residents in their own right, financially powerful as widows wielding their own resources.[65] In Ashmole we find several texts addressed to or about women. These include the Chaucer-attributed "Chronicle of Ladies" (a digest of the *Legend of Good Women*), the Lydgate-attributed "Complaint for my Lady the Duchess of Gloucester," and Lydgate's translation of Proverbs 31, the "Epistle to Sibille," an encomium to a virtuous wife that Anthony Bale aptly characterizes as "a distinctly materialistic, even capitalist, work of culture."[66]

A number of other textual groupings in Ashmole seem to target younger members of the hospital close—perhaps readers like the children of residents such as Beatrice Lurchon or Alice Markby-Shipley-Portaleyn. Ashmole features Lydgate's popular translation "Stans puer ad mensam" and excerpts from his "Pageants of Knowledge," as well as Scogan's "Moral Balade," a "mini-speculum principis" addressed to Henry IV's sons.[67] Such works extend parental discipline to children, boys in particular, within the mixed-age reading context.

All of the abovementioned texts might be considered works of conduct literature, broadly defined. In his recent work on the construction of late medieval married subjectivity, Glenn Burger evokes the generic multiplicity of conduct texts, noting that "textual genres and terrains that might once have been kept separate — sermons, exemplary stories, devotional literature, satire, *fin'amor* texts and practices, the *speculum principis*, biblical history, rhetorical manuals, debate, how-to collections, and wise sayings — can be brought together to produce innovative, hybrid models for female subjectivity and right action in the world."[68] I draw upon Burger's work to show how in Ashmole, texts for men, women, and children work individually and collectively to construct the "good wife" and her husband as "fully gendered and sexualized, yet still fully ethical, subjects."[69] The hospital close is a hybrid reading site that partakes of the religious and the domestic worlds, a uniquely fertile place for the gathering and reading of formative texts whose existence, as Burger shows, depended ultimately upon the translation of monastic disciplinary modes into secular practice.

Within the Ashmole manuscript, as within the hospital close and fifteenth-century culture at large, the worldly and the spiritual constantly mingle. Although this chapter highlights what we might consider the volume's more "secular" moralizing texts, we must acknowledge that such works always exist on a continuum with devotional and doctrinal works such as Lydgate's "Prayer to Our Lady" and "Prayer to St. Edmund," his "Invocation to St. Anne," and "A Holy Meditation." These poems emphasize Christian vigilance: worship of the Virgin and the saints, observance of mass and confession, and constant self-regulation. The "Holy Meditation" exhorts,

Lat not þy flesshly foule affecioun
þy soule putte far from hys dileccioun,
Looke by raisoun soo þou bridelde be
þat God Oure Lord ne be not wroþe with þee.[70]

The reward for this constant effort of self-regulation and attention to the social elements of religious practice will be heaven, the place every testator sought: "If þowe do þus, þanne shal þy soule weende / To hevens blisse whiche þat haþ none eende." Reading within the hospital close, whatever the text, might be a practice imbued with moral, spiritual, and social significance. Shirley assembled this manuscript to aid a range of readers in navigating the complex demands of life in this desirable yet demanding community.

## SECRETUM SECRETORUM:
### "A MIROUR TO LYVE" IN THE HOSPITAL CLOSE

The Ashmole collection opens with a partial translation of the prose *Secretum Secretorum*, a work that connects back to chapter 2 and the writings of hospital priest John Mirfield. The *Secretum* formed the basis for Mirfield's advice on dietary regimen in part 15 of his *Breviarium*, and it supplied the latter half of the *Florarium* chapter "De medicis." Both of these chapters were excerpted by fifteenth-century compilers: the "Regimen sanitatis" in five manuscripts and "De medicis" in BL MS Sloane 59. This medical collection belonged to King Henry VI's personal physician, John Somerset, who was a prominent patron of St. Bartholomew's Hospital.[71] The fact that the king's physician was reading a work issuing from St. Bartholomew's constitutes one salient link between the hospital's literature and the royal household.[72]

The popular *Secretum*, purportedly written by Aristotle for Alexander the Great, had a long history of translation from Arabic into Latin and various European vernaculars. The work's topics span the political, philosophical, moral, medical, and religious realms. Its medical contents were incorporated into many late medieval compendia that treated "the conservation of health through strict adherence to the Galenic principles of temperance and moderation."[73] Many other writers translated the work for readers outside church and university: the *Secretum* survives in at least nine Middle English versions. Given the work's ubiquity, it is not surprising that learned, inquisitive men such as Mirfield and Shirley encountered it. For both, the *Secretum* became a touchstone for their literary practices within the hospital.

In considering *Secretum* and the rest of Ashmole's contents, Joyce Coleman's influential theory of "public reading" provides a helpful paradigm for imagining how Shirley might have envisioned the uses of his final anthology. Coleman's focus on "court-oriented literature" available to "upper-middle- and upper-class individuals, most of whom would be literate" accords with our vision of Shirley's hospital reading community.[74] Coleman's corpus of texts, all of which constitute different sorts of "'rulebook' outlining in detail the conduct of various forms of group life, whether courtly . . . collegiate . . . or domestic" is likewise apposite for the Ashmole collection.[75] Among such texts, the *speculum principis* genre (of which the *Secretum* was the most popular example) had a central function within fifteenth-century communal reading contexts: "Read aloud in the chambers of the nobility and the bourgeoisie, they would lead to joint consideration of the relationships among self-governance, power, and rulership. . . . their inherent interest and intent could be realized only when these readers went on to discuss what they had read with others or shared in a group reading and discussion."[76] I suggest that one of the uses for the Ashmole anthology, with its collocation of moral texts, would have been just such reading aloud and discussion among friends in the hospital close. Shirley had a particular interest in the *Secretum*: his own translation of the work survives in BL MS Additional 5467, an anthology of his translations from French.[77]

Although the *Secretum* appears in fragmentary form in Ashmole 59, these chapters offer some key highlights of the text, casting the ruler as the repository for privileged knowledge who should embody largesse and forbearance, display wisdom and value scholarship, and live according to principles of moderation. Offering a "mirrour" and "forme" for princes, this text would have had utility for the hospital's lay literary community too. The masculine members of this community, embodying something of a microcosm of London's upper echelons, were well placed to appreciate its advice on equanimity and moderation. The form initially appears somewhat garbled, as Connolly explains: "Its text has been manipulated to incorporate an acrostic based on an alphabetical sequence. Shirley offers no comment or information as to the text's origins, though there may originally have been a table of contents and other preliminary matter which has since been lost; the text occupies a single quire which is now the first item in the manuscript, but the quire numbers indicate that this was not the original arrangement."[78] Shirley evidently did not intend to open the volume with this *Secretum* translation, but he did include it in a sequence that the extant book preserves, minus the original several quires.[79] At the start of the second quire, Shirley labels the volume an "Abstracte Brevyarye compyled of diverse

balades, roundels, virilayes, tragedyes, envoys, compleyntes, moralites, sto-
ryes, practysed and eke devysed and ymagyned as it sheweþe here folow-
yng."[80] Although the *Secretum* fits none of these generic categories, its unique
form as preserved in Ashmole gives it the quality of a digest fitting Shirley's
announced focus on "abstracte" or extracted texts.

In announcing its textual and translation history, the *Secretum* strikes
the titular note of secrecy, emphasizing the class privilege attached to the information being conveyed. The text is depicted as having been found by one

> Marmaduke þe sone of Patryke, þe sage of all langages. . . . And he trans-
> lated it owte of Greeke in-to Calddé and, affter þe requeste of þe Kyng of
> Arrabie, he translated it oute of Arrabeske in-to Latin. . . . And þus was
> þis boke translated in-to Latin, *nouȝt al, but such as is most profitable*
> *and gode [to] mans vnderstonding, for þestate and governaunce of princes.*
> *Þe whiche boke, with þe content, is nouȝt to shewe to comvne, ne to rede to*
> *every man opunly,* but secretly to kepe it and to rede it to-fore þestatly
> princes of þe worlde, þat may be a mirrour to lyve, and a directe fourme
> for hem and all þeire lieges, wysely to contynue.[81]

Here translation is depicted not as facilitating an expansion of audience, but
as an elitist process culminating with Latin: the present English version goes
unmentioned. Translation narrows the contents of the work to include
*"nouȝt al, but such as is most profitable and gode [to] mans vnderstonding,"* and
it further narrows the audience to a select group of "þestatly princes of þe
worlde." Despite (or perhaps because of) these elitist sentiments, the *Secretum* had already proved immensely popular among late medieval readers of
all sorts seeking the conduct advice that "a mirrour to lyve" might provide.[82]

Shirley's literary community included a number of readers intimately
familiar with "þestatly princes of þe worlde." He counted among his neighbors royal servants (William Cleve, clerk of the King's Works, and Joan Astley, Henry VI's nurse) and men who, like himself, had served under Richard
Beauchamp: Thomas Stokys and Thomas Portaleyn.[83] For such readers the
priorities of largesse and forbearance would also have been familiar values.
As the fourth section of the *Secretum* asserts, "þe prince is not comendable
but if he beo large to him-selff and to heos subjetz. But to my jugement,
seyþe Aristotle, I halde him moste noble kyng perseuerant, þat he þat is
large to him-selff and to heos servantz, he is moste worþy and beste liche to
to-longe endure" (208). Largesse might be the most vital quality for a king,

but it had to be used with intelligence and measure, lest by foolishly dissipating the kingdom, "he may lightly bring al to desolacion with-outen þat he purveye gode and convenyent remedy by ful weele avised provysioun" (210). The ruler must balance the need for generosity with wise expenditure: "If the king absteyne him and with-holdeþe him frome violent rape of þe moneye of heos subgettes, þat is a certayne token þat in hyme is verraye and gret bounté of vnderstnnding and plenté of perseuerant lawe, and pleine parfeccioun" (210). This section is typical of the text's advice at large, repeatedly emphasizing avoidance of excess and self-discipline. Such discipline will bear fruit not only in relation to "moneye" but also in the larger good will of the community, which recognizes in the well-regulated sovereign the qualities of "vnderstonding," "lawe," and "parfeccioun." Proffering advice that royal servants would recognize, the text also offers a model for well-regulated life in a communal context.

Readers with a connection to the Crown might see the *Secretum*'s emphasis on scholarship as applicable to their lord King Henry VI also: he had heeded the advice "to ordeine vniuersitees, studies, and scoles, for to leorne of þe noblest sciences to enriche þy reaumes by þeire cunninge, and beo to hem þeire preorogatyff and support" (221). In founding Eton School (1440) and King's College, Cambridge (1441), Henry had given more attention to "ordeine" and "support" scholarship than to any other aspect of statecraft, sometimes to the detriment of his reputation as a monarch. The medical section of this text, which begins by announcing that "þe conservacion of þy body is better þan any medecyne" (221), begins to unfold advice on "keping moderatly equalité and temperance" in eating (223), yet it is foreshortened by the loss of at least one quire. If the literary community of the hospital close had replaced Shirley's noble household, perhaps he envisioned sharing this idiosyncratic *Secretum* text, originally advice for a king, with others who had served the king or in the noble household and might, in retirement, have the time to reflect upon lessons learned in that setting.

## FORMING WIVES AND WIDOWS

Although the *Secretum* text has been disrupted, Shirley seems to have bound the extant twelve quires together as a whole as an intentional anthology. Given the volume's very large number of contents, I do not attempt to consider them comprehensively. In what follows I attend to two major thematic strands: formative texts for women and for children. Texts for and about women abound in the manuscript. The Virgin Mary features prominently as the model of feminine perfection, praised in several hymns and regaled in such verses as Lydgate's "A Valentine to her I love best," in which Mary, excelling mythological, Jewish, and Christian heroines, offers "Refuyt to synners þat for hir helpe calle / For mans helpe hir goodnesse excelliþe alle" (fols. 53r-v). Texts about secular women are also prominent in this volume: Shirley shared his love of Mary with an interest in other good women, both legendary and contemporary. Within Ashmole, the "Chronicle of Ladies" together with "Complaint for my Lady of Gloucester" and "Epistle to Sibylle" present complex visions of married female virtue.

Beatrice Lurchon, Alice Markby-Shipley-Portaleyn, Joan Newmarch, and Joan Astley were Shirley's neighbors and friends. These married women, their daughters, and other laywomen of the close would all have been potential readers of this volume. Ashmole's texts for women address the privileges and the pressures experienced by wealthy married women. These pressures may have intensified upon entry into the hospital close, as its matrons negotiated their domestic lives in constant awareness of the hospital's liturgical, educational, and charitable functions. More than simply leisure reading, Ashmole offers texts that instruct, analyze, and debate the question of women's virtue for consumption within this hybrid cultural context.

Veeman does not mention the hospital as the site for Ashmole's production, but she insightfully notes that Shirley's juxtapositions of texts embed in the volume a playful debate about women's virtue, which could have been shared by mixed-gender audiences. She observes that the collection presents a largely "positive" view of women but one that is also subject to variation. In one instance, Shirley pairs Lydgate's earnest religious "Invocation to St. Anne" and courtly lament "My Lady Dere" with his slyly misogynistic "Beware of Doublenesse."[84] The latter work, Veeman notes,

> satirizes the concept of women's faithfulness and truthfulness. The poem ostensibly praises women and finds in them no "doublenesse." However, as Shirley's headnote reveals, it is "a balade made by Lidegate of wymen ffor desporte and game per Antyfrasim" (f. 47v). The "desporte and game" of the poem is that it speaks in contraries, "per Antyfrasim"; a knowing reader is thus able to dispute each statement praising women.[85]

A similar dynamic operates within one of the sententious clusters that I consider below in my discussion of texts for young readers. Just after "The Pageant of Knowledge" and "Four Complexions of Mankind," Shirley inserts Lydgate's verse stanza "Four Things that Make a Man a Fool." In contrast to the first two texts, which transmit clerkly wisdom, "Four Things" is a comic stanza that ends by indicting women as worse culprits than "worship," "elde," and "wyne": "And bookis þat poetes wrot and radde, / Seyne wymen mooste make men to madde" (fol. 72r). Veeman suggests that by inserting "Four Things," Shirley "intentionally creates a debate centered around women's characters for the 'desporte' of Shirley's readers."[86] Veeman points to these interventions as evidence of Shirley's effort to appeal to a mixed-gender lay audience of varying levels of education and abilities.[87] Her suggestive arguments become even more resonant when we read the manuscript within the specific context of the hospital.

The volume's longer works on women also participate in this debate on female virtue. Ashmole offers multiple visions of the good woman in various settings, both mythological and historical. Whereas the "Chronicle of Ladies" depicts married female virtue as isolated suffering and self-abnegation, the "Complaint for my Lady of Gloucester" offers a double vision of virtue, in the innocent lady's victimization and in the loud voices of the "good wymmen" who defend her. Eschewing the model of "reproched womanhode," Lydgate's "Epistle to Sibille" places the good wife in control, emphasizing her wisdom and competence, her confident movement between the public and the domestic spheres. These visions of female virtue map a spectrum from "obedience" to "prudence," two qualities that Carolyn Collette considers the key attributes of the good woman in late medieval England: "The difference between Prudence and obedience is the orientation of agency: Prudence is a social virtue that supports the common good by actions that have public consequences; obedience is a private virtue that supports the public good by creating 'good' subjects."[88] Featuring women who manifest these qualities in varying degrees, sometimes to extremes, the Ashmole manuscript offers a range of subjects for its married female readers to emulate, pity, even laugh at. The matrons of the close were poised between public and private worlds: their comfortable homes were secluded and their pious activities centered in their favorite chapels, but public responsibilities persisted, including the management of far-flung estates, lawsuits, and difficult family members. The volume's diverse versions of virtue speak to the complexity of women's lives during and after marriage.

Ashmole's first extended vision of feminine obedience as suffering appears in the "Chronicle of Ladies," introduced as "þe nyene worshipfullest Ladies þat / in alle cronycles and storyal bokes haue ben founde of trouþe of / constaunce and vertuous or reproched womanhode by Chaucier."[89] In this digest of the *Legend of Good Women* with a few idiosyncrasies, all of the women are loyal wives except for the unmarried Thisbe (a loyal lover), and the verses condense their stories into brief accounts of their virtues, abandonments, and deaths.[90] Faithful suffering is the essence of love here: seven of nine die for their husbands' love, including four who commit suicide. The extent to which her suicide is tied to her identity as a faithful wife is particularly clear in the case of Queen Dido, Aeneas's wife:

> Sheo made him lord and sheo his humble wyve
> Wherby ellas sheo loste boþe ioye and lyve;
> For whane she wiste þat he was from hir goo,
> Vppon his swerde shee roof hir herte atwo.[91]

Although she began as "þis noble qweene of Cartage feyre Dido," her role as obedient wife subsumes this nobility and even her name, after she has "made him lord and sheo his humble wyve." However, the rhyme between "wyve" and "lyve" implies that in making this marriage she wrote her own death sentence.

Such a radical identification between marriage to a single man and a woman's very existence, with tragic consequences when that marriage was sundered, would be familiar to female readers immersed in the late medieval marriage system, which had transferred its ascetic modes into marital contexts.[92] However, as Shirley's readers also knew, not every woman remained married to one man for her whole life or viewed sexual dishonor as a reason for suicide, as did Lucrece, another "Chronicle" heroine whose story is abridged thus:

> It is grete right þat your bountee Lucresse
> Be putte in writing and alsoo your goodnesse,
> Wyff to þe Senatour gode Collatyne
> Which thorugh þenvye of RomaynTorqwyn

For yee to him wolde never applye,
He ravisshed yowe whereoff it was pyte;
With a Tyraunt ful soore ageinst youre wille,
He caused yowe for sorowe youre selff to spille.[93]

Lucrece embodies obedience to her husband, Collatyne, both in her refusal to "applye" (submit) to Tarquin's advances and in her suicide, presented here as the only possible outlet for the "sorowe" caused by rape.

Whereas Lucrece's self-annihilation represents the apotheosis of her "goodnesse" in this version, Shirley's laywomen neighbors who had experienced similar hardships did not necessarily respond as she did. In 1445, the recently widowed Alice Shipley was kidnapped and raped while a resident of the hospital: she immediately sought legal redress for the crime, going on to marry her final husband, Thomas Portaleyn, shortly thereafter.[94] Hospital close resident and widow Margaret Molefaunt (d. 1445), daughter of Joan Astley, had suffered a similar attack in 1438: she was abducted, starved, and raped while pregnant, shortly after her husband's death, by Lewis Leyshon, one of his personal servants. Having refused a forced marriage to Leyshon, Molefaunt petitioned Parliament for justice. King Henry VI endorsed her petition, but her assailant evaded the law and was never convicted.[95] Molefaunt may have sought out the hospital, where her mother resided and where her husband was already buried, as a place of "refuge" from her trauma.[96] Although Molefaunt had probably died before Shirley compiled Ashmole, her mother, Joan, was still living in the close. One may imagine that Joan, Alice, and the mature women of the neighborhood read the "Chronicle" with empathy, and with a grain of salt, knowing from experience that self-abnegation was not the only response to "reproched womanhode."

Whereas Dido and Lucrece experienced abandonment and shame in solitary grief, Alice Markby-Shipley-Portaleyn and Margaret Molefaunt sought support within the hospital close's female community. It is therefore striking that Shirley rounds out Ashmole's fifth quire with the "Complaint for my Lady of Gloucester," featuring a "reproched" and abandoned wife publicly supported by a host of other good wives. The poem, which Shirley had also copied in Trinity R. 3. 20, is introduced as a work by "a Chapellayne of my lordes of Gloucestre Humfrey" with the running title "Complainte made by Lydegate Of my ladye of Gloucester & Holand."[97] Lydgate's authorship has been disputed on stylistic grounds, but given

Shirley's intimate knowledge of the poet and his otherwise reliable attributions, and the fact that he offers the only witnesses to the poem, it seems probable that Lydgate composed this intriguing work.[98] Although Lydgate's authorship is not necessary to my argument, I will proceed with this assumption in my discussion.

The story of Jacqueline, Duchess of Holland, Hainault and Zeeland, who had married Duke Humphrey of Gloucester in 1423, was well known to hospital close readers. As nurse to the young Henry VI, Astley may have met Jacqueline herself in the early days of her marriage to Humphrey. Having annulled her second marriage in order to marry Humphrey, in 1425 Jacqueline found herself abandoned in her home city of Mons, at the mercy of her enemy the Duke of Burgundy, as Humphrey sailed back to England, where he soon embarked on an affair with Eleanor Cobham, Jacqueline's English lady-in-waiting and later his second wife.[99]

The short work, occupying fols. 57r–58v in Ashmole, written from the perspective of an unnamed "solytarye," does not describe Jacqueline in detail or even name her. Instead, it stokes desire for the missing duchess by lamenting her absence, casting her as the "faythfull truwe pryncesse" in contrast to Eleanor, the villainous seductress.[100] Lydgate had compared Jacqueline to virtuous ladies, including Hecuba and Lucrece, in his earlier poem "On Gloucester's Approaching Marriage" (copied in Trinity R. 3. 20 but not in Ashmole).[101] But her absence is the true subject of the "Complaint." In the solitary speaker's dream, he hears the clamorous sorrow of Jacqueline's female subjects, who desperately desire her return:

> And þus compleyning sore with pitee
> þe ladyes alle of þat feyre regyoun,
> Gode wymmen eke of hye and lowe degree,
> Gane maken ye gret lamentacioun
> And sayde O Lorde þou sende us nowe adowne
> Oure princesse which may stint al oure woo
> Whiche þat so longe haþe beo kepte us froo.[102]

The virtuous princess is wrongfully imprisoned, "kepte us froo" ("kepte" is Shirley's addition in Ashmole), but the chorus of "gode wymmen" serves as her advocates.[103] Whereas the historical Jacqueline had written a barrage of rhetorically astute letters to Humphrey and to Parliament seeking her husband's return and assistance, in the poem her goodness is defined through her invisibility and by the contrast to the wicked Eleanor, a "mermaid" accused of enticing the duke with her "fals incantaciouns."[104] Jacqueline's female devotees come to the fore in the poem, donning the mantle of womanly "pitee" to demand her release and vindication.

The good women of Lydgate's poem represent a fictionalized version of the London women who in 1428 had petitioned Parliament with letters demanding Jacqueline's return, as recounted in the St. Alban's Chronicle. The chronicle reports that the women's letters were critical of the duke, who was

> nolentem suam uxorem ab eflictione cercali ducens Borgundiae eripere, sed, ammore refrigerato, sic in servitute permanere sinerc; et quod aliam, adulteram, publice secum tenuerit.

> ———

> unwilling to tear his wife from the affliction of imprisonment by the Duke of Burgundy, but having fallen out of love, leaving her to remain this way, perpetually in servitude, and what is more, to conduct himself publicly as an adulterer.[105]

C. Marie Harker notes that "it is unlikely that Jacqueline's situation elicited a spontaneous protofeminist groundswell," but Lydgate's poem magnifies the women's intercession (and his representation of it) into a singularly efficacious rhetorical event.[106] As the poetic speaker wakes from his dream, he writes down the women's song:

> Þis dreme he wrote þus of hoole entent,
> Boþe of feyth and of his trewe affecioun,
> Three hundreþe thousande seyth fully assent
> Of suffisaunt people with inne þat regyoun;
> And eke right for gode conclusioun
> Alle þe meynee of þat worþy housholde
> Preyne vnto God þer for boþe yonge and olde.[107]

The petition to release Jacqueline that began as the expression of female "pitee" has, through the poet's earnest devotion, gained the support of "three hundreþe thousand," both women and men. Through the collaboration of female voices and poetic inscription, the poem suggests, "þat worþy housholde," by which he seems to mean the very realm of England itself, is moved to beseech God for Jacqueline's release. The Ashmole manuscript breaks off before the end of the poem (which is in any case not decisive, still lamenting that the duchess is "to longe aweye"). It leaves readers with a mental image of the collective prayer that these "good wymmen" have inspired the kingdom to utter. It is true that the competition between Jacqueline and Eleanor was lurid (and cautionary, after Eleanor's conviction for necromancy in 1441).[108] Yet more than its prurient descriptions of the hated Eleanor, Lydgate's evocation of a supportive group of women, whose concern for a scorned wife moves them to public speech, might have been particularly poignant for Shirley's female readers. Many of the close's widows viewed each other with affection rather than jealousy (Alice Markby-Shipley-Portaleyn and Joan Newmarch; Joan Astley and her daughter Margaret Molefaunt). The poem could be subject to many readings, but I suspect that its vision of mutual feminine support in the face of betrayal may have recommended its inclusion to Shirley here.

The "Complaint" offers a bifurcated vision of the good woman that ultimately celebrates women's ability to support and defend each other in public. Eschewing public drama and focusing on a single figure of married prosperity and domesticity, Lydgate's "Epistle to Sibylle" offers yet another vision. This poem too might have struck an inviting note for the matrons of the hospital close. The text, whose sole known copy survives in Ashmole, renders Proverbs 31:10–31, the account of the *mulier fortis*, into Middle English. The poem works within this particular reading context to construct a "good wife" who manages to be both self-restrained and publicly visible: a vision of "prudence," to recall Collette's category, as a "social virtue" with public implications. Anthony Bale has shown that the text powerfully celebrates secular domesticity while offering a kind of feminine *speculum principis*. Having uncovered much detail about the work's original addressee, the Norfolk householder and widow Sibylle Boys, Bale argues that "the poem addresses 'Sibille' through the culturally authoritative and stable voices of Scripture and Chaucer via Lydgate in a way reminiscent of the prestigious texts of statecraft being produced by Lydgate around this time for Henry V and Henry VI."[109]

This vision fits comfortably within the hospital close's mixed-gender reading context, in which both men and women, and indeed some married couples, such as Shirley and his wife, Margaret, or William Baron and his wife, Joan, could easily have shared the same book. Although Bale finds little significance in the manuscript's provenance, I wish to highlight this context as crucial for interpreting the poem.[110] It may be an accident that this is the only surviving copy, but its inclusion within this manuscript can be no accident. The work feminizes the edifying themes struck in the volume's other sententious texts, valorizing in domestic terms the idea of magnanimous self-discipline that constitutes a key strand in the manuscript's web.[111]

As Bale has rightly noted, the poem's thrust is secular: in a free translation of the Proverbs text, it emphasizes the wife's care for the household and her family. He argues for Lydgate's emphasis on the "worldly" over the "spiritual":

> her provision for 'hir servantz' (line 41), her resemblance to 'a shippe of marchandyse' (line 43, quoting Proverbs xxx.14) with her house 'full of stuffe' (line 46), her abilities 'in truwe pourchace' (line 47), her generous provision of alms (line 64, citing Proverbs xxxi.20) and virtuous teaching of her servants . . . prudent management of 'her childre' (line 100) and 'hir housbande' (line 101), and, finally, in Lydgate's envoy, her disposition to 'labour, avoydyng ydelnesse, / Vsinge her handes in vertuous besynesse' (lines 139f.). In celebrating the admirable pious wifehood practised by 'Sibille', the 'Epistle' also congratulates her on her wealth, her power, her authority, and her material success.[112]

This catalogue of concerns touches on several themes to which I will return. As Bale notes, the phrase "vertuous besynesse" is the poem's "refrain and its theme."[113] This phrase or some variant appears in all but one of the poem's twenty stanzas, marking the work's boundaries and the development of Sibille's portrait. The poem casts "vertuous besynesse" as a tool of discipline, the feminine force that brings order. This "vertuous besynesse" enables the woman to discipline her own body and soul, her household, her business dealings, and ultimately sloth itself—effectively merging the realms of the marital, the familial, the commercial, and the devotional.

It may be a coincidence that Shirley began copying the poem just below his bookplate stanza in the volume (fol. 59v) (see fig. 3.1). Whatever led to this conjunction, the poem's placement just after the bookplate visibly locates the "Epistle" within a context of shared mixed-gender reading. The work begins after the heading identifying it as "an Epistel made by þe same

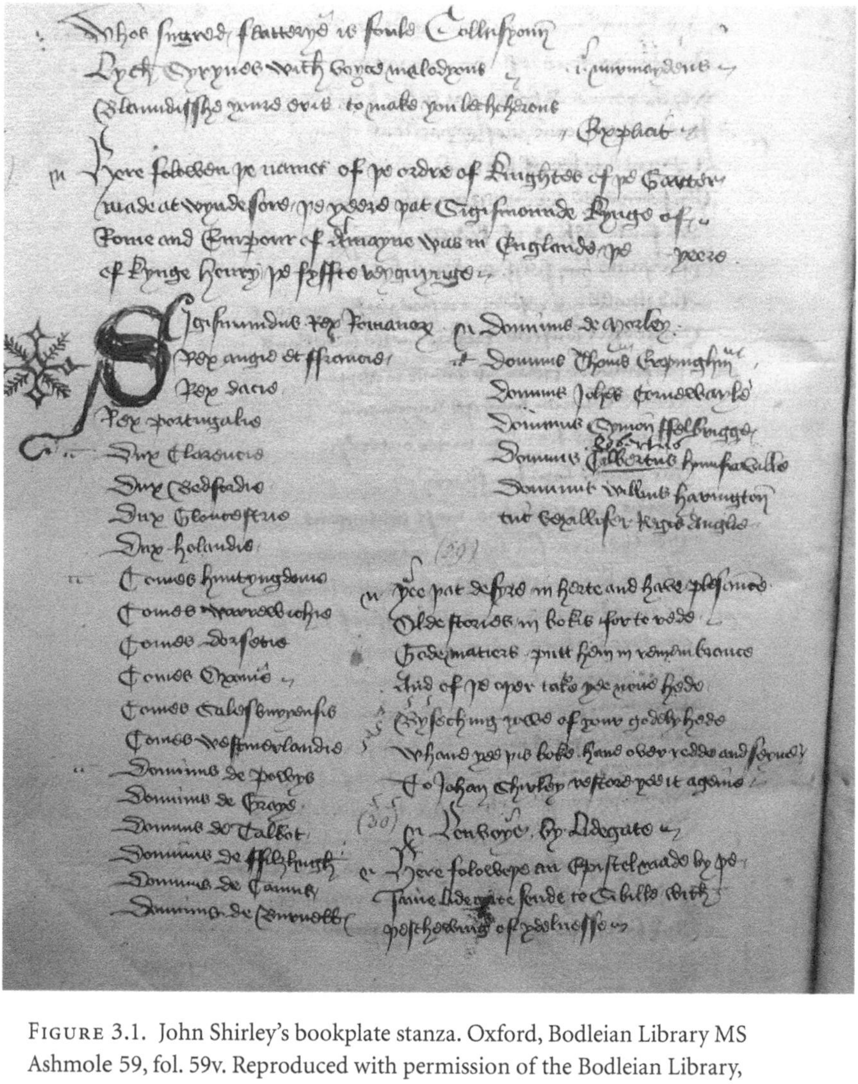

FIGURE 3.1. John Shirley's bookplate stanza. Oxford, Bodleian Library MS Ashmole 59, fol. 59v. Reproduced with permission of the Bodleian Library, University of Oxford.

Lidgate sende to Sibille with þeschewing of ydelnesse," giving us a first sight of the virtuous woman who inspired the text and who, in this new context, may inspire readers:

> The chief gynnyng of grace and of vertue
> To exclude slouþe is ocupacioun,
> Martha minystred to our lord Iesu,
> And Maria by contemplacioun,
> þeos boþe tweyne, of clene entencyoun,
> For to exclude al maner ydelnesse
> þeire labour sette in vertuous besynesse.[114]

From the first, "ocupacioun" is the woman's chief goal: "vertuous besynesse" is elastic enough to include "labour" of a spiritual or a worldly kind. As the poem unfolds, it becomes clear that the addressee, with her endless domestic duties, is more Martha than Mary. The wife's ability to banish sloth is continually praised: she is able "to gif ensaumple voyding ydelnesse," and her "femyninytee / Cawseþe slowþe from housholdes for to flee" (fol. 60r).

Not only is the virtuous wife an able helper to her husband in business, generating "worldely plenty" and "gret richchesse" for the family, but her "vertuous besynesse" generates both joy and strict discipline. Her version of "governaunce" is pleasurable rather than self-abnegating. Her husband "fyndeþe in hir so much souffisaunce, / Of wordely plentee fulsum habondance, / And in hir soule ful goostely gladnesse, / Ay most reioyssing vertuouse besynesse."[115] Here Lydgate's language of "suffisaunce" and "habondance," echoing Chaucer's Prologue to the Miller's Tale, minus the bitterness, suggests that "vertuous besynesse" is the very source of gladness and pleasure.[116] As Burger has argued, marital affection was linked in this period not only to procreation but also to "an ethic of care": "Marital affection first and foremost describes the care for the spouse that should take place—indeed, should develop and intensify—within the sacramental married state."[117] Even as it offers a source of joy for lord and lady, "besynesse" also functions as a means of guiding subordinate household members: "In cloþemakinge sheo shal eke besy be, / Wolle and flexsse vn-to hir servanteʒ dresse, / Sette hem on werke in vertuous besynesse."[118] The matron's "besynesse" sets the tone for the household, generating and structuring the industry of others.

Perhaps most striking within this particular reading context is the way in which "vertuous besynesse" becomes a means for the industrious lady of the house to control *herself*. In this way the poem evokes the social pressures and expectations borne by the substantial married woman or widow. In both the eighth and the twelfth stanzas, Lydgate's image of a "girdel" rings subtle changes on the biblical text. In the stanza depicting her industrious gardening, we see that

> Provydence did aye hir bryde[l] lede,
> Plauntynge amonge hir lousty fressh vynes,
> Whiche þat brought forþe delytable vynes
> *Vsinge a girdel aboute hir of clennesse,*
> *Her lyff tenbrace in vertuous besynesse.*[119]

The biblical verse depicts the wife as agent who "girds" herself: Proverbs 31:17 reads, "accinxit fortitudine lumbos suos" (she hath girded her loins with strength). In Lydgate's version the emphasis is slightly different: the beneficent force of "Provydence" directs the wife's activity, first with "did aye hir brydel lede" and then "Vsinge a girdel about hir of clennesse." The girding of the loins becomes a "girdel" of "clennesse," an instrument of purity that enfolds the wife both literally and figuratively as a providential force.[120] Although this initial mention of the "girdel" might be seen to reduce the wife's agency, the next mention restores it to her, again subtly complicating the biblical verse to make the "girdel" in question her instrument for mediating between public and private. Where Proverbs 31:24 reads "sindonem fecit et vendidit et cingulum tradidit Chananeo" (she made fine linen, and sold it, and delivered a girdle to the Chanaanite), Lydgate elaborates the stanza as following:

> Of golde and silke sheo made a ryche cloþe
> And solde it affter thoroughe hir providence,
> And for þat fame ful far in vertue goþe
> Sheo made a girdel of gret excellence
> For to represse þe mighty vyolence
> Of Canandus wilful wrecchednesse,
> *Sheo brideld hir with vertuous besynesse.*[121]

Claiming "providence" for herself as a forward-looking household value, she manages not only to sell her material "ryche cloþe," but also to make a metaphorical "girdel of gret excellence," an instrument of diplomacy against "Canandus wilful wrecchenesse." This "girdel" mediates between her control of others (perhaps difficult business partners, neighbors, and family members) and her own self-discipline, which remains central to her social position as wife.[122] As Burger notes, "the good woman and her social relations come into visibility . . . precisely by means of a careful attention to the body and its interfaces with the social."[123] In Lydgate's gendered use of "brideld" here, we may also recall the exhortation at the end of his "Holy Meditation," just a few folios earlier in the manuscript: "Looke by raisoun soo þou bridelde be / þat God Oure Lord ne bee wroþe with þee."[124] The same terminology works to connect religious with material self-discipline, yet here the powerful matron is bridling herself and others, not submitting obediently like Dido and Lucrece.

Within the hospital reading context, we know of several women who could have glimpsed themselves in the portrait of the industrious, substantial wife or widow. Other aspects of the wife's practice are notable in the hospital context, including her acts of charity and healing:

> To þe poure folke did hir almesdede,
> Hir armes oute a fer she gaue to reeche,
> Of colde in wynter hir meynee thare not dreede,
> For in suche cas sheo was a prudent leche,
> Alle hir servantes vertues ay to teche,
> Were twyes cladde, hem kepinge frome distresse,
> In somer and wynter by hir besynesse.[125]

Building upon the Proverbs description, this stanza casts the prudent matron as a font of charity as well as a "leche," a term with primarily medical overtones. Her "almesdede" becomes resonant within the hospital context, where widows like Beatrice Lurchon offered support to all categories of poor: bedridden hospital inmates and students, and also (in the residue clause of her will) "to pore pepyll most nedy, in mariages of pore maydenys of good name and fame, in redymyng and delyueryng of pore presoners out of prisons."[126] The term "leche" even reminds older women readers that they themselves, as widows, might become nursing sisters.[127]

Within the hybrid world of the hospital, as Lurchon's will reminds us, the practice and teaching of virtues has one ultimate goal: salvation. The Proverbs verse foresees a happy "last day" for the virtuous wife, and Lydgate adds an explicit emphasis on the attainment of heaven. He substantially augments 31:25 ("Strength and beauty are her clothing, and she shall laugh in the latter day") by asserting that the matron's "besynesse" will bring not only mirth, but spiritual reward:

> Of force, of clennesse and of honestee,
> And of fayrnesse made was hir vesture,
> Hir to defende in al adversitee.
> Of feyth, of trouþe, shal beo hir armure,
> And sheo shal love of entente moste pure,
> *Hir last daye of verray perfytnesse,*
> *Deservinge heven by vertuous besinesse.*[128]

Augmenting the biblical text to arm and clothe his matron in the virtues of "feyth" and "trouþe," he makes her "last daye" one not only of happiness but of perfection. Once again her "vertuous besynesse" appears as the engine by which her soul may confidently attain heaven. The work's constant awareness of the matron's reputation, in life and at the moment of death and beyond, is once again apt in the hospital setting, where female residents were intensely concerned with embodying virtue in life and after death, not only privately but in public ways: through commemorative torches on the hospital altars, and in funerary brasses, such as one featuring Alice with her first husband, that still lies embedded in the hospital church floor. Sutton points out that Alice Markby-Shipley-Portaleyn was praised in fulsome terms by her loyal second husband, who appointed her his executrix, "after her conscience without any rekenyng or accompte yeldyng or makyng therof to the bisshop ordenarie or any othir person, *for I trust hir more than all the worlde after.*"[129] Such husbandly esteem for his wife, whose authority exceeds even that of the bishop, echoes the praises expressed in Lydgate's poem, which Alice might have read from this very manuscript.[130] For Alice and other experienced "good women" of the hospital close, Ashmole provided a complex combination of reading materials, offering a range of potential models for crafting their evolving lives in this hybrid setting.

## EDUCATING CHILDREN:
## VIRTUE AND NURTURE FROM AUTHORITATIVE SOURCES

Just as the above texts construct a complex vision of feminine virtue, a number of other textual clusters contain material with particular relevance for instilling virtue in young listeners or readers. As Nicholas Orme has argued, the question of how medieval English children interacted with literature is a complex one. Children's literature is not always a distinct category, for a wide range of works could be "read or experienced" by young people.[131] Children might read or listen to texts; they might encounter works specifically written for them or consume works intended for adults.[132] In this section, I consider texts with a stated didactic function—some explicitly for children and some with a more general audience—that Shirley may have collected with the hospital close's young readers in mind. If we consider the close as an extended household, we can view educational reading as one of Ashmole's functions, in parallel to the "household book" or domestic miscellany.[133] I look at three notable textual sequences to suggest how these materials complement each other to instill the need and the means for living in community: one arguing for virtue above all, the second anatomizing its components, and the third showing how virtue may be embodied in a household context. In line with Edwards's argument about Shirley attempting to "emulate" court culture, many of the didactic pieces for youth were originally addressed to princes or other royalty, yet were translated easily into a gentry or bourgeois teaching context. In conduct texts, nobility becomes an attribute that may be embodied in behavior, not limited to those with noble blood.[134]

Several groups of short edifying texts seem particularly relevant to the hospital close's youngest members, whom we glimpsed above through the wills of their parents, grandparents and godparents. These children were girls and boys. Although some of the texts I consider below are addressed to male readers, others contain admonitions applicable to young girls also, particularly the last ones I consider: the *Summum sapientiae* (originally translated for Queen Margaret of Anjou) and "Stans puer ad mensam," a conduct poem that despite its masculine title, features the unisex subjects of "chylde" and "souerayn."[135]

In Ashmole, the sequence of secular didactic verses—starting at fol. 24v with Lydgate's retelling of Aesop's fable of the hound and cheese and

culminating with Lydgate's admonitory poem "Consulo quisquis eris"—
inculcates virtue in young men by instilling vigilance about language, its
use, and its interpretation. Sounding a preoccupation of the volume as a
whole, the texts obsessively cite authorities (some invented) and depend
upon biblical and historical exemplars.[136] This first cluster establishes virtue as an absolute requirement, especially through its longest text, Scogan's
"Moral Balade."

Shirley might have chosen Aesop's fable of the hound and the cheese
because it is the shortest of the seven that Lydgate translated. Its extreme
compression lends the story power.[137] This is the only manuscript in which
the hound and the cheese fable appears alone, with a ponderous title: "Here
begynneþe a notable proverbe of Ysopus Ethiopyen in balad by Daun Johan
Liedegate made in Oxenforde" (fol. 24v).[138] In two short stanzas we learn
the lesson of the hound who dropped the cheese in his greed for another:
the need to avoid covetousness.

> Who al þat coveyteþe, leseþe offte al in feere,
> A man al oone ne may not al purchace,
> Ne in heos armes al þe worlde enbrace,
> A meene is beste with good governaunce,
> To hem þat beon contente with suffisance.
> Þere is noman þat liveþe more at eese
> þane he þat cane with lytel bee contente.[139]

The emphasis on "good governaunce" and avoidance of greed resonates
strongly with the *Secretum Secretorum*, but on a more elementary and vis-
ceral level. Edward Wheatley argues that "the dog loses all he has, and 'all' is
the word with which Lydgate broadens the focus from the cheese to the
world."[140] With brevity and diction, Lydgate makes this fable into an urgently relevant teaching text for young and old alike.[141]

A focus on developing virtuous qualities at a young age comes to the
fore in Scogan's "Moral Balade," which Coleman aptly calls "a mini-speculum
principis."[142] Shirley carefully records the occasion of the poem's first performance, "at a souper of feorthe merchande in the Vyntre in London,
at the hous of Lowys Johan." This was the fourth quarterly meeting of the
merchants' company: the host, Lewis John, served, among other offices, as
the steward to the king's dowager queen, Joan of Navarre.[143] Scogan, tutor

to Henry IV's four sons, embraces the occasion to exhort the young men to virtue. Within the Ashmole manuscript, perhaps read communally within the hospital close, we can imagine the work taking on a slightly different yet still relevant meaning. The "Moral Balade" offers an uncompromising statement of the need for "vertuous noblesse," which warns noble hearers from taking virtue for granted, and in the hospital context makes such virtue accessible to the bourgeois reader. "Vertuous noblesse" is a goal, not an entitlement, and the poem uncouples status from conduct, as does the Wife of Bath's sermon, to which Scogan repeatedly alludes, noting at one point "þat lordshipe ne estate, / Withoute vertue, may not longe endure" (fol. 26r).[144]

The poem hammers home the need for instilling and preserving "vertue" in youth. Obsequiously calling himself "youre fadre called, unworthely," Scogan asks his adopted "sones," the young princes and dukes, to avoid emulating his misspent youth. Thus he posits a family group as the context for incorporating this wisdom: an extended family that would not be out of place in the hospital close. Scogan beseeches,

> My lordes dere, why I þis compleinte wryte
> To yowe, alle whome I love entierely,
> Is for to warne yowe, as I cane endyte,
> That tyme eloste in yowþe folely,
> Grevethe a wight goostely and bodely,
> I mene hem that to vyces list t'entende;
> *Þerfore I prey you lordes tendrely,*
> *Youre youþe in vertue shapeþe to dispende.*
>
> *Planteþe the roote of youthe in suche a wyse*
> *That in vertue youre growing beo alweye;*
> Looke ay, goodenesse beo in youre excercyse,
> Þat shal you mighty make, at eche assaye,
> Ffor to withstonde the feonde at eche affraye;
> Passeþe wisely þis paraillous pilgrymage;
> *Thenke on this worde and use it every daye:*
> *Þat shal yowe gif a parfyte floured age.*[145]

Scogan presents the prince's hoped-for growth in "vertue" as the remedy to his own dissolution. "It is entirely an exhortation to the royal princes to add virtue to their nobility," Robert Epstein argues. "The princes are Scogan's subject; his intention is to fashion poetically their ideal characters."[146] Scogan's emphasis on planting virtue at the "root," from which "a parfyte floured age" will grow, inspires his most powerful image, elaborated near the end in an organic tableau that connects "vertuous noblesse" to the routing of vice:

> Sithe, þere ageinst, þat vertuous noblesse
> Rooted in youþe, with goode perseverance,
> Dryveþe aweye al vyce and wrecchednesse,
> Al slogardrye, al ryote, and dispence;
> *Seothe eke howe vertue causeþe suffisaunce,*
> *And suffisaunce exyleþe coveityse:*
> Þus who haþe vertue haþe gret habondaunce
> Of wele, als far as raison can devyse.[147]

"Vertuous noblesse" combined with "goode perseverance" offers an organic remedy to all vices, particularly those involving laziness, a particular concern for the pampered nobility. Virtue is a capacious good that encloses all else, banishing the "coveitise" of which the preceding fable warned. That emphasis on "suffisaunce," on cultivating a virtue that will lead to personal and also social contentment and fulfillment, is central to this text and to the larger textual sequence. This stanza with its abhorrence of "Al slogardye, al ryote, and despence" also fulfills the poem's emphasis on industry or "besynesse," a term that is ultimately repeated three times, having first appeared in the following passage:

> Here may ye see þat vertuous noblesse
> Comþe not to yowe of youre auncestrye,
> But it comþe thorugh leofful besynesse,
> Of honest lyff, and noght of slougardery.[148]

This concern for "besynesse" in connection to virtue links Scogan's "Moral Balade" to the "Epistle for Sibille," in which it appeared as a refrain. Copied for young hospital readers, "besynesse" takes on a different meaning from when it was directed to the young princes. The hospital reading community was composed mainly of those who had earned their privileged place in its sanctuary through "besyness" of service or profession, rather than by heredity. One might think in particular of young Richard Joynour, the orphan ward of Master Wakeryng, who in 1436 had become part of the extended hospital family. Perhaps an industrious youth, Richard went on to become a successful grocer.[149]

It may be that Shirley placed the text he labels "Balade of Good Counsel" (an extract from Lydgate's *Fall of Princes*), directly after Scogan's "Moral Balade" in order to fill space at the end of a quire. Remaining in the ballad form, this text makes a transition from the absolute statement of virtue to an emphasis, which also becomes a touchstone in the edifying texts, on the need for careful speech and listening. Language, translation, and interpretation come to the fore in this short poem. If virtue is to be attained, care must be taken with language.

The balade, addressed to "Prynces" as an envoy to *Fall of Princes*, book 1, warns that although "some sey trouþe and some be deceyvable" (fol. 28v), princes must be discriminating, careful never to "gif ful jugement, / Or hasty credenes, withoute avysement."[150] As the refrain reminds readers (or hearers), "Þaughe some tale haue a feyre visage, / yitte may it conclude gret decepcyoun"; hence care must always be the rule in speaking or interpreting language. "Let folke be ware of al suche langage, / And kepe þeire tonges frome oblocucyoun."[151] Above all, "noble pryncess prudent of hye courage" must avoid flatterers: "Stoppe fast your eeris frome þeire bittur sovne / Beo circumspecte nought hasty but prudent.... And gif no credence withoute avisement."[152] The short extract conveys a powerful message for the young: the need for circumspection as a speaker and a listener, for careful parsing of advice.[153]

As the book proceeds, Shirley continues to excerpt Lydgate in order to anatomize virtue and teach the means to attain it in a household context. The next group of edifying short texts, starting a new quire with selections from "A Pageant of Knowledge," "The Four Complexions of Mankind," "Four Things that Make a Man a Fool," and the "The Saying of Wise Men," breaks down the rudiments of virtue and puts them into practice, a practice that comes into embodiment later in the conduct text "Stans puer."[154]

The "Pageant of Knowledge" might be seen as a rudimentary educational text: in its complete form it begins with the virtues and then describes the planets, astrological signs, and elements, the four complexions, the seasons, and the world's changeability. Ashmole contains a unique fragmentary version in which some verses appear out of order and most of the sections, including those describing the planets and the seasons, are missing.[155] Like

Scogan's "Moral Balade," this text has lost its connection to public performance, but we can imagine it being read aloud in the present manuscript. Although we cannot tell whether Shirley edited the text himself or used an incomplete exemplar, its truncation is suggestive for this cluster and the broader
volume. Minus the detailed information on the planets, the astrological signs,
four seasons of the year and mutable "dysposion of the world," the work loses
its learned detail and becomes an "abstracte" (Shirley's own term) emphasizing self-regulation and "nurture," appropriate for young people.

Some unique features in Ashmole 59 transform the text from a long
compendium into a more focused work. Shirley's heading emphasizes its
learned origins and offers the material as a culturally privileged, translated
work, perhaps worthy of memorization: "Here nowe foloweþe þe doctryne of many gret clerkes approved made in balade wyse and translated
oute of diuers langages in to Englisshe."[156] This version lacks the first two
stanzas, which would establish the different estates, and plunges the reader
into seven stanzas anatomizing Temperance, Justice, Prudence, Discretion, Reason, Plesance, Courtesy, and Nurture.[157] In outlining the various
virtues, the stanzas elaborate lessons learned from the previous sequence
of texts, unfolding these qualities as means of self-regulation in a communal setting. Whereas Temperance exhorts readers to "Reverence þe goode"
and "Punisshe paciently þe transgressiouns / Of men misruled," Justice
helps in the properly circumspect use of language treated in "Consulo
quisquis eris":

> Be truwe in rekennyng, sette no somme abak,
> And in þy worde late be no variaunce;
> Of thee be sadde demure of governaunce,
> Sette folk at rest and apees al trouble,
> Be ware of flatereres and of tunge double.[158]

The verse on "Rayson," a quality privileged in the earlier text, is especially
emphatic on how reason might function as a key to self-regulation:

> To rule man he be not bestyall,
> And þane him reson his owen doughter deer,
> Princis pryncesse moost soueren entier,
> *Þe bridell in man þe froward voluntee*
> Þat he not erre by sensualitee.[159]

Although the sense is somewhat garbled,[160] one may still discern the emphasis on reason as a check upon will, functioning as a "bridell": an image that any young reader or hearer would understand, and that we have seen in Lydgate's "Holy Meditation" and "Epistle to Sibille." It seems significant that the last stanza here (which thus receives emphasis in this version) describes Courtesy and Nurture: key terms in "Stans puer" also. "The Pageant" ends thus:

> Þis goode ladye called curteisye,
> And her sustre named is nurture,
> By þeire office longinge to genterye
> Lowly requeren til every creature,
> Als for and mighte and power may endure,
> With hole herte, body, wille, and mynde,
> To be contente with suche as þey fynde.[161]

As in Scogan's "Moral Balade," emphasis falls upon the combination of birth and work: here in a counterpart pair to "vertuous noblesse," courtesy and nurture work together to foster grateful sufficiency in the subject under formation.

The culmination of the manuscript's proverbial wisdom arrives with a group of two longer texts that reiterate and elaborate, by putting into practice, much of the earlier edifying secular content. Two texts with obvious relevance to the teaching of boys or girls, the *Summum sapientiae* and "Stans puer," stand out for their length and prominence near the end of the volume. Both are likewise translations. The *Summum* consists of 133 rhyme royal stanzas conveying maxims and proverbs from biblical and classical authorities: the advice is mainly secular, containing material that circulated in elementary schoolbooks of the period.[162] Proverbs formed the core of much grammar education, a means to teach Latin and conduct simultaneously.[163] It was not altogether unusual to include proverbs in a literary anthology: the *Summum* is also included in the Shirley-derived anthology BL MS Harley 2251.[164] Yet its combination with the foregoing material and its immediate conjunction with "Stans puer" seem unusual, suggesting not simply a desire to give proverbs a respected place within the book, but perhaps also an effort to appeal to a particular subset of young readers. This conjunction of "Stans puer" with proverbs is mirrored in a contemporary schoolbook, Oxford Bodleian Library Rawlinson MS D. 328, which also gathers the *Distichs* of Cato and Latin grammatical rules, among other pedagogically oriented materials.[165] This part of the Ashmole manuscript looks more like a teaching book than a literary anthology.

The *Summum*, a translation of Nicole Bozon's *Les proverbes de bon enseignement*, may have been commissioned either for or by Henry VI's young queen, Margaret of Anjou, close to the time of her crowning in 1445, when she was only fifteen.[166] Jenni Nuttall speculates that Margaret, looking ahead to her weighty responsibilities as queen and mother, asked for an English "sapiential text which supplied her with the wisdom of ancient authorities."[167] In Ashmole, the text might have served a similar function for young readers in the hospital close, both girls and boys. As Joseph Napierkowski notes, the proverbs tend to focus on "social harmony" and "social duties," including nineteen that warn against "abuses of the tongue."[168] The *Summum*'s rules for moral living text complement "Stans puer" in their emphasis on reason and self-control, careful speech and conduct, and generosity. The portrayal of Reason as a means of self-control takes us back to the Pageant of Knowledge and forward into "Stans puer":

> If yee desire worship and hounour
> An Emparour þis auctour wol yowe make,
> By raysoun calleþe him an Emperour
> þat cane him selff iustice and vndertake,
> Expelling vices and vertuous loore take,
> *Governe youre self and ruwel that heghe empyre,*
> *And soo yee may your hounor ay desyre.*[169]

As in many of the texts that I have considered in this section, for example Scogan's "Moral Balade," one becomes an "emperour" not via wealth, but through reason and discipline over one's own "heghe empyre," the self. Cascading from this exercise of reasoned self-rule is the mandate to control speech, expressed numerous times, as in the following warnings:

> Ofte it falleþe þat many a goode deede
> By offte seyers tourneþe to contrarie;
> Sume man byleueþe what þat ever is sayde,
> *By raison should he be mourningly*
> *Whane þat oþer laughe at his folye;*
> To scorninge wrecches causeþe gret debate
> In sundry places where þat he is ate.[170]

Again reason demands sobriety and care with words, and "offte [wrong] seyers" may easily turn good will to bad in company.[171] This tight link between "deede" and speech is reiterated throughout the stanzas, which continue to praise sober conduct and speech in contrast to rash speech and inappropriate actions.

The *Summum* is also notable for its repeated focus on almsgiving. Three stanzas in a row exhort charity, and one can see how this fundamental Christian virtue, central to life in the hospital, extensively documented in the hospital wills we have seen, would fit into guidance for young people living in its shadow. In a work for the young queen, and also young women and men living in the hospital close, these words from Tobias would resonate:

> If yee desire of God to haue grace,
> From þe poore folke voyde nouȝt þe visage;
> Par auenture þane wol oure lordes face
> Dyvert frome you to youre gret damage;
> Euer on pourayle sette welc youre courage,
> *Favour and socoure hem in necessite*
> *As kyndely nature oweþe by duetee.*[172]

Generosity to the poor is not only required for achieving God's grace but also recognized as basic to "kyndely nature" toward other people. To create the community of sympathy that the hospital required, one in which families and neighbors refrained from fighting, were not fooled by deceptive words, and remained satisfied with their "suffisaunce," required an overall effort to cultivate this sense of a circuit from human actions to divine consequence.[173]

The *Summum* moves seamlessly into the next text, Lydgate's translation "Stans puer ad mensam," a very popular work in educational and literary manuscripts alike. In his heading, Shirley draws attention both to its sententiousness and to the fact that it is a translation: "And here foloweþe next a doctryne of Curtesye cleped in Latyne stans puer ad mensam . . . translated in to Englysshe in balade wyse by Lidegate þe religious of Bury."[174] It is thus framed as a conduct poem for children, usually speaking directly to the child but occasionally about him or her in the third person, implying a multigenerational audience. The work begins here, "Dispose þy youþe affter my doctryne, / To all norture þy corage do enclyne" (fol. 98r), but it also includes passages generalizing about children's tendencies: "In children werre now mirthe, nowe debate, / In þeire quarell is no greet violence."[175] The poem might appeal both to children and their parents or advisors. A focus on children as readers and listeners is suggested by the envoy, where Lydgate implores his poem,

> Pray, *yonge childre þat þee shal see or reede,*
> Þaughe þat þou be compendyous of sentence,
> Of þy clauses for to taken heede,
> Which til al vertue shal þy youþe lede.[176]

Although the poem with its stated focus on the "table" may be understood rather narrowly as a courtesy text, phrases such as "all norture" and "al vertue" bespeak a more ambitiously formative purpose. In the context of the Ashmole miscellany, we may see the work as calling into embodiment the precepts and qualities theorized in the volume's earlier sententious texts that construct proper marital and familial relations.[177]

If we return to the full first stanza, we can appreciate the way in which "vertuous discipline" should take root (to borrow Scogan's metaphor) in mind, heart, and body:

> My dere chylde first þy self enable
> With al þyne herte to vertuous disciplyne
> A fore þy souerayne stonding at þe table,
> Dispose þy youþe after my doctryne,
> To all norture courage do enclyne.
> Ffirst whyle þou spekest be not reklesse,
> Kepe feete and handes and fingers stille in pees.[178]

Here the verse depicts the process by which advice becomes bodily *habitus*. When the childish reader or hearer receives these words of advice, it is up to him or her to put them into practice, to "þy self enable / With al þyne herte to virtuous disciplyne." Ability will come through that effort of "herte": in order to put into practice that "norture" already advertised by texts such as the "Moral Balade" and the "Pageant of Knowledge," the reader must internalize the advice in his or her "courage" and then express that resolve in speech and body ("fete," "handes," and "fingers").

"Stans puer" gives bodily expression to the virtues of courtesy and generosity described and theorized in the cluster's preceding texts. The poem repeatedly emphasizes good conduct before the "sovereign," but in a gentry or bourgeois reading context, the paterfamilias, the mother, or even the hospital master might occupy that authoritative role.[179] The coordination of expression, speech, and body must perform deference to this authority:

> Walke demurely by streetis in tovne,
> Advertyse þee of raysoun and wisdame.
> With dissolute laughtre þou do none offence[180]
> To-forc þy souereyn, ne in his presence.[181]

Here we have an urban scene and an embodiment of the virtues described in "Pageant" and the *Summum* proverbs: the controlled body that can appear in public as an advertisement of "rayson and wisdame." Laughter too must be disciplined before the sovereign.

Perhaps most salient within a volume that assumes a collective, mixed-age readership is the emphasis on generosity, relevant to individual households and to the hospital as an extended household within which neighbors lived, perhaps sharing goods, meals, and reading material. The table again becomes the site for the choice between greed and generosity: "þe beste morselles haue in remembraunce / Alle to þy selff do hem not applye / Part with þy felowe, þat is courtesye" (fol. 98v). Neither a child nor an adult reader living alongside the hospital could consider any property to be truly "alle to thyselff." Instead, children who might have read or listened to the texts in this book were being asked to embody ways of collective living that might further the goals of courtesy and charity, while echoing the communal and regulated practices of the hospital.

If we consider Ashmole 59 as an anthology for a hospital readership of mixed ages, statuses, and genders, then this collection begins to seem much less miscellaneous than it has in the past. By placing the volume in the context of the hospital close, a complex, heterogeneous literary community that Shirley grew to know well over the course of many years, we begin to see how this sophisticated translator and copyist used texts to envision a virtuous, disciplined, and generous community of readers, connected by affective ties both familial and spiritual.

Appendix to Chapter Three

Contents of Oxford, Bodleian Library MS Ashmole 59, fols. iv–134v.
Adapted from Margaret Connolly, *John Shirley: Book Production and the Noble Household* (Aldershot: Ashgate, 1998), table 3, 146–49.

| *Folios* | *Contents* |
|---|---|
| iv | motto and signature, Latin verses |
| iir | list of contents |
| 1r | *Secretum Secretorum* |
| 13r | Lydgate "Tragedy of Rome" [extract from *Fall of Princes* II] *DIMEV* 1904-2 |
| 15r | Lydgate "Tragedy of Princes" [extract from *Fall of Princes* III] *DIMEV* 1904-2 |
| 16v | Lydgate "Moral Epistle to King Jonas" [extract from *Fall of Princes* II] *DIMEV* 1904-2 |
| 17v | Gower "Balade of Good Counsel" *DIMEV* 4346-1 |
| 18r | Lydgate "Everything to his Semblable" *DIMEV* 6063-1 |
| 21v | Lydgate "Prayer to Our Lady" (Latin and English) *DIMEV* 4474-1 |
| 22v | Lydgate "Prayer to St. Edmund" *DIMEV* 3911-2 |
|  | Lydgate "Envoy to Henry VI, Life of St. Edmund" *DIMEV* 1535-1 |
| 24v | Lydgate "Isopes Fabules" (one only) *DIMEV* 6701-1 |
| 25r | Scogan "Moral Ballade" *DIMEV* 3465-1 |
| 27r | Chaucer "Gentilesse" *DIMEV* 5277-1 |
| 28v | Lydgate "Ballade of Good Counseyl" [extract from *Fall of Princes* I] *DIMEV* 1904-2 |
| 29v | Lydgate "Consulo quisquis eris" *DIMEV* 2156-2 |
| 31r | Lydgate "As a Mydsomer Rose" *DIMEV* 3058-1 |
| 33v | Lydgate "Horns Away" *DIMEV* 4169-1 |
| 34v | Lydgate "A Freond at Neode" (12 lines only) *DIMEV* 3034-1 |
| 35r | Lydgate "A Freond at Neode" *DIMEV* 3034-1 |
| 37r | Chaucer "Fortune" *DIMEV* 5803-2 |
| 38v | "Complaint of Venus" *DIMEV* 5590-3 [Chaucer] "Chronicle" *DIMEV* 1666-1 |

| 39v | Lydgate "Ballade at the Reverence" *DIMEV* 176-1 |
| 41r | Lydgate "Amor vincit omnia" *DIMEV* 1160-1 |
| 43r | "Versus philosoforum" (Latin) |
| 44v | Lydgate "Invocation to St. Anne" *DIMEV* 5824-1 |
| 45v | Lydgate "My Lady Dere" *DIMEV* 1230-1 |
| 47v | Lydgate "Doublenesse" *DIMEV* 5793-2 |
| 49r | Lydgate "A Holy Meditation" *DIMEV* 244-1 |
| 52r | Lydgate "Valentine to Her I Love Best" |
| 54r | Lydgate "Ballade to Henry VI on his Coronation" *DIMEV* 3554-1 |
| 56r | Lydgate "On verbum caro factum est" *DIMEV* 6819-1 |
| 57r | [Lydgate] "Complaint for my Lady of Gloucester" *DIMEV* 159-1 |
| 59r | Lydgate "Tragedy" [extract from *Fall of Princes* III] *DIMEV* 1904-2 |
| 59v | Garter List *IMEP* IX [2] |
|     | Shirley "Bookplate" *DIMEV* 6840-1 |
| 60r | Lydgate "Letter to Lady Sibille" *DIMEV* 5232-1 |
| 62r | Lydgate "Mumming at Bishopswood" *DIMEV* 3497-1 |
| 64r | "Invocation to Our Lady" *DIMEV* 1715-1 |
| 65r | Lydgate "Invocation to St. Denis" *DIMEV* 4070-1 |
| 66r | [Lydgate] "Quia amore langueo" *DIMEV* 2461-1 |
| 67r | St. Augustine "Verses on the Mass" *DIMEV* 3813-1 |
| 67v | Against Swearing *IMEP* IX [3] |
| 68r | Anchoress of Mansfield, "Hymn on the Five Joys" *DIMEV* 1713-1 |
| 68v | Lydgate "The Pyte to the Wretched Synner" *DIMEV* 4102-1 |
| 69r | Lydgate "Deus in nomine tuo" *DIMEV* 1563-1 |
| 70v | Lydgate "A Pageant of Knowledge" *DIMEV* 939-1 |
| 71v | Lydgate "The Four Complexions of Mankind" *DIMEV* 4168-1 |
| 72r | "Four Things that Make a Man a Fool" *DIMEV* 6798-1 |
|     | Prophecy (Latin) |
|     | "The Saying of Wise Men" *DIMEV* 5155-1 |
| 73r | "Devout and Virtuous Words" *DIMEV* 5584-1 |
|     | "Thou that wear the crown of thorns" *DIMEV* 5862-1 |
|     | "Love gentle Jesu" *DIMEV* 509-1 |
|     | Augustine, prose text (Latin) |

74v        Chronicle of England (Latin)

75r        Lydgate "The Kings of England sithen William the Conqueror"
           *DIMEV* 5731-1

77r        Thomas of Canterbury, prose text (Latin)

78r        Prophecy *DIMEV* 6299-1
           Prophecy (Latin)
           Counsels of St. Isidore *IMEP* IX [4]

83r        [Augustine] "Contemptu Mundi" *IMEP* IX [5]
           "Why is this world beloved that false is and vain" *DIMEV* 6670-1

83v        Words of Jerome (Latin)

84r        Prophecy of Jerome (Latin)

84v        Sybil (Latin)
           [Lydgate] "Summum Sapientiae" *DIMEV* 5502-1

98r        Lydgate "Stans puer ad mensam" *DIMEV* 3588-4

99v        "The Chronicle of the Three Kings of Cologne" *IMEP* IX [6]

128v       Prester John continuation *IMEP* IX [6]

130v       "The morow of screfte" *IMEP* IX [7]

131v       Recipe (Latin and English) *IMEP* IX [A1]
           Recipe for the stomach *IMEP* IX [9]

132r       Recipe for a cough *IMEP* IX [10]

132v       "Treatise on Egyptian Days" *IMEP* IX [11]

134r       Prayer *DIMEV* 1544-2

134v       One stanza rhyme royal ("Thou be wise dread thine own conscience")
               *DIMEV* 5819-1
           Lydgate "Deus in nomine tuo" (one verse only) *DIMEV* 1563-2
           Recipe for sciatica *IMEP* IX [12]

# FOUR

# Collaborative Devotional Reading at St. Bartholomew's and St. Mark's

John Shirley may have been the most famous bibliophile to reside at St. Bartholomew's Hospital, but he was not the only accomplished bookmaker living and working there at mid-fifteenth century. Augustinian brothers also produced books for use within their houses. In this chapter, I consider several volumes copied by Shirley's friend John Cok, fifteenth-century brother of St. Bartholomew's, London, and by sixteenth-century brothers John Colman and William Haulle of St. Mark's, Bristol. These Augustinian scribes copied their Latin, Middle English, and bilingual collections for a range of hospital residents: clerical and lay, male and female. Their manuscripts suggest the generativity of hospitals as sites for collaborative reading, a spectrum spanning individual study, shared devotional performance, and reading aloud, among other modalities. Cok copied the volumes that are now British Library MS Additional 10392 and Gonville and Caius MS 669*/646. Colman's volumes include Oxford Bodleian Lyell MS 38 and Oxford St. John's College MS 173. Haulle copied the book that is now Bristol Public Library MS 6. Building on bibliographical and intellectual histories of the Augustinian Order, I place these volumes into conversation with each other to show how their scribes imagined devotional reading as a means to build varied programs of ordered communal life in the hospital setting.[1] These hospital-produced volumes demonstrate the permeability of their institutions as lay-clerical spaces, settings for the practices of penance, meditation, and charity that priestly canons and lay residents might share. At other moments, their books speak to the distinctiveness of Augustinian identity in tandem with the Rule of Augustine's requirements. Sometimes these impulses are visible within the same multifunctional volumes.

For these scribes and their audiences, reading in the Augustinian hospital becomes a practice constitutive of communal religion. Such an approach coexisted with the individualized practices of "lay asceticism" that Amy Appleford attributes to hospital close resident William Baron, one of John Shirley's bookish lay neighbors.[2] In her study of Baron's devotional collection, now Oxford Bodleian MS Douce 322, Appleford argues that Baron collected death-focused devotional texts, such as *Pety Job* and *Learn to Die*, in order to "cultivate inner asceticism: a private conversion and spiritual withdrawal from everyday life, fueled by reimagining daily vicissitudes in eremitic terms."[3] This book's clustering of death-focused texts with other Middle English devotional guides, including Rolle's *Emendatio vitae*, which articulates an eremitic identity, is striking. I agree that *Pety Job*, a verse meditation on Job's frailty and the wretchedness of human existence, ultimately stresses "the conviction that ascetic suffering is, in the end, productive."[4] As MS Douce 322 suggests, and as I have shown in my work on late fourteenth-century texts such as *The Abbey of the Holy Ghost* and *Fervor Amoris*, many late medieval English readers sought out texts to assist them in turning away from active toward contemplative lives inflected by monastic and eremitic practices.[5] On the evidence of this manuscript, Baron and like-minded readers may have viewed the hospital close as a place conducive to intensive meditation upon death, becoming "isolated in their spiritual identities by the mortified interior dispositions they learned to cultivate through death meditation."[6] Although Baron lived in the hospital close, he chose to be buried in the London Charterhouse, the institution most closely associated with the "mortified contemplative life" to which Appleford contends he aspired.[7]

The configuration of texts in Baron's anthology may promote a Carthusian-inspired spiritual isolation, but a self-isolating reading practice was not the only variety of devotional reading available at St. Bartholomew's. I focus in this chapter upon volumes that construct individual and shared reading within a larger set of social and communal practices. The Augustinian hospitals of St. Bartholomew's and St. Mark's offered unique sites for reading: with their hybrid status as religious institutions and "parishes," hospitals allowed contemplative and eremitic modes of piety to coexist within a penitential framework that constantly reminded lay and clerical readers of their duties to each other. In the volumes that I consider, awareness of death may serve less as an occasion for self-abjecting meditation than as a spur to self-reformation and a goad to the performance of charity. These books prod readers to make tribulations productive for themselves and for the poor, the ever-present objects of the hospital's charity.

The hospital volumes that I consider here combine languages, genres, and modes for multiple possible users or audiences. Multilingualism becomes especially salient in the Latin/Middle English volumes from St. Mark's, but each of the books under study bears the mark of a multilingual community. Christopher Baswell's comment on earlier multilingual French/Latin manuscripts helps to theorize the uses of these books: "In that most adaptable and intimate of archives, the codex, where varying dependencies on sight, touch, and sound can yield varying, if always interrelated, experiences of language and text, 'multilingualism' needs to be understood not as a descriptor but as a constant and active presence."[8] These miniature archives of hospital practice sometimes combine languages to invite readers into varied forms of collaborative reading. Cok's Middle English devotional collection, which Shirley annotated in Latin, makes meditative and eremitic modes of devotion available in English; Shirley's annotations suggest his interest in Rolle's advice on resisting worldly temptations and carving out a spiritual life with his community in mind. Cok's MS Additional 10392, a Latin collection, invites clerical and lay users, perhaps including Shirley, into a shared Latin devotional space, with an emphasis on the collective participation of priest and layperson in penitential practice.

John Colman of St. Mark's also copied both Latin and Middle English, sometimes in close proximity within the same volume. His early Latin production, MS Lyell 38, collects texts with specific relevance to Augustinian life, including Rolle's Latin *Emendatio vitae*, which appears in this context as a professional disciplinary text in conversation with the Rule of Augustine. Yet in another volume, now St. John's MS 173, Colman combines English and Latin texts within the same booklets, as does William Haulle in the multilingual MS 6, a volume with similar characteristics. I suggest that rather than mapping a hierarchy of clerical or lay reading according to language, the bilingual booklets offer a spectrum of practices and modes of reading (including reading aloud and preaching) for hospital readers pursuing differently regulated, intersecting devotional lives. I read these surviving books as "intimate . . . archives" of relationships among canons and between canons and laity within the hospital.

## John Cok:
### Shared Reading and Spiritual Life in the Hospital

John Cok was an Augustinian priest and brother of St. Bartholomew's, London by 1421. In this section I seek to understand how Cok's work as scribe and compiler extended his priestly practice within the hospital and possibly shaped his relationship with Shirley. Cok and Shirley knew each other: Shirley names Cok as an executor in his will.[9] Although Cok offers some information about himself in the cartulary, we find few of his chosen details corroborated elsewhere. He commonly refers to himself in his books as "frater" (brother), yet Shirley is the only one who explicitly calls him a priest.[10] He includes "Sir John Wakering maister of the forsaid hospitall of Seynt Bartilmew Sir John Cok prest and his broþer professed" among the small group of friends and family he asks to "assiste comforte help and councell" in the execution of his testament.[11] We find Cok's hand as both scribe and annotator in numerous surviving books, large and small.[12] His most famous institutional work is the great hospital cartulary, which he copied along with several other scribes, and Cok also copied smaller, more personal collections. One such book is a collection of Latin religious texts (BL MS Additional 10392), dated 1432. A. I. Doyle suggests that the volume "probably belonged to the hospital."[13] Cok also copied a collection of Middle English devotional works (Cambridge, Gonville and Caius MS 669/*646). At some point, Shirley owned and annotated this vernacular volume.

In keeping with the larger pattern of contemporary English Augustinian manuscripts, which tended to be "personal compilations," these two small volumes are unique collections.[14] The Additional collection contains all Latin texts with one exception, a short proverb in English, copied on the last leaf.[15] In contrast, the Caius volume's contents are all English—a meditation on Christ's passion, Rolle's *Emendatio vitae* and *Form of Living*—with two brief Latin extracts from *Piers Plowman* on free will and poverty.[16] Shirley engaged with the English texts in Latin, annotating the volume with his characteristic "videte" and "nota per Shirley." Whereas the English volume seems more narrowly focused on individual meditation and self-transformation, the Latin collection is varied and compendious, a multifunctional priestly collection with many possible users. I look first at the Caius volume, then more extensively at the Additional volume to suggest that together these two books demonstrate the complementarity of the eremitic and the penitential, the ascetic and the communal, as modes of lay devotional reading within the hospital.

### Gonville and Caius 669*/646: Shirley Reads Rolle in the Hospital

In its selection of a Middle English Passion meditation, Rolle's *Emendatio vitae* and *Form of Living*, the Caius volume collects three popular works transmitting the contemplative and eremitic teachings that appealed to many Londoners at mid-fifteenth century. Cok probably copied the volume during Shirley's residency in the hospital close, which began in the 1430s and lasted until his death in 1456.[17] Cok copied the three Middle English devotional texts in a textura hand, and the book is punctuated with gold letters, blue lombards, and other decorations.[18] Cok may have copied the volume as a gift for Shirley, Simon Horobin notes.[19] Jeremy Griffiths raises the possibility that it was a commercial commission, and G. H. Russell supposes that it was made as "part of his [Cok's] clerical vocation."[20] "If we accept the suggestion that the Gonville and Caius manuscript was copied by Cok as a gift to Shirley, then it may be that the volume reverted to Cok upon Shirley's death," states Horobin.[21] Whether or not the Caius collection was originally intended for him, Shirley owned and used it, for it contains his autograph and numerous annotations.

As a whole, the Caius volume offers a series of complementary directives on self-regulation, reading, and meditation applicable to many possible readers. While the *Meditations* provide material to ponder, the *Emendatio* and *Form* offer frameworks for ordering religious life and practice, suggesting strategies and moments for meditation. All three texts traversed the porous lay/clerical boundary that the hospital tended to dissolve to some extent in its welcome of regular and secular clergy along with lay residents of different ages and sexes. The translated *Emendatio* and *Form of Living* offer definitions of professional (priestly and anchoritic) religious life and practice that in the fifteenth century moved via linguistic translation or manuscript transmission into the realm of lay devotion.[22] *Emendatio* traces a twelve-step path from renunciation to contemplation, beginning with "conversion," a turning from the world, and culminating in "contemplation" of God. Hugh Kempster calls *Emendatio* a work of "contemplative 'pastoralia,'" a phrase evoking the text's hybrid nature and potential appeal to a wide range of readers.[23] *Emendatio*'s "systematic and relatively brief" quality probably contributed to its popularity among priests, as well as nuns and lay readers of both sexes.[24]

Whether Shirley commissioned Cok to copy this volume of spiritual works or received it as a gift from his friend the hospital canon, its creation and annotation testify to a collaborative literary relationship between the two that unfolded within the space of the hospital. Can we view the volume as an extension of Cok's spiritual guidance of Shirley? We do not have enough evidence about their friendship to assert this, but we can certainly detect the relevance of the volume's three texts to lay life in the hospital. The *Emendatio* bridges lay and priestly states, the worldly and spiritual lives. The work's hybridity suits the hospital, where even lay residents living in private apartments within the close might be in contact with the hospital's devotional routines and personnel, participating to varying degrees in the institution's mediation of spirit and flesh. Shirley's readerly engagement with the text may be linked to his life in the hospital context, perhaps marking the desire to seek an ordered religious life in a space connected to yet separate from the business of the city. Shirley's notae may indicate, in Marleen Cré's terms, "what he wanted to come back to when he read the anthology again, what he wanted to point out to other readers."[25] Although I remain cautious of overinterpreting Shirley's annotations, his notes around passages related to conversion, collective self-discipline, and virtuous love of God suggest that these themes were salient to him as he navigated life in the hospital close.

Throughout his Middle English *Emendatio* text, Shirley annotated passages of direction and exhortation, moments where Rolle spells out the shape of the holy life. The initial difficult "conversion" from a worldly to a spiritual life begins when the sinful subject realizes that self-amendment is the only way to prevent an unprepared death. Rolle's text opens with a warning not to delay conversion away from sin, "for deþ wiþouten mercy sodeinly steliþ away synneful, and bitternes of peynes falliþ unwarly on hem þat for sleuþe turnen here, ne we mowe not nombre hou many worldely liuers to moche fals truste haþe bygylyd, for hit is grete synne to trust to Goddis mercy and ceese not of synne."[26] Shirley adds a "nota per Shyrley" to this sternly penitential passage, with its warning of "sleuþe," the mental laziness that may allow "worldely liuers" to believe, wrongly, that God will forgive them. Although the reader of the vernacular *Emendatio* may not literally be leaving the world, he must embark on this journey ready to amend himself on both a physical and a mental level.

In his discussion of conversion, Rolle highlights the danger of being pulled back into the worldly desires after committing to flee from them. Shirley too remains alert to this danger, drawing attention with his "videte" mark to the exemplary story of "þe man, þat men seyd had lyfyd a wondire streit lyf fyftene ʒeer, and after, he fylle in synne wiþ his seruauntys wyf"[27] (see fig. 4.1). For, as Rolle adds (and Shirley annotates a few lines later), "alle newe bygynnyng most fle alle occasions of synne and wiþdrawe worde, dedis, and syʒtys þat may stere to any yuel. For þe more unleful any þing is, þe raþer it is desiryd." The flight from the world must be accompanied by a concerted discipline of body and speech, for it may not include the luxury of complete isolation. The reader of Rolle's text remains in a mixed community, where sexual temptations may still assault him. These essentially penitential directives would complement the ministrations of priestly advisor that we will find in Cok's Latin devotional book, MS Additional 10392.

As a reader who had left the immediate world of the city for the pleasant communal retreat of the hospital close, Shirley may have been receptive to Rolle's advice on entering into a newly ordered mode of living focused more on God than on worldly reputation or pleasures. In his marginal annotations to the *Emendatio*, Shirley attends to the need and the difficulty of leaving behind worldly pleasures and reputation. This process is a gradual one. In the discussion of spiritual poverty, Shirley marks Rolle's assertion that those willing to leave behind care for worldly worships will ultimately win grace. It is "leeful" to keep "oure necessaryes while we lyuen," Rolle asserts, "but þei ben the lesse worþ, þat þei dar not suffre for God to be pore or nedy, or to haue defauʒte. But bi grace, ʒit þei mow com to hiʒe lyuing in vertues and to heuenly contemplacioun, ʒif þei leue þe grete occupacyouns and wordely offices or besinesse."[28] Although spiritual beginners may not be able to "suffre for God to be pore or nedy," the withdrawal of concern for "grete occupacyouns" may be enough to start the reader on the path to an essentially different orientation, a reconceptualization of "hiʒe lyuing" that depends upon "vertues" rather than material wealth. Shirley's attention to spiritual virtue in this text runs parallel to the focus on forms of courtly, feminine, and youthful virtue that we saw anatomized in his final autograph collection, MS Ashmole 59.

Rolle's "ordenaunce of living" values not radical asceticism but constant mindfulness of God. His directives are not particularly ascetic; instead, they focus on the inner orientation of mind and spirit. Daily practice

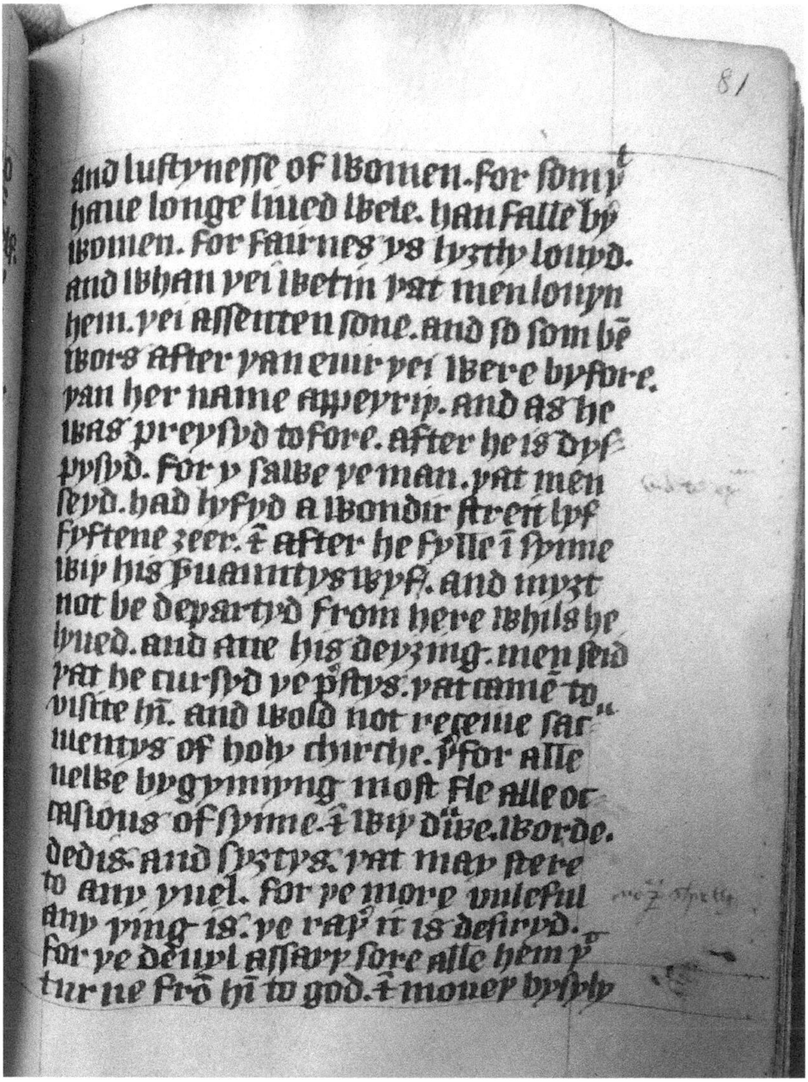
81
and lustynesse of women. for som þt
haue longe liued wele. þan falle by
women. for fairnes þs lyȝtly louyd.
and whan þei weten þat men louyn
hem. þei assenten sone. and so som bē
wors after þan eur þei were byfore.
þan her name appeyriþ. and as he
was preysyd tofore. after he is dys
pysyd. for þ salue þe man. þat men
seyd. had lyfyd a wondir streit lyf
fyftene zeer. & after he fylle ī synne
wiþ his seruauntys wyf. and myȝt
not be departyd from here whils he
lyued. and atte his deyȝing. men seid
þat he cursyd þe prestys. þat came to
visite hī. and wold not receiue sac
mentys of holy churche. ffor alle
newe bygynnyng most fle alle oc
casions of synne. & wiþ dīuē worde.
dedis. and syȝtys. þat may stere
to any yuel. for þe more vnleful
any þing is. þe raþer it is desired.
for þe deuyl assayþ sore alle hem þ
turne frō hī to god. & moueþ bysyly

FIGURE 4.1. John Shirley's *videte* annotation to *Emendatio vitae*. Cambridge, Gonville and Caius MS 669*/646, p. 81. Reproduced by permission of the Master and Fellows of Gonville and Caius College, Cambridge.

should be moderate and God-focused: "In mete and in drynke be þou skars and discrete. Refuse no mete þat is leful to use, and þe whils þou etyst and drinkest, late not þe mynde of God þat fediþ þe passe from þin herte, but worschip and blesse God atte euery morsel, þat þin herte be more in God þan in þi mete."[29] Shirley marks this passage with his nota, perhaps indicating appreciation of this advice. As a resident of the hospital close who had left behind the hubbub of the city yet remained at the center of a lively lay community, Shirley may have been attracted to a disciplined mode of living, a life of "discrete" piety in a space organized around the worship of God. To reside in the hospital close was to remain perpetually aware of the need to keep one's "mynde" on God. It is certainly possible that he shared his book, with its annotations, with members of his reading circle.

Attaining a perfect love of God is the goal of any individual Christian journey. Nicholas Watson argues that in *Emendatio* "love of God should be reverent, not abject . . . it is only love for Christ, not the fear of hell . . . which is strong enough to make conversion from the allurement of this life permanent. Thus a penitential attitude alone cannot be enough, and the reader must go on to the more advanced states described in the later chapters."[30] Although Shirley did not extensively annotate the latter sections of his *Emendatio* text, his notes suggest interest in the text's promise of spiritual bliss and rest to virtuous lovers of Christ. He flags the question of who will be chosen by God to receive bliss. In the long chapter of "þenking on þe passion," Rolle anticipates this rest will be

> ȝouyn to som þat ben ordeynyd of God, to loue hym more: not for any
> oþer good dedis þat he doþe more, or for he suffreþ more, but for he
> louiþ more. Þe which loue is brennyng in swettnes and in al þing it sekiþ
> rest. So noman may sette hym self as bi traueile to do so or so, as he
> coueytiþ hym self such degre or such, but he schal haue suche degre as
> God haþ chose hym to. For som men þat men wenen ben in þe upper,
> ben in þe lower, and some men be holdin but in the lest degre, and ben
> in þe hiȝest.[31]

Placing his nota next to "he schal haue such degre as God haþ chose hym to," Shirley highlights the possibility that at a certain point, one's efforts to love may result in a profound rest untouched by others' judgments. This rest is not dependent upon "good dedis" but upon the quality of one's love.

When he arrives at the chapter on the love of God, he continues to flag this link between "vertue" and "loue," as in the following passage: "A singuler ioye it is of þe loue euerlastinge, þat bindeþ louers wiþ bondis of vertues, and rauischeþ hem aboue alle wordeli þing, vp to þe place of blys."[32] Although the love is "singuler," the "louers" of this passage are plural. This passage suggests something important about spiritual life in the hospital: each individual lover of God remains linked by "bondis of vertues" to others in the community whose support is necessary for spiritual progress. We lack much evidence beyond Shirley's will about his devotional practices, yet his ownership and annotations of this volume suggest there may have been a spiritual side to his literary life in the hospital. These annotations may reflect his experience of the hospital close as a place where neighborly sociability was inflected by penitential reading, "discrete" piety, and reflection on the links between virtue and love within a lay community.

## BL MS Additional 10392: Shared Augustinian Time and Space

Although we have few details of brother John Cok's life, we can tell from his books that Cok was an individualistic scribe with a varied output. His bookmaking was, to cite Jean-Pascal Pouzet's categories, "liberated from the constraints of remuneration or profit . . . freer to depend on individual talent and craftsmanship and on the deployment of that talent in time and space."[33] Cok notes within the cartulary that he began his career apprenticed to the goldsmith Thomas Lamport: by 1418 he had turned to scribal work for hospital master Robert Newton.[34] In all of his varied books, Cok shows a keen eye for "craftmanship" in both design and decoration.

Pouzet's phrase "time and space" is suggestive for my investigation, for I contend that MS Additional 10392, Cok's Latin anthology, emerged from the Augustinian time and space of the hospital. The manuscript itself organizes time through prayer and space through its close attention to layout, mise-en-page, and illustration. The book's varied contents range from catechetical materials to multiple long theological works, such as the pseudo-Augustine *Speculum peccatoris*, explorations of conscience, including the pseudo-Bernard *Tractatus de interiori Domo*, and dialogues on the religious life, such as Hugh of St. Victor's *Soliloquium de arrha anime*. These three texts frequently traveled in Augustinian contexts, and among Augustinian spaces the hospital presents an especially propitious location for individual and shared reading by religious and laity.[35] As David Harry has suggested of the popular pseudo-Bernardine *Meditationes*, which influenced the *Tractatus de interiori domo* and traveled together in manuscripts with the *Speculum peccatoris*, Cok's collection suggests a similarly hybrid purpose: offering material for "private devotional reading" and "a range of practical textual tools for a priest."[36] The central section features an extensive sequence of prayers, including the *Fifteen Oes*, the Psalters of Jerome and the Virgin, and the litanies of the saints. Near the end of the manuscript, we find a set of eight beautifully drawn and colored hand diagrams designed to guide meditation.

These meditation hands, like many of the book's contents, visibly suggest possibilities for individual and shared use. In this small but wide-ranging book, Cok stages in textual and visual form the individual and communal rhythms of an Augustinian hospital priest's religious life. How might Cok have designed and used this book to engage with others, including other priests and laypeople such as Shirley? Shirley knew Cok as a priest, and the Additional manuscript's extensive penitential and pastoral materials suggest that Cok used (and perhaps shared) the book for a range of priestly purposes.

We may assume that as a hospital brother, Cok followed the Augustinian Rule: as a priest-brother, he probably had primarily liturgical (and obviously scribal) rather than pastoral responsibilities. Unfortunately there are no extant statutes directing the priestly brothers' conduct for St. Bartholomew's. In York's Hospital of St. Leonard, episcopal visitation directives of 1364 direct priest-brothers to adopt pastoral responsibilities as chaplains, such as hearing confessions and administering the sacraments to the sick.[37] Yet Cok's precise relations to resident laity remain obscure. Despite his prominence in the hospital (or perhaps because of it, Barron suggests, in his busy role as rent collector), Cok appears in external documents only in Shirley's will.[38]

Cok evidently took pride in his book, with frequent signatures and references to himself, at the head of the table of contents, and throughout, as in a note on fol. 124r, where he writes "quod Johannes Cok qui scripsit istum librum" in red at the close of the prayer of St. Edmund.[39] Such visibility enhances the teaching role that he has implicitly adopted as compiler, copyist, and annotator. I suspect that he created this book to serve as a kind of priestly *vade mecum*, to be used and shared with Augustinian brothers and perhaps also with laypeople, such as Shirley, to whom he may have administered sacraments and spiritual advice. The book features a broad, unique combination of texts for catechetical/confessional use, private study, shared performance, and meditation. One of the volume's most striking features is the way Cok punctuates the book with techniques of schematic display, including lists, tables, rubrics, and diagrams. Many of the longer texts are intended for study, laying bare the theological questions of professed religious life. They are framed by texts elaborating the elements of the catechism, demonstrating highly structured prayers, and depicting programs of meditation. One may imagine lay residents with less Latin knowledge than Shirley also engaging with this book, hearing portions of texts read aloud in translation, seeing key passages marked with rubrics and notes, or performing familiar prayers, such as the *Fifteen Oes*. In this volume, Cok visualized and performed the care of souls, extending its penitential imperatives into programs of prayer and meditation to be shared with a range of readers in the hospital community.

## PENITENTIAL FOUNDATIONS: LISTS

Pastoral care grounded in the regime of penance provides a basis for MS Additional 10392. This foundation is not surprising given the Augustinian Order's pastoral focus, especially within the hospital, where priest-brothers and chaplains might minister to a range of people: fellow clerics, ill and poor patients, and residents who treated it as their parish. Cok's Latin volume opens with a full seven folios of lists (fols. 2v–5v). These enumerate pastoral and penitential information: the seven vices and their remedies, the cardinal virtues and their effects, the five sheddings of Christ's blood, the properties of the Host, the effects of Christ's passion, to name a few. Nicole Eddy finds these lists "repetitive" and even "sometimes contradictory" in their details, bespeaking "an encyclopedic, rather than synthesizing, impulse."[40] But Cok's schemes show greater sophistication than might seem apparent at first. Cok strives to be comprehensive in this book, but not without discernment. At the start of his manuscript, Cok created lists that would enable him to consult foundational information necessary for performing the pastoral role. In the case of the virtues and vices, Cok's techniques of display speak to the idea of the hospital as a spiritually curative space.

As I noted in the Introduction, the image of the priest as a spiritual physician whose authority derived from Christ was familiar in late medieval religious culture. In the space of the hospital, which combined care for the physically vulnerable with prayer and counsel for patrons and community, the priest's role as spiritual healer became heightened. It is thus striking that Cok has structured his lists of virtues and vices in terms of diseases and cures, drawing attention to the healing aspect of his pastoral role and in relation to the curative power of Christ's sufferings.[41]

From the start of this section of the manuscript, we find connected folios that suggest not only an emphasis on spiritual healing but also the dynamism of Cok's pastoral practice. In moving from delineating the vices and how virtues might cure them, to visualizing them as diseases, to suggesting how envisioning Christ's passion might begin to cure them, Cok's method of display suggests that he regarded penance as a guided progress through memorization, association, and reflection. Turning to the third set of lists on fol. 2v, we see the seven vices and the virtues that "cure" them (e.g., pride is cured by humility, envy by charity) (see fig. 4.2). Directly to the right, Cok has copied the seven sacraments and their effects (e.g., baptism cleanses the infant, confirmation strengthens those who are struggling). Carrying on to folio 3r, we see these fundamentals of Christian knowledge placed within a curative frame: on the left column, the second list connects the vices to physical ailments: pride to inflammation, envy to fever, anger to frenzy, and so on (see fig. 4.3). To the top right, another list delineates how the vices are "cured" by Christ's passion ("Septem vicia christi passione curantur"). Such a scheme was common in penitential literature and sermons of the period, as Siegfried Wenzel has detailed. Sermons often pictured "the deadly sins healed by Christ in various ways," preeminently through the Passion: "his wounds, his bloodshedding, and his last words on the Cross are all set against the seven deadly sins."[42] In Cok's scheme we see that Christ inclining his head on the cross cures pride, his side wound cures envy, his carrying of the cross cures laziness, and so on. McCann's comment about the medical valences of the penitential psalms is relevant for these texts also, where "the medical register is used as part of an overarching structural presentation of penance."[43] By constructing the book not only textually but also visually as a vehicle for interaction between priest and penitent, Cok fashions an artifact that reflects the hospital's function as a crossroads of spiritual and physical care.

## *SPECULUM PECCATORIS*: SELF-CONTROL IN COMMUNITY

Although it may seem counterintuitive to imagine a densely written Latin volume as accessible to anyone other than clerical readers, even some of the

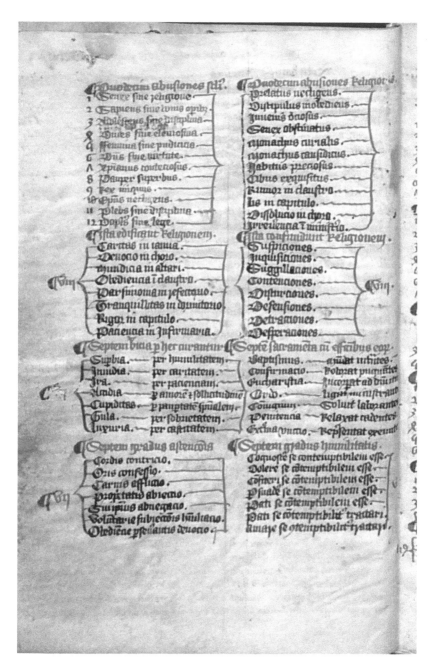

Figure 4.2. List of vices and virtues. © The British Library Board, MS Additional 10392, fol. 2v. Reproduced with permission.

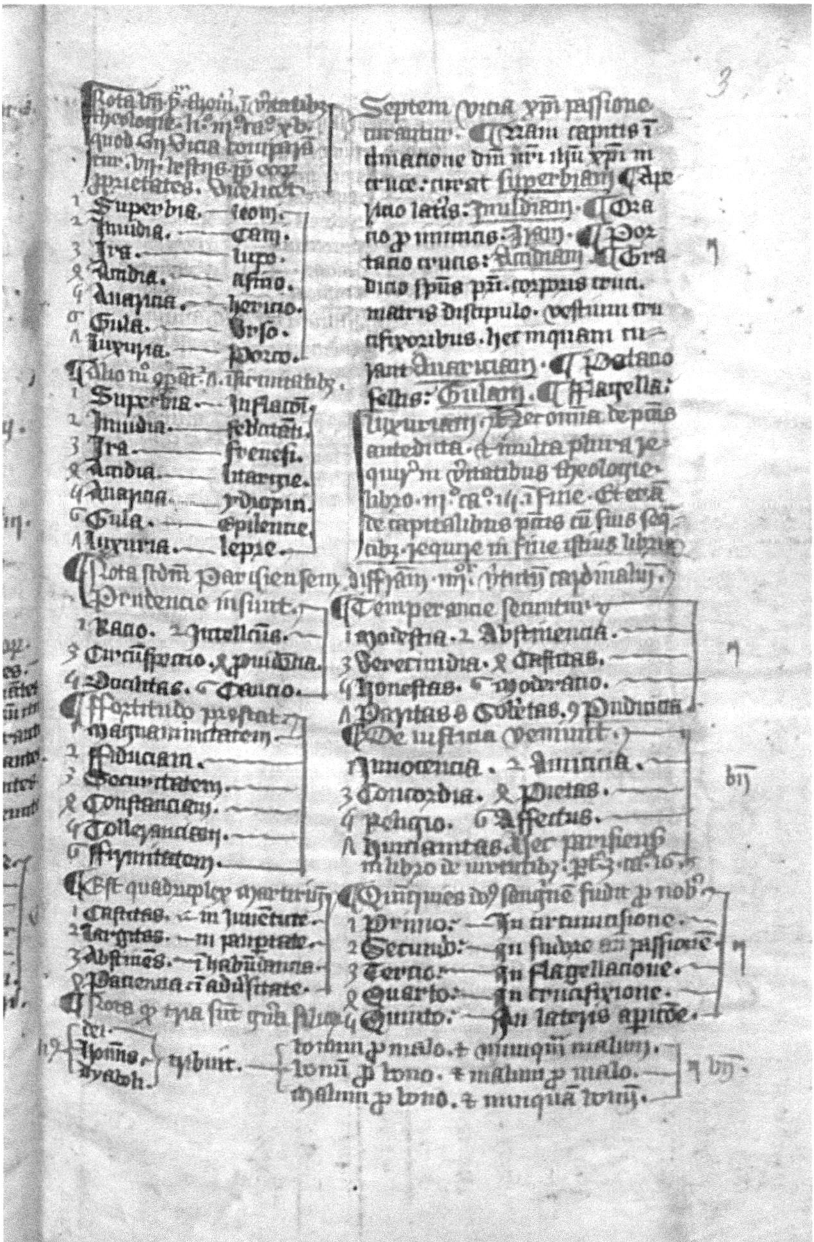

FIGURE 4.3. List of vices and their "cures." © The British Library Board, MS Additional 10392, fol. 3r. Reproduced with permission.

lengthier penitential and theological works included in this codex may have reached a range of users in the hospital setting. The popular pseudo-Augustine *Speculum peccatoris* runs from fols. 47r to 50v. This work, composed for priests and later translated into French, German, and English, expounds Deuteronomy 32:29: "Utinam saperent, et intelligerent, ac novissima providerent" (O that they would be wise and would understand, and would prepare for their last end).[44] Over eight chapters, the *Speculum* explicates the need for self-purification in the face of imminent death. Many of its exhortations are relevant to all Christians (as evidenced by the text's wide translation), and might have supplied priests with material for confessional conversations or sermons. At other moments the work targets clerical readers, calling attention to reading, study, and the superiority of contemplative life.

Cok's annotations, regular but not copious, suggest a two-fold interest: on the one hand, marking out rhetorically striking passages with general hortatory value, and on the other hand drawing attention to passages relevant to fellow priest-brothers living in community. Examples of the first type include the following, early in the text, where he annotates this lament:

> Heu, heu, paucorum est ista uirtus: pauci sunt qui salutarem Domini saluatoris sententiam sapiant. Pauci sunt quibus est ante oculos propriae fragilitatis cognicio, corruptibilis carnis fetor, peccatorum recordatio, instantis mortis meditacio, fetentis gehenne putei consideracio.
>
> ———
>
> Alas, too few attain this virtue. There are few who taste the wisdom of the Lord our savior. There are few who have before their eyes the knowledge of their frailty, the stink of the corruptible body, the memory of sins, the meditation of approaching death, the consideration of the stinking pit of hell.[45]

The text is punctuated by verses, which Cok differentiates with paraphs and with the phrase "nota versus" marked by a blue paraph. One such verse, on the value of renunciation, might equally fuel a homiletic exhortation to penitents or a private reflection by hospital brothers:

> Vive Deo gratus toto mundo tumulatus, Crimine mundatus, semper transire paratus. O quam beatus vir, cujus anima circa huiusmodi studium euigilat! Quam prudenter sapit et intelligit, ac nouissima prouidet.[46]

Live grateful to God, but dead to the world, cleansed from sin, always ready
to depart. O blessed is that man whose heart still watches in contemplation, how to be wise, how to understand, how to prepare for the end.

This verse exemplifies the sort of "self-mortification" that Appleford finds
salient in William Baron's book and spiritual profile. Although such an emphasis does not characterize the entire volume, these verses would be appreciated within the hospital, where patients, brothers, and lay residents had in
varying degrees willingly separated themselves from the world to participate
in an ordered life conducive to wisdom, understanding, and the ordered
preparation for death. Such passages might be relevant for clerical teaching
of laity, perhaps even in ad hoc translation, and for private contemplation,

In the *Speculum*, imagining oneself "dead to the world" does not necessarily translate into self-isolation, for the text also contains advice to religious living in community. Cok annotates sections targeted to regular religious who might also have shared the volume. Addressing the sinful monk,
the final chapter targets the "origin of the vices" with particular reference to
claustral foibles. Cok annotates the following critical passage, which highlights numerous lapses in religious conduct:

Velox ad mensam, tardus ad ecclesiam; potens ad potandum, eger ad
cantandum, peruigil ad fabulas, sompnolentus ad uigilias; prouus ad lo-
quendum, mutus ad psallendum; promptus ad iram et detraccionem,
piger vero ad oracionem; invidie amator, proximi persecutor.[47]

Quick to table, late to church, ready to drink, but reluctant to sing; watchful
for tales; sleepy at vigils, good at speaking, silent at psalms; quick to anger
and insult; truly lazy at prayer; a lover of envy; a persecutor of neighbor.

This passage singles out some of the major duties of the cleric, whether monk
or canon, pinpointing the cloister as a site of potential dereliction. Although
Cok attributes this text to Bernard, it is notable that the phrase "persecutor
proximi" essentially reverses the first line of the Rule of Augustine, the rule
Cok shared with his confrères at St. Bartholomew's: "Ante omnia, fratres
carissimi, *diligatur deus, deinde proximus*, quia ista sunt praecepta principaliter nobis data."[48] By highlighting this passage in *Speculum peccatoris*, Cok

was perhaps reminding brothers who shared the book of their paramount duty within religious community. All of the passages I have mentioned relate to the need for self-discipline, in a penitential, contemplative, or regular mode, and the various annotations might assist Augustinian confrères in identifying important concepts in the work, whether using it to counsel laity or for private reflection.

## THE FIFTEEN OES: INDIVIDUAL PENITENCE AND COLLECTIVE PRAYER

The central section of Cok's little book is composed mainly of prayers and excerpts from devotional texts. This section forms an embedded prayer book that, rather like the books of hours that proliferated in standardized formats, might have served as a bridge between liturgical and private reading. This section builds on the penitential foundation with prayers that intensify the connection between the penitent and the suffering Christ. Cok's rubricated copy of the *Fifteen Oes* devotion offers one striking example of such a prayer. It seems likely that he shared this section of the volume with both confrères and Latin-literate lay readers, for this devotion was universally popular and commonly included in books of hours.[49] Attesting to its use by lay readers within the hospital close, we know that close resident Joan Newmarch bequeathed a copy of the *Fifteen Oes* to her children and grandchildren.[50] In the Additional manuscript, Cok's unusual rubrication has a complex function. His notes visually encourage an individual reader to perform a connection between sacramental penance and meditation. In their addition of a plural voice, they shape the performance of the *Fifteen Oes* as a collective prayer.

The section of prayers marked "in honore passionis oraciones" (prayers in honor of the Passion) contains the *Fifteen Oes*, popularly attributed to St. Bridget of Sweden. Cok also adds marginal notes in red summarizing the prayers using a first-person plural "we" voice. Although it is typical to rubricate the Pater Noster and the Ave Maria prayers that punctuate the recitation of the *Fifteen Oes*, Cok's marginal annotations seem unusually schematic compared to other manuscript examples that I have examined.[51] The *Fifteen Oes* links each stage of Christ's passion to a stage in the individual penitential life. As Duffy notes, the prayers constitute "pleas of mercy to a merciful Saviour . . . whose suffering forms an enduring bond of endearment and tenderness between him and suffering humanity."[52] He also makes the point that despite the fifteenfold structure of the prayers, their fundamental structuring principle is Christ's seven words from the cross.[53] This sevenfold scheme refers back in an answering fashion to the scheme of the seven vices that forms a key framework for Cok's book.

The first prayer begins with Christ's betrayal, condemnation, and buffeting, ending with the petition, "Da mihi queso ob memoriam harum antem crucem tuam passionum ueram ante mortem meam contricionem, puram confessionem, dignam satisfaccionem et omnium peccatorum meorum remissionem" (Grant me before my death true contrition, a sincere and entire confession, worthy satisfaction, and the remission of all my sins). Cok's annotations reiterate the petitionary content: for example, on fol. 112v he annotates the first "O" as follows: "hec petimus ueram contricionem, puram confessionem, & dignam satisfaccionem" (here we beg for true contrition, pure confession, and worthy satisfaction) (see fig. 4.4). The second prayer visualizes the start of the Crucifixion, describing how Christ's torturers "crudeliter te distraxerunt in longum et latum crucis tue" (stretched thy Body on the cross, pulled thee from all sides, thus dislocating thy limbs). It ends with the petition "deprecor te . . . ut des mihi timorem et amorem tuum" (grant me the grace to fear thee and to love thee). Cok annotates the prayer as follows on the right margin: "hic petimus timorem & amorem Domini" (here we beg for fear and love of the Lord).[54] These annotations condense and reinforce the petitions, which respond to the image of Christ's suffering, in effect stressing how the reader should *perform* the prayer. For a reader in a hurry it might be possible, though not as efficacious, to take a shortcut by reading out only the red annotations, thus still performing the prayers' essential content.

In her study of the *Fifteen Oes*, Rebecca Krug argues that the prayers place their reader in an intimate conversation with Jesus, allowing the supplicant to quote and appropriate Christ's words from the cross in such a way that prayer is transformed from "a solitary imaginative exercise" into a dialogue with Christ himself.[55] The idea that the *Fifteen Oes* scripts not only an exchange between an individual reader and Jesus, but also a shared or collective prayer, is suggested by Cok's repeated use of the first-person plural, indicating "we beg" rather than "I beg," the singular form used in most of the prayers themselves. This emphasis on a shared experience of prayer suggests to me that Cok shared this section of the book with other readers, laypeople probably among them. As a final example, I take Cok's annotation to the twelfth prayer, which supplicates Jesus, "Scribe queso pie

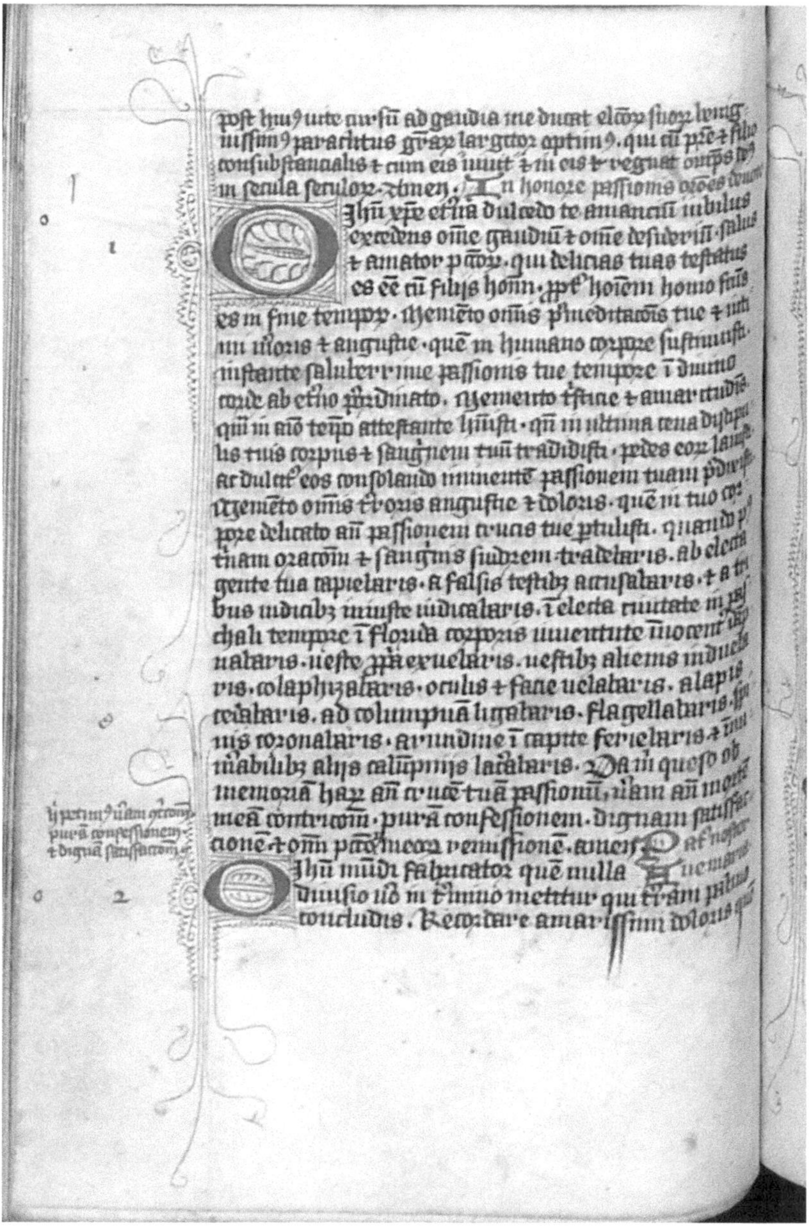

FIGURE 4.4. John Cok's annotation to the *Fifteen Oes*. © The British Library Board, MS Additional 10392, fol. 112v. Reproduced with permission.

Ihesu omnia uulnera tua in corde meo preciosissimo sanguine tuo, ut in illis legam tuum dolorem et amorem, ut in graciarum accione usque in finem uite mee iugiter perseruerem" (Write all thy wounds upon my heart with thy most precious blood so that I may read in them thy sorrows and death and persevere in giving thanks until the end).[56] The marginal annotation reads, "hic petimus ut perseuerare possimus in graciarum accione usque ad finem" (here we beg that we may be able to persevere in giving thanks until the end). Cok might well have used the prayers for his personal devotions, but the annotations' plural voice strongly suggests that these prayers were copied and annotated in a shared spirit, so that even a single reader, whether Cok himself, one of his confrères, a chaplain, or a lay resident, might envision him- or herself performing them in the context of a religious community. Cok's "we" includes not only all Christians but the "we" of the hospital: brothers and sisters, ill and poor patients, and lay residents alike.

DIAGRAMS: MEDITATION

The most visually striking section of Cok's volume comes near the end: a set of eight hand diagrams, designed to guide meditation. These appear near the end of book, but they do not occupy a booklet unto themselves. They are beautiful examples of the *manus meditationis* image, carefully drawn and lettered, decorated with colored flourishes and scrolls. These hands are conventional in many respects, and we find analogues to two of them in another volume with an Augustinian provenance (BL MS Harley 4987). Yet I have not encountered another manuscript featuring so many hand diagrams. Cok has set out eight of them: four left hands, lettered in black, followed by four right hands, lettered in red.[57] The arrangement of the hands leaves room for readers to ponder all of the left hands first or match each left hand to a right, for each pair of left and right hands exists in a responsive relationship.

Unlike the MS Harley 4987 analogue that places the right and left hands together, Cok has placed all of the left hands first, followed by all of the right hands: a reader is thus faced with both sequential and paired possibilities for reading and meditation. If we read the first and second left hands together on the opening, we find the nighttime meditation ("Meditatio Nocturna") on fol. 178v (see fig. 4.5) paired with a meditation on the fear of the lord ("Timor Domini") on fol. 179r (see fig. 4.6). The nighttime

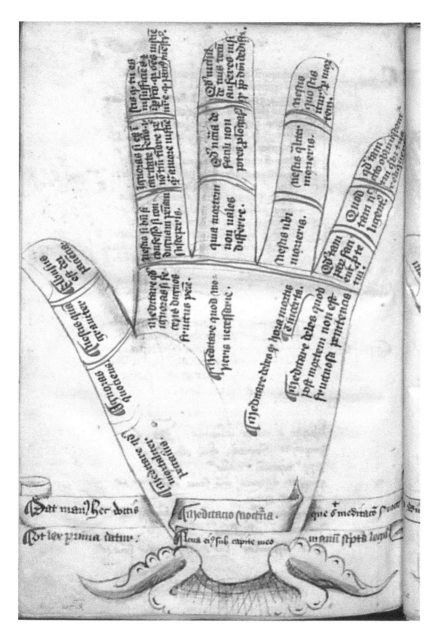

Figure 4.5. Nighttime meditation. © The British Library Board, MS Additional 10392, fol. 178v. Reproduced with permission.

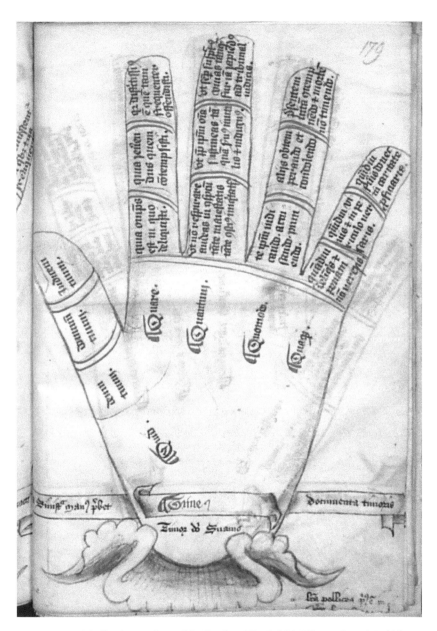

Figure 4.6. Meditation on fear of the Lord. © The British Library Board, British Library MS Additional 10392, fol. 179r. Reproduced with permission.

meditation guides meditation on death and the individual's lack of knowledge about it or control over it. To take a few of its exhortations, the fourth finger of this hand warns readers, "Nescis ubi morieris" and "Nescis qualiter morieris" (You do not know where you will die; You do not know how you will die). The little finger warns, "quod post mortem non est fructuosa penitencia" (that there is no fruitful penance available after death). In productive visual conversation with the nighttime meditation, on the recto side, meditations on the fear of the Lord are introduced by the scroll at the wrist: "Sinistra manus prebet documenta timoris" (The left hand shows a lesson of fear). As Geneviève Hasenohr has noted, the five reasons and ways to fear God (why, how, how much, in what way, for how long) abbreviate a standard procedure laid out in manuals for the examination of conscience.[58] This manuscript continually reminds readers that fear of God is integral to the healing regime of *Christus medicus*: in Augustine's words, "Timor Dei sic vulnerat, quomodo medici ferramentum" (The fear of God wounds like the knife of the physician).[59] In Cok's ordering, the reflection on death and one's lack of control over it is strongly congruent with reasons to fear God, the ultimate arbiter of death and the benevolent yet dreaded father of all.

Continuing chronologically through the book, the next opening reveals the third and fourth left hands. The hand described as "of the devil" appears on fol. 179v (see fig. 4.7). The hand teaching readers how to cast out demons appears on fol. 180r (see fig. 4.8). These too share thematic congruity and even a potentially sequential relationship. The verso page offers examples of sinful humanity in thrall to the devil. The wrist scroll reads, "Manus dyaboli est sinistra, huius v digitos" (The left hand is the devil's, of which there are five fingers). The legend above the index finger reads, "Dyabolus demonstrat sanctorum opera et exempla ut homines ad peccata alliciat" (The devil shows the works of the saints and examples to entice men to sin). On each segment appears an exemplary figure and his sin: Peter's sacrilege, Paul's persecution of the disciples, and David's adultery. The implication is that these three were tempted by the devil, and that readers would know of their eventual repentance. On fol. 180r, the facing page in Cok's manuscript, the left hand reads, "in manu dei deiccio demonum" (in God's hand is the casting out of demons). This hand offers tools for resisting the devil or treating others assaulted by sin: the middle finger lists "Obedientia ad mandatos et precepta ecclesie; iudicia iudicare omnia; compassio proximorum in aduersis" (Obedience to the commandments and teachings of

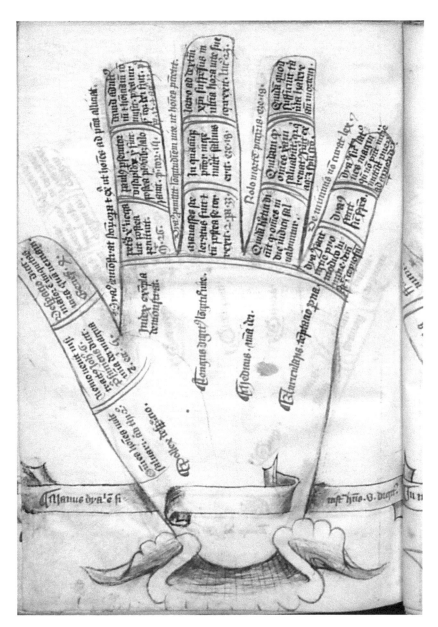

FIGURE 4.7. Hand of the devil. © The British Library Board, British Library MS
Additional 10392, fol. 179v. Reproduced with permission.

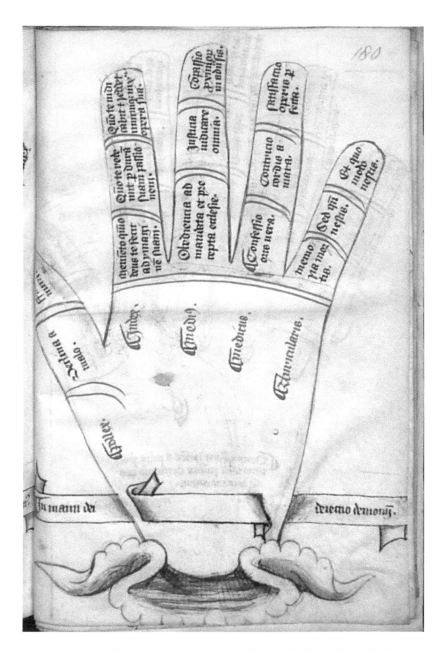

FIGURE 4.8. Hand for casting out demons. © The British Library Board, British Library MS Additional 10392, fol. 180r. Reproduced with permission.

the church; the judgment to judge everyone; compassion for neighbors in difficulties). This hand includes the stages of confession, while the little finger reminds readers once again, recalling the first set of hands, of the uncertainty surrounding death.

Cok probably took his examples from a source that paired the left and right hands together on the same page or on the same opening, as does BL MS Harley 4987, fol. 121v, which pairs the nighttime meditation and the daytime meditation on the same leaf (see fig. 4.9). One can therefore imagine another way of reading Cok's book: moving ahead by a few folios in order to pair left and right hands. In response to "Meditatio Nocturna," Cok's fourth and final red hand on fol. 182r bears the title "Meditatio Diurna," as in the Harley volume (see fig. 4.10). This hand directs meditations on a wide range of concepts and images, enumerating some aspects of religious practice that one *can* control in life. The thumb advises grateful meditation on God's creation: "beneficia dei creacionis ex vili spermati" (the favor of God's creation from a lowly seed). The pointer advises reflection upon one's evil deeds: "tot mala que fecisti que commisisse non debuisti uel ommittere denegare potuisti" (how many evils you have done, which you should not have committed or should have been able to refuse or omit); the little finger directs meditation on the anticipated spectacle of the Last Judgment. A reader familiar with other versions of these images or texts might have known to look for the conventionally matching hand: the Harley MS 4987 scribe has used exactly the same text in pairing nighttime and daytime meditation hands on the same page.

In the second pair of hands in Cok's book, left and right also relate closely to each other: the second left hand on fol. 179r offers reasons to fear God; the second right hand on fol. 181r enumerates the five reasons for loving God (see fig. 4.11). For example, *quomodo*, the third finger, advises loving God "in desideriis cordis et deuotione," "in iubilacione laudis et oracione," and "in emulatione virtutum et operatione" (in desires and in devotion of the heart, in jubilation and in prayer of praise, in the imitation and in the work of virtues). If we recall the first prayer of the *Fifteen Oes*, which asked that "we beg for the fear and love of God," we can see how this hand diagram might extend that prayer into a more fully developed meditation, for which the reader had already prepared by envisioning Christ's betrayal and suffering at length. The scribe of the Harley analogue also paired the fear and love of God hands on the same page.[60]

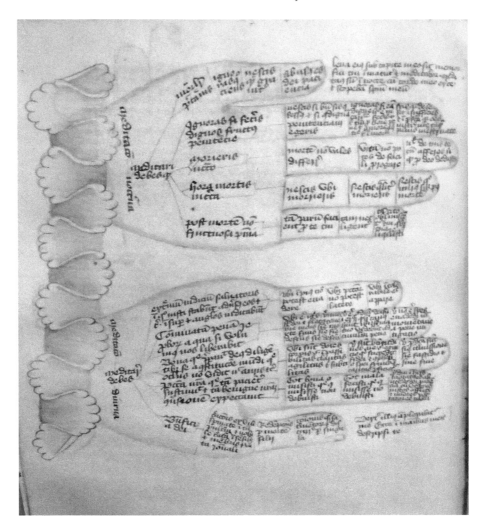

FIGURE 4.9. Nighttime and daytime hands together. © The British Library Board, MS Harley 4987, fol. 121v. Reproduced with permission.

Working with the same logic of paired black and red hands, if we return to the third left hand (fol. 179v), the hand of the devil, we can appreciate its mnemonic function in a different way when it is paired with the third right hand on fol. 181v (see fig. 4.12). For this hand depicts the five fingers of the "manus ecclesie": mirroring on the index the same figures of sinfulness but with the reassurance that "nullo peccato est desperandum"

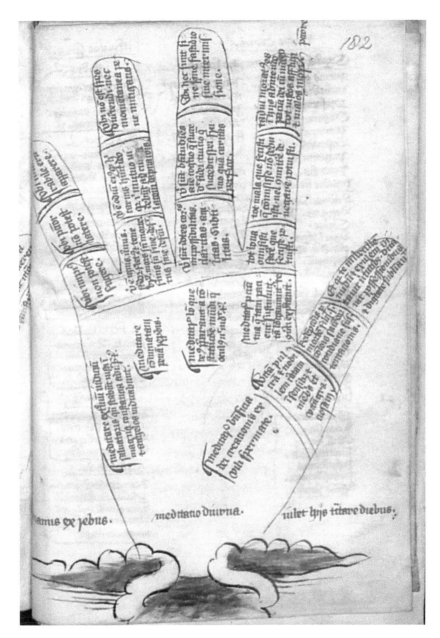

FIGURE 4.10. Daytime meditation. © The British Library Board, MS Additional
10392, fol. 182r. Reproduced with permission.

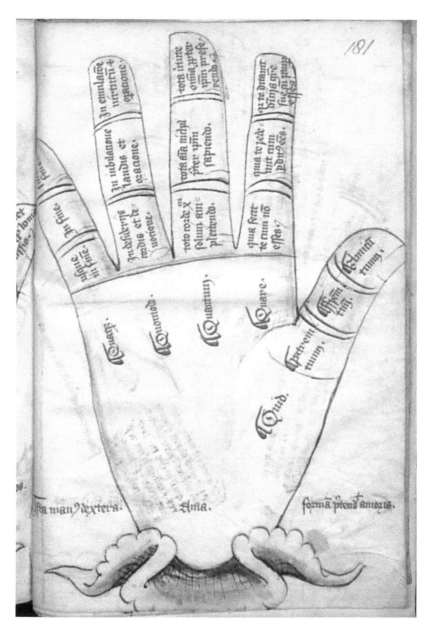

FIGURE 4.11. Reasons to love God. © The British Library Board, MS Additional 10392, fol. 181r. Reproduced with permission.

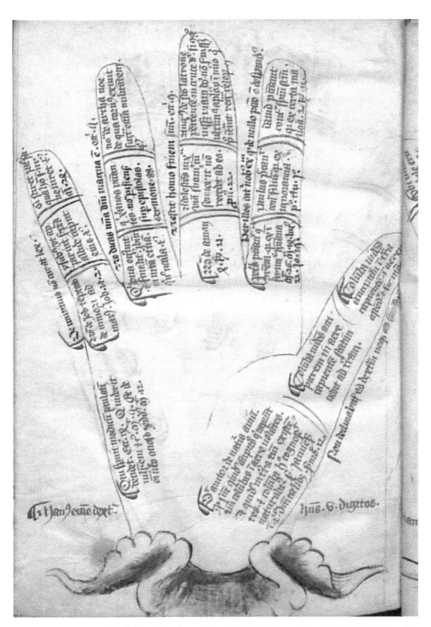

FIGURE 4.12. Hand of the Church. © The British Library Board, MS Additional 10392, fol. 181v. Reproduced with permission.

(no sin is to be despaired of ). Here again we find Peter sinning against the Father out of human weakness, Paul against the Son out of ignorance, and David against the Holy Spirit out of malice. This hand reassures readers that despite the enormity of their sins, these figures will be saved through participation in the Church.

My speculation about possible lay use of the hand images is complemented by the evidence of several *manus meditationis* pictured in late medieval English parish churches. One such image is recorded in a 1480 list of properties from the church of St. Stephen Walbrook in London, and a painted panel *manus* survives in the parish church of St. Mary in Bishops Cannings, Wiltshire. The St. Stephen Walbrook list also includes painted tables of catechetical information, a combination of material that parallels the progression of pastoralia found in Cok's compilation.[61] The location of these *manus* panels in parochial settings offers an instructive parallel to their inclusion in Cok's book, for in both cases the diagrams may have been intended for mixed lay and clerical use. In this unique Latin volume, Cok used numerous techniques of display to structure and enhance penitential performance, and in doing so he may have had not only himself but other readers in mind: fellow priest-brothers and laypeople to varying degrees. Cok created a compendium that would function flexibly: as an adjunct to pastoral care, an aid to personal study, and a tool for devotional performance by a range of users.

## SCRIBES OF ST. MARK'S HOSPITAL AND THEIR BOOKS

Both John Cok, brother of St. Bartholomew's, London, and John Colman, brother of St. Mark's Hospital, Bristol, copied Rolle's *Emendatio vitae* (Cok an English version, Colman a Latin version).[62] Like Cok, Colman was a prolific copyist within his hospital. Colman too showed concern for how clerical and lay practices might overlap within the hospital's hybrid space. Yet whereas Cok's Latin devotional volume seems designed for shared clerical and lay use, Colman's annotations to the Latin *Emendatio* in MS Lyell 38 work to define the professed brother's religious discipline in strict distinction from secular life. Colman and his hospital brother William Haulle were both canons of St. Mark's by 1498, and both copied devotional Latin/ English anthologies.[63] As I show in the final section of this chapter, Colman's MS 173 and Haulle's MS 6 prove the most hybrid books of all, inviting alternating, shared forms of devotional practice by priestly and lay readers, male and female.

St. Mark's of Bristol was a relatively small institution, yet it was just as deeply imbricated within the civic community as were St. Leonard's and St. Bartholomew's. St. Mark's maintained close relations with lay benefactors, extended control over its own parish and chantries, and welcomed selected students and retirees within its precincts. As I noted in my Introduction, the 1259 charter included a commitment to housing twelve poor scholars who would serve in the choir.[64] Choristers and students remained at St. Mark's up to the end: several "childern" and "queresteres" are recorded at the 1539 suppression.[65] Some poor scholars evidently became lifetime brothers of the house: Thomas Tiler testified in 1496 that he had been "brought furth in the said place of Gauntes from yowth."[66] The hospital's educational function influenced its character as a scribal community. St. Mark's evidently housed "more than a song school," in Doyle's estimation, and its leaders must have imparted scribal training, for the scripts of several brothers from this period look very similar to each other. In particular, Doyle notes similarity in the "informal Secretary style" of MS 173 and MS 6.[67] Doyle speculates that both books could have been copied by Colman, and Jessica Lamothe's recent discovery of Haulle's signature in MS 6 identifies him as its copyist.[68] One could easily mistake Haulle's hand for Colman's, and indeed as Doyle notes, we must allow for the possibility of multiple scribes contributing to the same books.[69] In MS 173 and MS 6, Colman and Haulle created kindred anthologies with similar pastoral priorities: both work to guide priestly and lay readers in overlapping, collaborative devotional practices. The two hospital brothers may well have cooperated on writing these volumes and perhaps others.

The priests of St. Mark's took seriously their supervision of local laity, whom they viewed as their parishioners, much as the priests of St. Bartholomew's ministered to residents of the hospital close. We find evidence of the hospital's concern for pastoral care in the community in records of controversies over jurisdiction with the neighboring Abbey of St. Augustine and its parish church of St. Augustine the Less. In 1426, the master and brethren of St. Mark's accused the vicar of St. Augustine of arrogating the hospital's rightful spiritual services and revenue by ministering to and burying people who lived within the hospital precincts, taking obventions that belonged to the hospital.[70] Not only concerned with the rights and benefits of burial, the hospital asserted its right to another life-cycle event: women's purification after childbirth, typically a parochial prerogative. In the same letter, the hospital claims that the vicar, not content with removing bodies from the hospital's own burial ground, had also maliciously appropriated the right to purification and its attendant payment:

> quamdam Sibillam Huchyns infra saepta domus predicti conuersantem a purificacione post partum pro eam in dicte domo siue hospitali facienda subtraxit et solicitauit subtrahi ne fecit cerero quoque siue candelam et vestem vocatam 'a chrysmar' in dicto domo offerendam ac cetera . . . dicte purificationis obueniencia et ad dictos religiosos viros.

---

> William drew away and enticed Sibilla Huchyns from purification after childbirth, which should have been done in the said hospital, and kept the candles and the garment called a "chrysmar," which should have been offered in the said hospital, and other obventions arising from the said purification belonging to the religious of the said hospital.[71]

Supporting the hospital's claims, the consistory court ruled in its favor, requiring the bodies restored to the hospital cemetery, the lost tributes paid, and all the elements of the purification ceremony restored: chrysmar, hundred shillings, and candles. The hospital's insistence on its right to spiritual jurisdiction and pastoral care as well as monetary payment demonstrates the importance of lay parishioners to the hospital's life. Hospital master and brethren felt responsible for (and entitled to) supervising lay spiritual life cycles.

In the late fifteenth and early sixteenth century, a period of economic good fortune that David Harris Sacks calls "the last flowering of Bristol's late medieval prosperity," St. Mark's Hospital continued to develop close relations to local laity and clergy by welcoming them into the community in various ways.[72] The wills of two local men affiliated with the hospital express concern with personal commemoration and with furthering the institution's mission of "changing the earthly into the celestial and the transitory into the divine," a phrase from the hospital's chantry foundation document of 1351.[73] Thomas Swayde (d. 1495) was the rector of St. Andrew's Church who had evidently retired to the hospital in his old age. In his will he names Thomas Tiler, hospital master, as his executor.[74] Swayde asks to be buried in the church of the hospital of St. Mark "ante imaginem Sancti Marci" (before the image of St. Mark).[75] He implies in his bequests that he wishes his own clerical identity and practices to be carried on by the hospital's brothers, giving eleven pounds sterling to purchase a cloth (perhaps an altar cloth) and a silver basin, which might have been used for church services. Finally he asks that the "ornamenta" (ornaments) and "utensilia" (utensils) from his room be used in the service of the hospital, perhaps envisioning turning "the earthly into the celestial" for the benefit of the community in which he spent his final days.

Another layman devoted to the hospital in this period was the well-off Walter Wralltesley (d. 1502). Although he hailed from Worcester and donated money to a local church in his will, he asks to be buried in the chancel of St. Mark's hospital church next to his wife, who had predeceased him.[76] He too asks Master Tiler to be his executor and gives generously to the master and brethren of the house. In addition to bequeathing significant lands in Somerset to the house, Wralltesley leaves a silver goblet and his horse to the master, six shillings eight pence to each brother, and twenty shillings to the "clerk of the church." Whether Wralltesley lived in the hospital or became linked to it through his wife, who had elected burial there, the house figured prominently in his devotions at the end of his life.

John Colman, Tiler's successor as master, continued to foster close relations between the hospital and local clergy and laity. These relations were extended through the sharing of religious books with fellow priests.[77] Colman had personal relationships with other Bristol rectors, including one John Bradley, to whom he gave a Latin devotional collection (now Bodleian MS Bodley 618).[78] Colman was a prolific copyist and annotator in his own right. Building on the foundations that Doyle and Erler have laid, I show how Colman's and Haulle's devotional books respond to the particular challenges of living, studying, and working in the early sixteenth-century Bristol hospital.

## EMENDATIO VITAE IN BODLEIAN MS LYELL 38: AUGUSTINIAN STRATEGIES FOR PRIESTLY READERS

Although St. Mark's was closely tied to Bristol's larger civic life, Colman's work as a scribe and annotator in a book for hospital brothers makes the case that worldly attractions should exert no sway upon canons committed to a disciplined religious life. Oxford Bodleian MS Lyell 38 is a parchment book, dated to the first half of the sixteenth century, containing Rolle's *Emendatio vitae* and *Expositio super novem lectiones mortuorum*.[79] Colman certainly copied the first text and perhaps the second too. His copying and annotation of the *Emendatio* foreground the Augustinian priority of "docere verbo et exemplo" for clerical readers. With annotations and emendations, Colman inserts himself into the reading process as a coteacher with Rolle, particularly addressing those newly converted into religious life and suggesting how his clerical confrères might guide each other. He focuses on passages that advise rejection of worldly matters, emphasize moderation and personal purity in a communal context, and offer signposts for beginners in religious discipline. Colman's annotations assert the distinctiveness of the professed Augustinian identity and demand adherence to its discipline. This insistence may be related to the presence of lay residents in the house and a need for brothers to remain conscious of the distinctions between canons and laity.

Colman may well have been master of the house when he copied and annotated the *Emendatio* text, for he served as master from circa 1517 until the house's suppression in 1539.[80] (As Doyle notes, Colman's changes often reference the 1510 printed version of Rolle's *Emendatio*.)[81] Whether or not he was already master, Colman's annotations transmit his authority and experience to readers, shaping a rigorously Augustinian clerical reading practice. In the first chapter, on conversion, Colman indicates concern with turning definitively from the world. He annotates the same passage that John Shirley had marked in his English *Emendatio*, on the dangers of succumbing to fleshly temptation after successful renunciation. Yet Colman's annotations advocate a radical break from the world, a *contemptus mundi* that treats all material goods as "vanities of the world" to be scorned. Colman too is attentive to the danger of falling into bodily sin, placing a maniculum next to the passage describing the man who after fifteen years of continence sinned with a servant's wife; Shirley placed his nota next to the same section in his Middle English copy (see 4.13). However, Colman, working with a slightly different version of the text, highlights the danger of sin rather than acknowledge its attractions, as Shirley did when marking the passage that reads, "for þe more unleful any þing is, þe raþer it is desiryd [desideranda]." Colman's text reads, "res est magis illicita, eo amplius

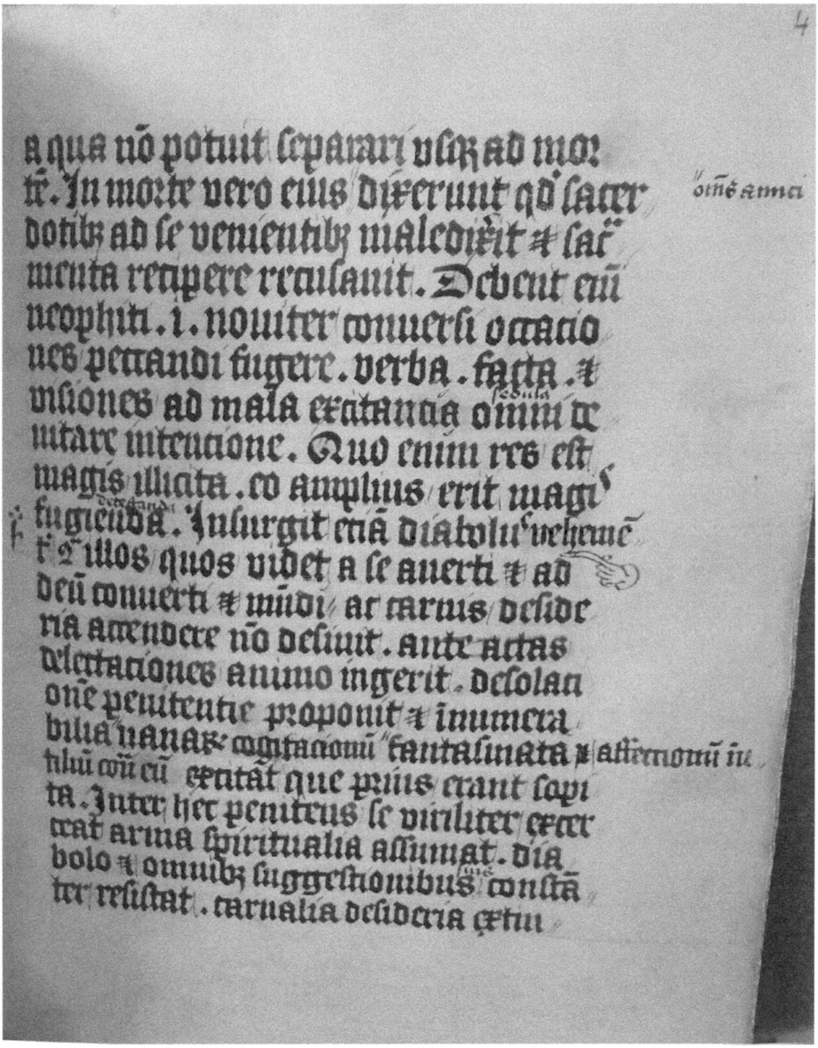

FIGURE 4.13 John Colman's annotation to *Emendatio vitae*. Oxford, Bodleian Library MS Lyell 38, fol. 4r. Reproduced with permission of the Bodleian Library, University of Oxford.

erit magis fugienda" (the more illicit a thing, the more it should be fled).[82] He adds "detestanda" over the line, in accordance with the 1510 print reading. Colman amplifies his version of the text, which differs from many other manuscript witnesses, by rendering the illicit not only forbidden, but despised, rejecting rather than acknowledging the pull of the world upon the regular canon.[83]

Colman's readings are in keeping with an Augustinian tradition of viewing spiritual conversion as a radical bodily separation from the world. The *Expositio* on the Rule of Augustine (one of the contents of St. John's College MS 173) develops this idea at length. The Rule's command "Et sit vobis anima una et cor unum in Deo" (Let all be united, one mind and one heart, in God) calls forth a gloss emphasizing the Augustinian brother's withdrawal from the world into God:

> Fili, da mihi cor tuum. [Proverbs 23] Prius in corde et voluntate trahimur ad Deum. Ergo si corpore separamur a seculo, corde et anima iungamur Deo. Vt possimus dicere veraciter: Mihi autem adherere Deo bonus est. Nam qui adheret Deo, unus spiritus est.
>
> ———
>
> Son, give me your heart. First we must draw the heart and will toward God. Thus if we separate bodily from the world, we are joined heart and soul to God, so that we may truly say, It is good to join with God. He who joins with God is united in spirit with Him.[84]

In the Lyell annotations, Colman exerts a similar pressure on would-be clerical readers of the *Emendatio*, encouraging a decisive break from worldly desires and entanglements. It seems important to Colman, as to the *Expositio* author, that this break should take place as a part of a communal effort in which a brother strives to keep himself spiritually and physically pure, supporting fellow brothers through gentle correction.

The *Emendatio*'s chapter on *contemptus mundi*, though short, is enhanced in Colman's copy by numerous annotations highlighting rejection of worldly things. He seems particularly concerned that his readers notice Rolle's exhortations to suppress greed (cupiditas) in order to encourage love of God. Colman brackets the following aphoristic statement on fol. 5r: "Quanto ergo profundius cupiditatem expellis, tanto magis diuinum amorem gustabis" (the more deeply you expel greed, the more profoundly you taste divine love). Rolle's dramatic address to the wayward soul, which begins "O misera anima, quid in mundo queris" (O miserable soul, what do you seek in the world) is marked by a maniculum at its climax, upbraiding the soul who heedlessly follows "ruinous things" (res perituras), not realizing that they will lead to nothing: "Sed scio ubi habitas, ubi sedes est Satane, qui oculos tuos cecauit et per prestigia sua tibi illudit, ut cuperes fugienda, amares odibilia, permanencia contempneres" (But I see that where you are is the seat of Satan, who has blinded your eyes and for his own sake fooled you, so that you desire fleeting, hateful things and condemn permanent ones).[85] Colman adds a further expression of detest for the world in a heading at the top of the next folio, 5v: "Omnia vanitas honor diuicie et potestas" (honor, riches and power are all vanities). This heading draws attention to the subject of the discussion, the deception of souls by material goods "per diuicias, per dignitatem, per voluptatem, per potestatem, per honores." These evils link wayward souls to sins in bonds that may only be dissolved at death, Rolle warns, "sed tunc nimis tarda solucio, quibus non restat nisi cterna cruciacio" (but for those who are late to the payment, there remains only eternal suffering). Colman's early flurry of annotations foregrounds the rigor required in the Augustinian clerical life.

Within the loving religious community, the challenges of tribulation must be borne in patience. Colman flags the value of suffering tribulations with an array of annotations: he marks with his signature flower the statement, "Ideo immittuntur tribulaciones, ut nos ab amore mundi reuocent et ne grauius in alia vita puniamur" (tribulations are allowed so that they call us away from worldly love, lest we be more gravely punished in the next life).[86] Within the context of patience, fraternal correction comes up: "Multi pacientes uidentur, quando non impugnantur. Sed statim, cum leuis flatus (non dico iniurie sed correcionis) eis attigerit, mox mens eorum in amaritudinem et iram se vertit" (Many seem patient when they are not criticized. But suddenly when the soft breath [I mean not of injury but of correction] reaches them, they turn their minds in bitterness and anger).[87] At this point in the manuscript, Colman flags his concern for the exercise of patience in community, where the voice of "correction" could be misinterpreted by those resisting it. Colman brings a characteristically Augustinian focus on teaching to the fore and cautions readers to be receptive to his suggestions.

This annotation, highlighting concern for fraternal correction, is in keeping with a strong Augustinian focus on helping brothers in religion. The *Expositio* on the Rule contains a seventh chapter on fraternal correction. The Rule compares the erring brother to a suffering wounded man:

Magis quippe innocentes non estis, si fratres uestros quos indicando corripere potestis, tacendo perire permittatis. Si enim frater tuus uulnus haberet in corpore suo quod uelit occultare, dum timet secari, nonne crudeliter a te sileretur, et misericorditer indicaretur?

―――――

Yours is the greater blame if you allow your brothers to be lost through your silence when you are able to bring about their correction by your disclosure. If your brother, for example, were suffering a bodily wound that he wanted to hide for fear of undergoing treatment, would it not be cruel of you to remain silent and a mercy on your part to make this known?[88]

This is the communal ethos in which Colman draws attention to Rolle's comment: Rolle's "soft blast" of "correction" alludes to the merciful voice that the *Rule* musters to heal the wound of sin in the soul.

Rolle's text is self-consciously organized around principles of spiritual progress, and copyist and annotator Colman is aware of Rolle's emphasis on forward, upward movement in the spiritual life. Throughout his *Emendatio*, Colman marks passages that offer definitions of important concepts, and his annotations suggest the progress that a reader might make in understanding or practicing them. Amid Rolle's discussion of prayer, for example, Colman's annotations encourage and track a reader's movement through the section, beginning with a maniculum to mark a comforting start: "Si enim pure oraueris, auxilium habebis" (If you pray purely, you will find help).[89] As the discussion continues, he marks off another of Rolle's encouraging comments with the maniculum: "Multum confert ad stabilitatem cordis obtinendam crebris oracionibus insistere, psalmodiam deuote cantare" (It contributes greatly to obtaining stability of heart to persist with repeated prayers and to sing psalms devoutly).[90] In this chapter, Rolle alternates appealingly between encouraging directives and statements on the efficacy of prayer, such as the promise that "in oracione demones uincimus et eorum insidias" (in prayer we vanquish demons and their evils).[91] Colman highlights the promise of success and pleasure that Rolle hopes his readers will feel in the process of prayer, marking with his flower the passage reading, "Sic profecto in nobis mira affluencia bonitatis diuine inuenitur, quia ex intimis medullis cordis nostri exurget amor Dei" (So it is accomplished that the amazing flow of divine goodness is found in us, for the love of God surges out of the innermost part of our hearts).[92] Here Rolle evokes the possibility of generating "amor Dei" through prayer, a sense of unity that the prayerful reader may attain by following this set of directives with discipline. Colman's *Emendatio* offers a carefully annotated plan for achieving spiritual transformation within community, in which he himself remained textually present to his canon-brothers as teacher and coadvisor with Rolle.

## OXFORD ST. JOHN'S COLLEGE MS 173: A MIXED DEVOTIONAL COLLECTION

Two turn-of-the-century male devotees of St. Mark's Hospital, cleric Thomas Swayde and layman Walter Wralltesley, became part of the hospital community at the ends of their lives. Widows also gravitated to the hospital during Colman's mastership. Mary Erler observes that sometimes widows retired to male houses, some of which "must have had a local tradition of welcoming such sojourns, stays which could be supported both by the occasional presence of other retired women and by male spiritual direction. It may be significant, too, that the house at which these three women lived was a hospital."[93] Given the prominence of widows within English hospitals, I believe that this choice of institution was indeed significant. The bilingual books copied by Colman and Haulle stage a collaborative form of Augustinian reading for priestly and lay readers, including women residing in the hospital.

An ethic of teaching, practicing communal worship, and sobriety is made explicit in the self-consciously Augustinian St. John's College MS 173, a volume that gathers Latin and vernacular texts to make these ideals available to brothers and lay readers, who might well have shared this book. Colman combines English and Latin within the same volume and even within individual booklets, taking an eclectic approach to the reformation of the self with a range of patristic and medieval spiritual guidance.[94] Many of the texts, some attested in other Augustinian contexts, define religious life for novices, notably the Rule of Augustine and its accompanying *Expositio*, selections from David of Augsburg's *Formula novitiorum*, and Peter Damian's *Institutio monialis*.[95] Colman has organized MS 173 into several booklets: one of these combines Latin and English texts and thus seems particularly suggestive for defining the boundaries and the elasticity of an Augustinian reading model for religious and lay readers.

Another contemporary bilingual spiritual anthology survives from St. Mark's Hospital (Bristol Public Library MS 6). This codex, copied by William Haulle in 1502, likewise gathers a range of texts to guide priestly brothers and lay residents in embodying the communal discipline and continual charity essential to life in the hospital. Erler has insightfully studied this codex in in detail.[96] The collaborative ethos of MS 6 parallels that of MS 173, suggesting that Haulle shared not only similar handwriting but also pastoral priorities with Colman, which is logical given their shared milieu and small brotherhood.

In some respects we may see MS 173's approach to collaborative reading as parallel to that of brother John Cok's Latin collection, MS Additional 10392. Not only collecting Latin works, such as sermons, that might be translated and read aloud to lay readers, but also including English devotional works, Colman takes a further step toward inviting lay residents to use and internalize the volume's texts. The volume encompasses works both ascetic (pseudo-Augustine, *De contemptu mundi* and *Sermo ad fratres in eremo* 56) and inclusive (Augustine's Sermon 350 and the Middle English text "be it knowen to good crysten peple").[97] As Erler has shown of a later booklet (fols. 133r–43v), Colman gathered and ordered texts with a "mixed" readership in mind: Augustinian brothers and the lay widows under Colman's spiritual direction. The source from which Colman took some of his material, Syon monk Thomas Betson's printed book *A ryght profitable Treatyse*, articulates a desire to appeal "to religyous people as to the laye people." Erler remarks, "It is hard to escape the conclusion that these traditional assignments to audience were being largely disregarded as directives and that by the opening of the sixteenth century the categories of lay and religious reading were everywhere elided."[98] The volume's other bilingual booklet runs from fol. 27r to fol. 34v. Its Latin and English texts offer varied admonitions, potentially relevant both to clerical men and to lay women. In this booklet as in the volume more widely, Colman seems to recognize the different religious practices and capabilities of clerical and lay readers, offering advice that in some cases might have allowed them to converge.

The bilingual character of these booklets allows us to view the relationship between English and Latin as dynamic, to understand multilingualism as "a constant and active presence," in Baswell's formulation. We need not assume that Latin texts were intended only for clerical users or English texts only for laywomen.[99] Despite the enduring association between women and vernacularity, scholars of medieval and early modern Latin have amassed considerable evidence of women's abilities to read and write in Latin.[100] As Carole Meale memorably suggested, Lady Alice West's reference in her 1395 will to "all the bokes that I haue of latyn, englisch and french" "should caution us against any rigid association of women with a particular language."[101] Late medieval English women owned and gifted Latin religious books. For example, the London vowess Margery de Nerford (d. 1417) bequeathed to the Priory of Holy Trinity Aldgate a volume "de omeliis evangeliorum" (of homilies on the Gospels) that she claimed had belonged to her "father." This is almost certainly a reference to her spiritual father, chaplain William de Bergh, who had owned a book by the same description.[102] As Erler points out, such a book of homilies might have been used either for preaching or reading.[103] We see a similar kind of sharing between priestly father and pious widow in St. John's MS 173.

Nerford's bequest suggests that women gained access to Latin texts through varied means, including hearing them read aloud or reading independently in selective ways. The English and Latin texts in the MS 173 booklet are not laid out as Latin "originals" and vernacular translations, nor are Latin texts grouped with English counterparts on similar subjects, as in some earlier bilingual manuscripts targeting both lay and clerical audiences.[104] In MS 173 the Latin and English texts appear side by side. They include harrowing visions of the soul after death, celebrations of communal charity, inclusive daily devotional routines, and exhortations to study. Although Colman offers no explicit rationale for the booklet's organization, I view this booklet as a miniature "archive" accessible in different ways to lay and clerical residents through collaborative reading.

As Erler has shown, the resident widow with a probable link to this collection was Joan Regent, widow of William Regent, a former sheriff and mayor of Bristol.[105] Regent came to reside in the house between 1499 and 1504, making her will in 1510. In her will she calls John Colman "my gostly fader," indicating that he was her spiritual advisor.[106] She shows her devotion to the hospital in multiple ways: asking to be buried "in the mydde of the Gauntes qwere in Bristoll," leaving forty pounds to the house and ten shillings to each brother, gowns to Master Tiler and Colman, and establishing a fund of twenty nobles to support a yearly "solempne obite atte Gauntes aforesaid for my soule and my husbondes William Regent's soule, our children's soules and for all Cristen soules." Erler speculates that the forty

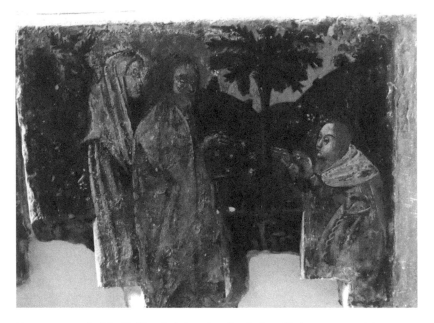

FIGURE 4.14. St. Mark's Hospital chapel wall painting: Christ appears to Mary Magdalene. Author photo. Reproduced with the kind permission of Bristol City Council.

pounds may have been spent on wall paintings to adorn the hospital chapel, originally located in a chamber with squints to the altar. The subjects are the Nativity, Christ's resurrection, and Christ's revelation to Mary Magdalene on Easter, flanked by another woman who may be the Virgin Mary (see fig. 4.14). Erler suggests that Regent might have gifted the wall paintings, featuring prayerful female subjects, to the hospital.[107] The bilingual books copied by St. Mark's scribes shape daily devotional practice in ways that would have complemented the liturgical devotions performed in the chapel and perhaps enhanced Regent's sense of spiritual kinship with the Magdalen and the Virgin.

In an intriguing booklet that appears early in MS 173, Colman collects a series of Latin texts and one English text that offer alternating and complementary visions of religious practice for a mixed readership. The booklet's first text comes from Peter Damian's Letter 66, advising a widow newly converted to monastic life. This extract from the letter imagines the sinful soul's terrified apprehensions as it leaves the body. The next several texts include selections from sermons or entire sermons enumerating the dangers of ingratitude, commending charity, and praising study. These sermons contain advice ranging from the general to the very specific, and the booklet comes to rest on a note of radical inclusion, with the English text "Be it knowen to good crysten peple that desyren to come to euerlastyng lyf dyligently to kepe thyse v poyntes." This apparently unique work offers streamlined advice on devout living, strategies that might enable readers to die confident of heaven, rather than living in terror of hell, as in the first text.[108] I suggest that the volume's clerical and lay readers might have used and shared these texts in a range of ways.

Although the extract from Peter Damian's letter lacks a gendered address, the full letter offers guidance to a widow (Countess Blanca) who had recently entered religious life.[109] Much of Peter's letter is devoted to celebrating her conversion to spiritual marriage with Christ, the "veri sponsi" (true bridegroom).[110] Such an origin makes this text appropriate reading for devout laywomen in the hospital, but this selection is penitential and unisex rather than celebratory and feminized.[111] At the moment the "anima peccatrix" (sinful soul) has left the body, it experiences fear and anxiety in contemplating the torments of hell: "quanto amaro terrore concutitur, quantis mordacis consciencie stimulis laceratur" (the bitter terror that buffets it, and of the biting stings of conscience with which it is afflicted).[112] The soul painfully regrets rashly enjoying the things of the world and bemoans the loss of heaven: "inter tam breue spacium adquisisse potuit leticiam seculorum omnium. Deflet in se propter tam breuis illecebre voluptatem, inerrabilem perpetuae suauitatis prodidisse dulcedinem" (in so short a time it was able to capture all the world's enjoyment; it weeps that because of this brief thrill of pleasure, it will forfeit the unspeakable delight of everlasting sweetness).[113] Colman may have envisioned reaching either Augustinian confrères or resident laity with this terrifying scenario. Peter Damian's original addressee, though she remains elusive, was probably a woman literate in Latin. St. Mark's resident widows may not have possessed the ability to decipher the entire text, yet its Latin is relatively easy, full of vocabulary (e.g., "seculorum omnium" and "illecebre voluptatem") that lay readers might recognize at sight. Or we may imagine a priestly advisor translating the text aloud for a lay learner, reading it to her as Peter Damian might have read to his spiritual charge.

The following sequence of Latin sermon extracts and sermons likewise casts a wide net in its appeal to pious readers. Whereas the extracts from Bernard of Clairvaux warn of ingratitude and temptation, Augustine's Sermon 350 on charity offers an expansive picture of religious observance to men and women, one not defined by knowledge or study.[114] Whereas clerical brothers might have read the sermons aloud or privately, Colman could have read them in the vernacular to Joan Regent or other women, for sermons notated in Latin were often delivered in the vernacular.[115] The first Bernard extract warns of the threat ungratefulness presents to spiritual life in community. The "karissimi" addressed in this extract, from Bernard's sermon "De septem misericordiis," were doubtless monastic brothers. Yet the text's message, on the need for communal gratitude in order to achieve grace, would have been relevant for any reader in the hospital context, for the seven works of mercy were the very foundation for hospital life. Ingratitude, Bernard warns, "vias obstruit gracie" (obstructs the ways of grace). He laments the danger of laughter and idle words to the spiritual fate of his listeners, warning that those who "diuine gracie immemores et ingrati . . . deserantur a gratia" (are unmindful of and lack gratitude for divine mercy . . . will be abandoned by grace).[116] Bernard's admonitions to practice communal piety and decorum, which recall the advice of the *Speculum peccatoris* copied by John Cok, would resonate with brothers and with laywomen under their spiritual care.

The presence of Augustine's Sermon 350, the booklet's following text, is striking: this work not only offers a welcoming vision of charity but also sets forth both male and female models for readers to emulate. Perhaps Colman had both confrères and female residents in mind as readers, offering a communal vision of charity that both might enact. From the start, the sermon holds out charity as the *sine qua non* for righteous Christian living: "Divinarum Scripturarum multiplicem habundanciam, et latissimam doctrinam, sine vllo errore comprehendit, et sine vllo labore custodit, cuius cor plenum est caritate" (All the varied plenty and wide-ranging teaching of the divine scriptures may be grasped, and kept without any difficulty by that person whose heart is full of charity).[117] Some versions address "brothers and sisters," and some "fratres" only, but MS 173 contains no specific address formula, making the text available to readers of any gender.[118] Although an understanding of "divine scriptures" is of course desirable, this sermon maintains the greater importance of love, following Christ's commandment to the apostles to "love one another" (John 13:34–35). As the author later rearticulates, charity trumps study: "Si ergo non vacat omnes diuiunas paginas perscrutari . . . tene caritatem, vbi omnia pendent: ita tenebis quod ibi didicisti; et eciam quod nondum didicisti" (If there is no time or leisure to pore over the sacred pages . . . hold onto charity, on which they all depend. In this way you will hold onto what you have learned there; you will also get hold of what you haven't yet learned).[119] In this particular manuscript context, this statement might offer comfort to readers without the time or ability to read the longer, more technical Latin texts.

The communal focus suggested by the reference to the apostles is reiterated in a typically Augustinian mode several times, with the author's focus on "behavior" (moribus), the insistence on conduct as the index of charity: "Ille itaque tenet et quod patet et quod latet in diuinis sermonibus, qui caritatem tenet in moribus" (Those who keep a grip on charity in their behavior, have a grasp both of what is revealed and of what is concealed in the divine writings).[120] Thus charity is made a precondition, even possibly a replacement, for learning. It is also ideally a quality that can be recognized by others and imitated.

This sermon offers not only male but also female biblical exemplars of charity. The author declares charity "in Abel per sacrificium grata, in Noe per diluuium secura . . . *Casta in Susanna erga virum, in Anna post virum, in Maria preter virum*" (acceptable in Abel through his sacrifice, safe as Noah through the flood. . . . *Chaste in Susanna toward her husband, in Anna after her husband, in Mary apart from her husband*).[121] The female trio embodies the married, widowed, and virginal stages of wifely charity, making their respective forms of chastity into the women's most powerful statement of love. This section would have obvious relevance to women readers who might have passed through all three stages. It is ambiguous which Anna is referred to here, but the author may intend the pious widow Anna of the Purification episode. This would be a fitting touch in the context of hospital devotion, for Anna's prayerful widowhood formed a contemporary model, as we saw in chapter 1, for women who retired to hospitals.[122]

To follow this expansive, multigendered account of charity with a sermon narrowly focused on learning and retreat from the world seems jarring at first. The final Latin text, the pseudo-Augustinian *Sermo ad fratres in eremo*, offers a rigorous vision of religious life that rejects worldly pleasure for study and internalization of scripture.[123] The *Sermo ad fratres in eremo* 56, attributed to Augustine, was in fact part of a collection written during the fourteenth century and circulated by Augustinian friars advocating for their priority over the canons as followers of the Augustinian Rule.[124] St. Mark's was an establishment of canons rather than friars, but we have seen in Colman's choices of texts and annotation practices in MS Lyell 38 an inclination toward asceticism when addressing clerical readers. Perhaps Colman introduced this text, which is also attested in library lists from Leicester and Thurgarton, in order to reassure brothers who shared this tendency that a devotion to study was welcome in the house. Again, Colman may be working to reinforce a sense of distinction between canonical and lay identities, even within the space of a book that shapes both.

The sermon takes avid reading as its keynote and argues that internalizing the word of God keeps the religious subject pure: "ille qui in corde suo abscondit eloquia Dei, non peccat" (he who hides the word of God in his heart, does not sin).[125] In contrast to the prior text, the emphasis here is on study as the key to charity, on the words of God as true sustenance to the spiritual man. This sermon offers a bracing call to study that in the context of this manuscript seems intentionally placed between the expansively welcoming sermon on charity and the final text delineating the five points that all pious "peple" may embody daily.

At the end of the booklet awaits a disarmingly simple English text, addressed "to good Crysten peple that desyren to come to euerlastyng lyf dyligently to kepe thyse v poyntes."[126] This text, which has not been found elsewhere, offers a brief devotional routine for the lay penitent. Its abbreviated routine and English language target a lay, perhaps female reader, yet the address "to good Crysten peple" potentially enfolds everyone in the hospital community. Although the text uses the medieval universalizing "he" to describe its reader, women readers who considered themselves good Christians would have found its advice relevant to their lives. The text's emphasis on heartfelt devotion and regard for the poor may indeed have been tailor-made for hospital readers. All are invited into fail-safe routines for daily devotion, beginning with prayers upon waking that recognize God with a Pater Noster, and by doing so "make a couenant and purpose with God to kepe his commandements truly þe same day to deye. And this shalbe his fyrste oblacion of the whych al seyntes in heuen shal joye."[127] The next step is going to church: not just passively sitting, but actively engaging in penitential reflection:

> Not rennyng ouer hastely, but so grete deuocyon, as yf he to eche of þe Pater Nosters sholde kysse on of his blessyd woundes and prynte his mouthe there uppon. And doynge this he heryth masse truly, and receyuth gostely with the prest þat sayeth masse þe holy sacrament in to his herte. And he shal fare þe bettyr al þat same daye, by cause God wyl make a dwellyng place in his sowle.[128]

This text offers a short devotional routine for a layperson, demanding a deliberate performance of prayers with deep reflection on the Passion and imagined physical contact with Christ via repetition of the Pater Noster. In this fashion, the reader invites God into his or her soul: an internalization comparable to that offered in works such as *The Abbey of the Holy Ghost*.[129] Yet at the same time that she invites God into her soul through devout reflection, she must perform outward works of charity as well. The third point involves prayerful and reflective eating of meals, at which the pious subject should

> saye deuoutly his grace or one Pater Noster and one Ave. And in ony wyse he must geue almysse at hys table to hym þat askyth it in þe name of God. And yf he be of power, ones in þe woke he shal calle a pore man to his table. And then he receyueth thus our Lord Ihesu hymself, and therefore God wyl putt hym at his heuenly borde in euerlastyng lyf.[130]

Here the work of mercy, feeding the poor, is made a foundation of everyday practice through the giving of alms or feeding the poor. And although such munificence may not be within every reader's means, the mandate to give alms is constant, making the text appropriate for residents of the hospital, where alms had been distributed regularly from its foundation.

Writing this practice into the "five points" required every day effectively creates a lay rule for hospital dwellers, who if they read nothing else in a day might profitably consult this text. When the addressee is doing "werke or besynesse," he or she is adjured to keep God in mind at all times, speaking ill of no man, so that "*he lyueth a heuynly lyf in erth*, and þe sayntes in heuen ben gladde of hym and a byden with desyre after his comyng."[131] Thus the reader may envision both inviting God into her heart and becoming part of a heavenly community on earth, a lay version of monastic community. Such a vision counteracts that terrifying scenario, in the booklet's opening text, of the sinful soul invited into the company of demons.

The day ends as it began, with a bedtime prayer whose practice will enable readers to avoid the terrible regret plaguing the "anima peccatrix" of the booklet's first text. It advises, "And then goyng to bed he shal seye iij Aues upon his knees, praying Our Lady þat she wyl kepe hym frome his ghostly enemy and from all euyl, and then he shal reste þe better and be clenlyer and ryse deuoutlyer to the worshyppe of God. Lyue as thou wolde deye."[132] The living soul is invited into a simple yet demanding program that counteracts the first text's frightening vision and offers a plan that any hospital resident might embody. To enhance the text's proffered advice, Colman has placed marginal marks of emphasis in two places: a *nota bene* next to the advice for "whan he gooth to churche" (see fig. 4.15) and his characteristic dotted flower next to "þe sayntes in heuen ben gladde of hym and a byden with desyre after his comyng" (see fig. 4.16). These annotations flag the reader's most important duty (disciplined worship), and her ultimate reward (belonging to the company of saints). These two facets of the text would be equally important for either Augustinian brothers or laywomen readers.

## BRISTOL PUBLIC LIBRARY MS 6:
### LATIN AND ENGLISH, EXEMPLARY LAITY

In 1502, Colman's brother William Haulle copied another bilingual devotional miscellany, now Bristol Public Library MS 6. This complex volume also targets clerical and lay readers within the hybrid Augustinian space of St. Mark's Hospital. The volume is remarkable for its kindred pastoral priorities to MS 173, and its dating makes it possible to speculate that it too could have been used in the spiritual guidance of Joan Regent. One finds a broad division in the book between Latin texts for male clerics and English works for laywomen. Yet at certain key points the boundaries of language, gender, and role seem to dissolve in textual combinations that may encourage lay readers to embrace the suffering and charity essential to the hospital context.

Erler highlights a codicological and thematic division within the book, whose first section features Latin expositions of liturgical sequences, perhaps for novice brothers, and whose latter half contains English works directed at pious laywomen, including a form of confession for a woman and a treatise on the discretion of spirits: "The manuscript's polyglot nature speaks of the realities of a priestly working life in a linguistically complex

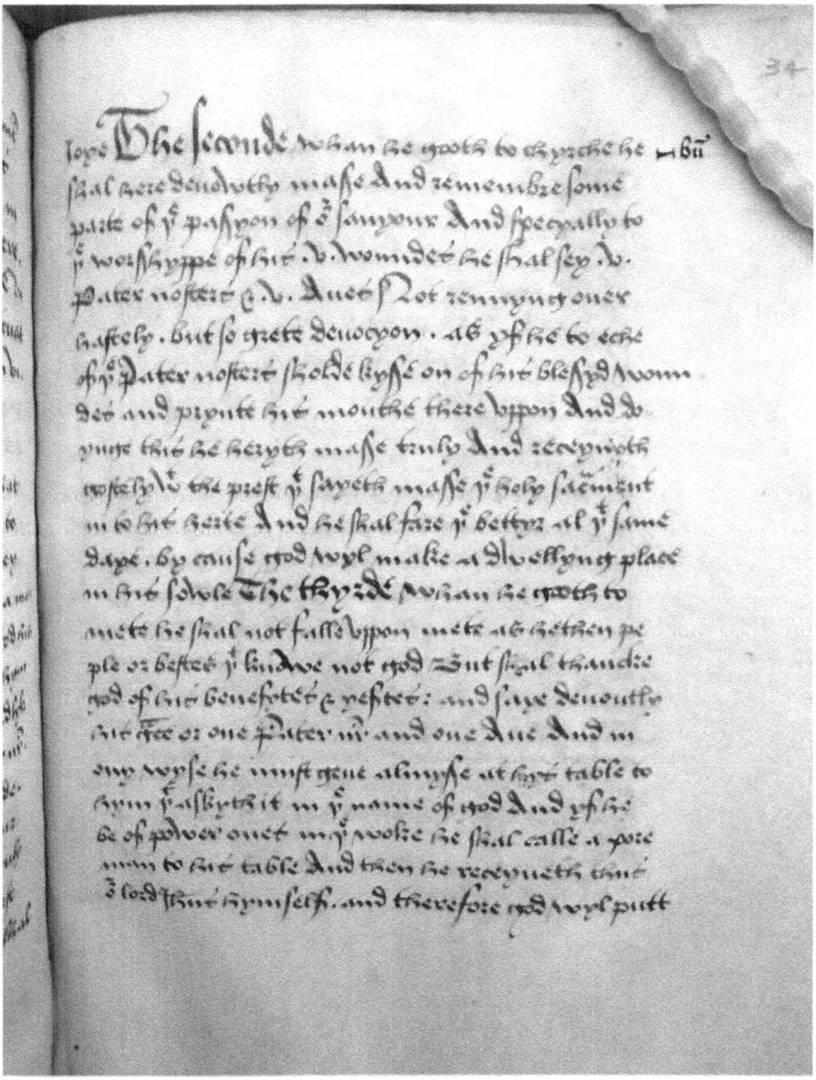

The seconde whan he goeth to chyrche he
shal here deuoutly masse And remembre some
parte of y passyon of o sauyour And specyally to
y worshyppe of hie v woundes he shal sey v
pater nosters & v Aues Not renny ouer
hastely but so grete deuocyon as yf he be seke
of y Pater nosters sholde kysse on of hie blessyd woun
des and pryute hie mouthe there vppon And b
pursse thus he herytt masse truly And recey
wostfully the prest y sayeth masse y holy sacrement
in to hie herte And he shal fare y bettyr al y same
daye by cause god wyl make a dwellyng place
in hie soule The thyrde whan he goth to
mete he shal not fall vppon mete as heithen pe
ple or bestes y knowe not god But shal thanke
god of hie benefotes p resftes and saye deuoutly
hie thre or one Pater nr and one Aue And in
any wyse he must geue almysse at hys table to
hym y askyth it in y name of god And yf hie
be of power ouer any noble he shal calle a pore
man to hie table And then he recey veth thus
I lord thus hymself and therefore god wyl putt

FIGURE 4.15. John Colman's *nota bene* annotation. Oxford, St. John's College,
MS 173 fol. 34r. Reproduced with permission of the President and Fellows of
St. John's College, Oxford.

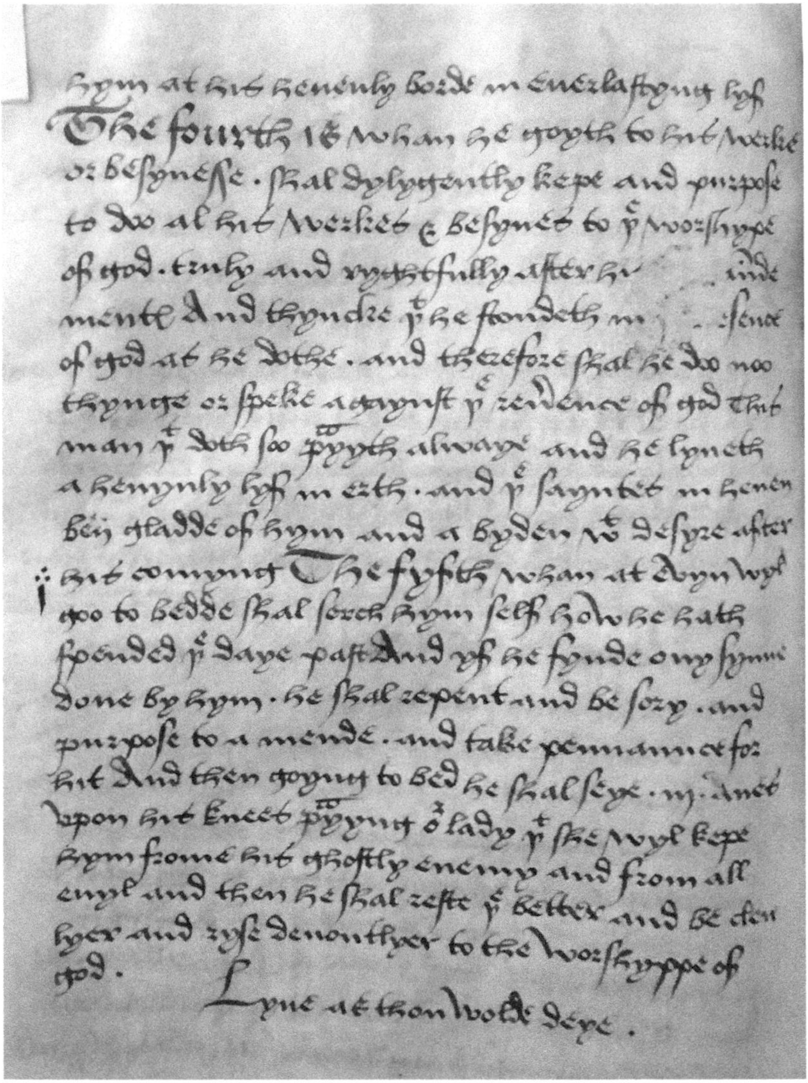
hym at his hevenly borde in everlastyng lyf
The fourth is whan he goyth to his werke
or besynesse. shal dylygentely kepe and purpose
to do al his werkes & besynes to þe worshype
of god. truly and ryghtfully after h[illegible] inde
mente And thyncke þt he stondeth in [illegible]sence
of god at he dothe. and therfore shal he do noo
thynge or speke agaynst þe reverence of god That
man þt doth soo pyyth alwaye and he lyveth
a hevynly lyf in erth. and þe payntes in heven
ben gladde of hym and abyden wt desyre after
his comyng The fyfth whan at evyn wyl
goo to bedde shal serch hym self how he hath
spended þe daye past And yf he fynde ony synne
done by hym. he shal repent and be sory. and
purpose to amende. and take penaunce for
his And then goyng to bed he shal seye. iij. aves
upon his knees pryyng our lady þt she wyl kepe
hym frome his ghostly enemy and from all
evyl and then he shal reste þe better and be clen
lyer and ryse devoutlyer to the worshyppe of
god.
Lyue as thou wolde deye.

FIGURE 4.16. John Colman's dotted flower annotation. Oxford, St. John's College, MS 173 fol. 34v. Reproduced with permission of the President and Fellows of St. John's College, Oxford.

climate. More unusually, it allows us to ask about the practices implicit in spiritual direction. Was the manuscript's perusal shared between priest and penitent?"[133] Either Haulle or Colman (Regent's "gostly fader") might have used the English portion of the volume to advise lay female spiritual charges. Yet as in the MS 173 booklet examined above, parts of this section blur the Latin/English boundary and the divide between clerical teacher and lay learner, offering the lay reader spiritual independence within the hospital context. Preceding the form of confession, the treatise on discretion of spirits, and the form of life for a hermit, we find an English text on tribulation just before a Latin text on almsgiving. This conjunction of these two texts seems particularly fitting in the hospital context. Both texts outline a concerted yet moderate program of religious discipline for the lay reader, defining spiritual practice as a combination of suffering and charity, the two essential experiences of the hospital.[134] The tribulation text argues that even a small amount of tribulation, if borne with true meekness, may outshine the most ascetic practice:

> Tribulacyon is the best thyng that any man may haue yn this world, ffor yef there hadde be any better thyng in thys world than tribulacioun, oure Lord God wolde haue yeven hit to his owne son, for he suffred the grettest tribulacyon yn this world that ever dyd any creature. Also a man may desire in meke sufferaunce of a lytell tribulacyon more meryte than he shuld do, and he did faste xxx yere brede and water, and by the same tyme livede as devoutly as did Mary Magdaleyn. Also yef Oure Lady and all the seyntes of heven prayde for a man, yet all they shuld nat gete hym so mych mede as he shulde gete hym self by meke sufferance of a litell tribulacyon.[135]

Here we see individual tribulation defined as a "litell" but significant imitation of Christ's profound sacrifice. It is notable that the work cites Mary Magdalen and Our Lady as the primary examples of devout living and intercessory prayer, given their prominence in the hospital chapel paintings that Joan Regent might have commissioned. Here the saints appear as textual models, complementing their visual representation in the chapel. Yet the text's emphasis falls ultimately on the reader's own self-sufficiency: through "meke sufferaunce of a lytell tribulacyon," she takes her place on a continuum of suffering stretching from Christ, through the poor seeking alms at the institution, to her own moderate forms of self-denial.

Elite laywomen such as Regent had come to the hospital to learn from Augustinian teachers how to pursue disciplined lives of prayer in retirement. As she uses the English text to install a regime of humility that parallels the Rule followed by the canons, the reader may show with her body the effects of this discipline:

> By mynde of thi afautes and for shame of thi synne, be dismayed to loke proudelych; walke wyth a lowe chere, a meke mouth and a sadde vyssage. In hygh worshippes haue grete mekenes. Thogh thow be of hygh power, restreyne hyghnes yn thy hert, let nat worshyp yeven to the of God make þe proude; the hygher thow art yn dignyte, the lower by mekenes make þu the.[136]

Leaving behind the "hynes" and "worshyp" of her worldly state, her bodily practice in the hospital space demonstrates her mindfulness of "afautes" and "shame." Self regulating in gaze, walk, speech, and visage, she not only emulates canonical conduct but also potentially becomes a model for her fellow laywomen.

The "six profits of tribulation" text treats the experience of tribulation as an opportunity to experience kinship with saintly models and to teach others, rather than primarily as an ascetic or self-isolating practice. This outlook on tribulation seems essentially different from the emphases that Appleford posits in her study of the tribulation- and death-related texts used by pious lay hospital-dweller William Baron. We find in MS 6 the opposite of a "perfectionist lay religiosity" focused on teaching "practices of interiorization and self-mortification designed for the perfected few."[137] Instead its texts counsel readers to *avoid* the extreme asceticism that might encourage spiritual pride or self-absorption. In connection with the tribulation text, immediately following appears a short Latin text, in Christ's voice, urging genuine outward-directed charity.[138] Christ assures readers attracted to ascetic practices that he would be better pleased with small, sincere demonstrations of neighborly love. Significantly in the hospital context it begins, "Da pauperibus unum denareum in vita tua cum bona voluntate, et hoc mihi plus placet quam si dares post mortem tuam aureos in monetam compositos" (Give a penny to the poor during your life out of good will, and this will please me more than if you gave mountains of gold coins after your death).[139] The reader's charity is tested through suffering neighborly unkindness rather than through imposing self-discipline: "Sustine pacienter et dulciter unum verbum durum et opprobriosum a proximo tuo, et hoc magis mihi placet quam si disciplinares corpus tuum cum tot virgis quot possunt crescere per vnum diem in tota terra" (Bear patiently and sweetly a hard difficult word from your neighbor, and this will please me more than if you disciplined your body with all the rods that may grow in one day on the whole earth).[140] The physical care of others, "the poor and the sick," pleases the speaking Christ more than if the reader were to fast for three days on bread and water. Increasingly lurid self-punishments are detailed, then disavowed, in favor of a moderate, genuine love of Christ and neighbor.

Placed between the praise of tribulation and directions on the proper handling of temptation,[141] this text offers in simple Latin a lesson on proper spiritual orientation for lay hospital readers. Perhaps it was intended to dispel some assumptions that such readers might have had: that large post-mortem gifts would improve their spiritual condition after death, or that secretive self-punishments would improve their standing in Christ's eyes. In concert with Colman's efforts at defining an inclusive, temperate form of devotion for confrères and lay readers, this text concretizes a practical approach to the charity celebrated in Sermon 350, copied into St. John's College MS 173. It is tempting to imagine Colman and Haulle collaborating in the planning and the execution of these two complex anthologies.

These two bilingual booklets create striking combinations of inward- and outward-looking devotional texts. Capable of being read aloud, silently, collectively or individually, these texts define readers' routines, utterances, and acts in the terms of Augustinian community, grounded in charity. This charity was never monolithic, and sometimes it was expressed with difficulty. The Augustinian books of Cok, Colman, and Haulle offer textual shape to clerical and lay lives in hospital community. These lives required penitential discipline, the embrace of tribulation, and constant awareness of Christ's suffering as mirrored in the plight of the poor. Real boundaries existed between priestly and lay practices, and the books I have considered both reinforce and blur these boundaries. Hospital scribes used their skills to teach readers "verbo et exemplo," perhaps giving some hospital residents the ability to teach each other in the process.

# FIVE

# Poverty, Charity, and Poetry

## *Critique and Reform before the Dissolution*

English hospitals were uniquely affected by and in some cases uniquely responsive to the intertwined religious and political changes of the 1530s and 40s. These decades saw Henry VIII's break with Rome in 1534, the dissolution of the religious houses in a gradual process from 1536 to 1540, and the abrogation of the chantries beginning in 1545. The same period witnessed a flurry of national and local attempts to manage the rising tide of poverty, assisting the "deserving" while punishing the "undeserving" poor. In 1530, a royal proclamation, "noting that the number of vagabonds and beggars was rising every day, ordered local officials to punish all vagrants and physically able beggars found outside of the hundreds where they were born or had lived for a period of 3 years." In 1531 a new national statute authorized "licensed begging" within strictly defined areas, with punishments for those who begged outside their designated regions.[1] This chapter considers how critiques of hospitals, from the late fourteenth through the mid-sixteenth century, intersected with concerns about religious practice, endowment, and poor relief. These issues remained linked throughout the period, up to and beyond the Dissolution, for the early critiques (both lollard-reformist and establishment-bureaucratic) anticipated later suggestions for hospital reform, in some cases presaging the new configurations that hospitals took after the Dissolution. Hospitals became particular flashpoints for the intersection of poverty, charity, and religion during this long period. Amid these fifteenth-century critiques, new institutions founded in this period had begun to take on different forms, as secular individuals and groups began to found smaller, more selective institutions with often onerous and specific requirements for residents.

Even as turn of the sixteenth-century London saw the foundation of the Savoy, a new model hospital built on European humanist principles, a chorus of literary/satirical voices in the 1520s and 30s combined reformed religious perspectives on purgation and intercession with concern about poor relief and the increase of "vagabonds" besieging the metropolis. Simon Fish's radical *Supplication for the Beggars* (ca. 1529) carried forward the earlier lollard argument for disendowment and intersected with governmental proposals for poor relief that involved hospital reform, albeit with few concrete results. The last section of this chapter offers an extended consideration of Robert Copland's little-studied poem, *The Hye Way to the Spyttell Hous* (ca. 1536). This work, which has not been adequately understood in the context of hospital history, offers a nuanced view of St. Bartholomew's contemporary predicament and expresses a complex understanding of the hospital's historical role and possible future in the city.

## LATE MEDIEVAL CRITIQUES OF HOSPITALS
## AND PROPOSALS FOR REFORM

Well before England had any inkling of an official Reformation, the late fourteenth-century lollards' critiques of purgatory and the religious orders held important implications for hospitals.[2] Margaret Aston has argued that "poverty was a continuous theme—if not an obsession—in Lollard writings."[3] Although it stemmed from an antipathy toward the religious orders that was not shared by most, the lollard position on disendowment as a means of poor relief dovetailed with more mainstream concerns. Orme and Webster argue that the lollard plan for disendowment "would not have been acceptable to the authorities in England, lay or clerical, but it provoked (or reflected) a measure of public concern."[4] A preoccupation with aiding the poor in gospel-authorized ways appears in the lollard Twelve Conclusions, circa 1395, and in a more developed form in the lollard disendowment bill presented to Parliament in 1407 or 1410. Both documents propose aiding the poor through the institutional means of almshouses, while decrying ecclesiastical control over such houses and the intercessory prayer that undergirded the charitable economy of hospitals. The Seventh Conclusion criticizes prayer for the dead as the "false ground" of alms:

special preyeris for dede men soulis mad in oure chirche preferryng on be name more þan anothir, *þis is þe false ground of almesse dede, on þe qwiche alle almes houses of Ingelond ben wikkidly igroundid*. . . . preyere meritorie and of ualue schulde ben a werk proceding of hey charite, and charite accepte no persones . . . us thinkis þat þe giftis of temperel godis to prestis and to almes housis is principal cause of special preyeris, þe qwiche is nout fer from symonie. Another skil: for special preyer mad for men dampnid to euerlasting peyne is to God gretli displesing. . . . Þe correlari is: þe preyere of ualue springand out of perfyth charite schulde enbrace in general alle þo þat God wolde haue sauid, and leue þer marchaundise now used for special preyeris imade to mendynauns and possessioneris and othere soulis prestis.[5]

Whereas intercessory prayer had always been a central hospital function, lollards decry "special preyeris" as a "false ground of almesse dede," literally an unstable foundation for "alle almes houses of Ingelond." The lollard idea of predestination nullifies the benefit of special intercessory prayer, since, as the author argues, "þe preyere of ualue springand out of perfyth charite schulde enbrace in general alle þo þat God wolde haue sauid," but the identities of the "sauid" souls are known only to God.[6] Not only are endowments to priests and almshouses tantamount to "symonie" because they exchange material goods for spiritual work, but the "marchaundise" given over to specialized priests makes them a burden upon the "puple." The conclusion renders the entire basis for hospitals and chantries illegitimate, but without removing the possibility that such institutions could be reformed.

In the vein of reforming and bolstering the realm's almshouses, the Seventh Conclusion mentions "a bok þat þe kyng herde þan an hundrid of almes housis suffisede to al þe reme, and þereof schulde falle þe grettest encres possible to temporel part."[7] Although this reference is vague, its reference to the "encres . . . to temporel part" begins to link the strategy of clerical disendowment to the support of almshouses, a proposal that appears full-blown in the Disendowment Bill of 1407–10. The bill proposes disendowing the clergy in order to free up money to endow "c houses of almesse and euery houvs c marcis with londe to feden with all the nedefull pore men and no coste to the tovne but only of the temperaltes morteysed and wasted amonge provde worldely clerkes."[8] Hudson argues that the proposal's careful language and specific proposals mark "the high point of legitimate

Lollard activity in the fifteenth century," manifesting a confidence in the movement that should be taken seriously, even though the Disendowment Bill was apparently never taken up.[9]

Most strikingly and presciently for the later history of English hospitals, the petition implies a severing of almshouses from religious supervision. It proposes that these one hundred new almshouses should be funded from the king's disendowment of "bisshopes, abbotes and priours, yoccupyed and wasted provdely withinne the rewme." Instead of the religious who have historically misgoverned hospitals, secular rulers should run these new institutions: "and euery house of almesse c marcz, *by oueresiht of goode and trewe sekulers, because of preestes and clerkes that now have ful nyh distroyed all the houses of almesse withinne the rewme;* and also for to ordeyne that euery tovne thurhoute the rewme shulde kepe alle pore menne and beggers which mowe nat travaylle for her sustenaunce, after the statut made at Cambrigge."[10] The statement that almshouses (in which hospitals are notionally included) have been mismanaged by religious leaders and should be taken over by "goode and trewe sekulers" does not seem to have been taken seriously by Parliament at the time. (Later the proposal clarifies that it is not advocating the dissolution of existing hospitals.)[11] Yet the proposal for management of hospitals by secular masters anticipates arrangements put into place during some English hospital refoundations of the 1540s. At St. Bartholomew's, the lollard suggestion would be fully taken up when by 1546 the refounded hospital came to be governed by prominent citizens and funded by taxpayers. The insertion of hospitals into the growing sixteenth-century debate over managing "pore menne and beggers which mowe nat travaylle for her sustenaunce" anticipates later complaints by authors Simon Fish and Robert Copland.

In 1414, probably taking a cue from lollard efforts, but without acknowledging them, the House of Commons proposed formal visitations and inspections of the nation's hospitals.[12] The petition named the familiar categories of unfortunates as deserving of hospital care: "veigles hommes & femmes, lazers hommes & femmes, hors de lour senne & memoir, poveres femmes enseintez, & pur homme q'ount perduz lour biens & sont cheiez en grant meschief" (old men and women, leprous men and women, poor pregnant women, those who have lost their senses and memory, and men who have lost their goods and fallen on hard times).[13] The petition lamented that such people were now dying from lack of care by corrupt clerics who diverted their rightful alms: "plusour hommes & femmes ount moruz en graunde meschief, pur defaute d'eide, vivre, & socour, al displesance de Dieu, & peril de lour almes qu'ency gastent & expendent les biens d'icelles povere hommes & femmes en autre oeps" (many men and women have died in great misery through lack of help, livelihood and succour, to the displeasure of God, and bringing peril to the souls of those who thus waste and put the goods of the same poor men and women to other uses).[14] The petition, like the lollards' Seventh Conclusion, invokes the displeasure of God as a warning to the king, but it argues for the restoration rather than the abolition of endowments and alms as bases for the support of hospitals.

Although the king pledged to make the "ordinaries" investigate all the royal hospitals and also vaguely promised that all other hospitals would be subject to "correction & reformacion solone les Leies de Seinte Esglise" (correction and reformation according to the laws of Holy Church), little came of these statements.[15] For when the Commons raised the issue again the following year in a detailed petition, proposing deadlines for the ordinaries' reports and for the promised "reformations" and threatening to revoke the jurisdictions of officials who failed to fulfill these duties, the king merely referred to the previous statute: "Soit l'estatut eut fait garde & mys en deu execution" (Let the statute be kept and duly executed).[16] Rawcliffe suggests that Henry V's concern for a war effort that depended upon Church support made him reluctant to advance the petition, given the possibility of angering the clergy.[17] Not until royal interests found a reason not only to reform but to *dissolve* the hospitals would his descendant Henry VIII take decisive action to change royal policy.

## Changing Hospital Foundations in the Fifteenth Century

The above parliamentary critiques of English hospitals were informed by other contemporary complaints about maladministration. Although it may be an overstatement to say that "financial mismanagement and outright corruption were endemic among English hospitals of all types in the later medieval period," some hospitals, including London's St. Mary of Bethlehem, run by an embezzling warden, were clearly diverting resources away from the poor.[18] Rawcliffe argues that many large urban hospitals in the later period devoted more funds to the work of commemorating the dead, that practice anathema to the lollards, than they did to caring for the poor.[19] Yet many of the older London foundations were singled out in this period for being well run. St. Thomas's, Southwark; St. Mary's, Bishopsgate; and St. Bartholomew's had been chastised by clerical visitors in the fourteenth century, but each of these received approval and in the fifteenth century "for the 'grete comforte' offered to paupers and unmarried pregnant women, who were rarely welcomed at provincial hospitals."[20] The city of London took particular interest in the administration of St. Mary's, which treated the insane, and attempted (sometimes in conflict with the Crown) to make sure that the hospital benefited Londoners.[21] As Barron and others have noted, these administrative efforts anticipate the civic takeover of several London hospitals in the sixteenth century. Yet even as some of the large older houses continued to prosper, the trend toward founding large hospitals had already ended by the later thirteenth century.

Changes had been afoot in English hospital and almshouse foundations for some time by the fifteenth century. Many late medieval and early Tudor hospitals and almshouses developed qualities that carried over into the post-Dissolution period: these included an emphasis on receiving and selecting the "deserving" poor, an enhanced intensity (in some cases) of prayer requirements for residents, and an increased emphasis on regulating their conduct.[22] Official distinctions between the "worthy" and "unworthy" poor had begun to be instituted after the devastation of the Black Death, which was followed by the Ordinance of Laborers in 1349 and additional statutes in 1351 and 1388. These statutes attempted to distinguish between the "worthy" (widows and children, the sick, the maimed, and the old) and the "unworthy" poor or "sturdy beggars" capable of working and therefore not deserving of alms.[23] Miri Rubin has argued, based mainly on evidence from the Hospital of St. John in Cambridge, that such changes had begun to be felt as early as the late thirteenth and early fourteenth centuries, as increasingly secular founders and patrons began to move away from donating indiscriminately to the sick and poor toward founding private chantries and supporting carefully chosen retirees and scholars.[24]

In contrast to the large ecclesiastical and royal foundations of the twelfth and thirteenth centuries, most later medieval foundations were smaller, founded by secular individuals or groups. These founders began to show greater discrimination toward prospective residents, requiring them to be "respectable" and often to perform more intensive rounds of prayer, sometimes manual work.[25] The pregnant, the very young, the infectious, and the poor were not welcomed at these houses, which catered primarily to the "elderly and disabled."[26] Among the most famous examples, with surviving statutes and exceptional buildings, are Alice Chaucer's foundation at Ewelme (founded 1437, with statutes from 1448–50) and Henry Chichele's almshouse at Higham Ferrers (founded 1427). Colin Richmond has detailed life at Ewelme with its exhaustive instructions for prayer, public and private (including five daily visits to the almshouse church): "In addition to the formal routine of prayer, the almsmen were to go to church every day 'whanne they mowe best therto attende,' where they were to say for the king and the founders 150 Aves, fifteen Pater Nosters, and three Creeds, that is, three times 'oure lady psawter, a psawter conteyning thryes Aves with Pater nostris and 3 Credis.'"[27] The almshouse at Higham Ferrers combined slightly less burdensome liturgical requirements with work, including gardening.[28] Intimating a connection between the almshouse and later forms of civic regulation, Richmond notes Ewelme's "house of correction aspect," which limited almsmen from leaving the premises and suspended their wages if they went abroad.[29]

Despite the secular founders and overseers of these new late medieval institutions, their extensive liturgical requirements argue against wholesale secularization during this period.[30] The requirements of many late medieval almshouses may prefigure reformed worship in another respect, Orme and Webster suggest. Fifteenth-century records often record a twice daily attendance at services, "anticipating Cranmer's reform of English worship in 1549, which reduced the divine office from eight services to the two of matins and evensong—a reform which may well have been influenced by practices like those of the hospitals."[31] As I show in chapter 6, when I consider the changed liturgical requirements of St. Bartholomew's and St. Mark's, reformed hospitals stood at the forefront of an altered civic piety, their rules converging with the everyday practices of newly Protestant citizens who retained memories of the older institutions and may have viewed the provision of charity as largely continuous with the old ways.

## TUDOR HOSPITAL INNOVATIONS AND CONTINUED CRITIQUE

Even as turn-of-the-century London saw further extension and innovation on the traditional hospital model, the 1520s and 30s gave rise to critiques combining reformed perspectives on purgation and intercession with

concern about the surge in poor needing relief. In turn, Robert Copland offered a more thoughtful critique of the hospital with attention both to its
past and its future. As the great pox swept Europe and England, even many
large hospitals were obliged to turn away patients. Contemporary observers
such as Bishop John Fisher lamented (in 1509), "How many lye in stretes
& hye wayes full of carbuncles & other vncurable botches, whiche also we
dayly perceyue at our eye greuous to beholde, how many be crucyfyed in
maner by intollerable aches of bones & Ioytnes with many other infyrmy-
tees."[32] In response to such suffering, which he too lamented in his 1509
will, King Henry VII envisioned three new hospitals to be built in London,
York, and Coventry.[33] Only one of these materialized: London's Savoy, an
experiment that innovated on a traditional model. The Savoy, inspired by
the renowned Hospital of Santa Maria Nuova in Florence, exemplified the
Italian influence on English policy, as did the founding of the College of
Physicians by Cardinal Wolsey in 1518.[34] The Savoy's main buildings seem
to have been in place by 1515, the year the hospital's statutes were written.[35]
It was traditional in many ways (dedicated to the Virgin Mary and St. John
the Baptist, featuring open wards with chapels), but much was revolution-
ary in the Savoy's approach to hygiene and medical care, which drew upon
Italian practices. The poor were admitted only one at a time, bathed and
provided with gowns, and a physician and surgeon came to examine sick
patients every day.[36] What might have been an incipient trend was damp-
ened by Henry VII's death, Henry VIII's break from Rome, and the subsequent piecemeal dissolution of England's hospitals. Although the Savoy
was dissolved in 1551/52, its statutes may in turn have influenced the rules
of the refounded St. Bartholomew's Hospital.[37]

Over the next several decades, a chorus of critics voiced growing
concern with the question of how the Church should intervene in the
treatment of the poor and unfortunate. This concern was concurrent with
antipoverty proposals and legislation in this period of crop failures and increasing rural and urban destitution. Yet another parliamentary bill of
1512 proposed the "reformacon & amendment" of hospitals to care for ill
people dying in the streets, address the problem of vagrancy, and discipline hospitals that were raising funds by selling false indulgences and letters of confraternity.[38] "Concern about begging was probably accentuated
because people seeking help for themselves were joined by more aggres-
sive solicitation of alms for charitable institutions," McIntosh argues. "As

hospitals put greater pressure on their proctors to bring in specified sums each year, competition over territory and income mounted."[39] Despite widespread support for such reforms, this proposal languished and was eventually superseded by Henry's dissolution of the religious houses and the Chantry Acts, which would result in the closure rather than the reform of many hospitals.[40]

Of the early sixteenth-century religious reformers, the most radical and comprehensive critic of hospitals was Simon Fish, whose *Supplication for the Beggars* appeared in 1529. In his own petition to Henry VIII, Fish implicates hospitals in a scathing critique of purgatory and alms linked to prayers for the dead. The influential *Supplication* cites the hospital as a primary symptom of traditional religion's failings, a metonymy for the problematic Catholic provision of charity.[41] Fish opens his tract by speaking for the "true" beggars, a litany of unfortunates lining up closely with the traditional groups cited by past petitioners. The petition begins:

> Most lamentably compleyneth theyre wofull mysery vnto youre highnes youre poore daily bedemen the wretched, hidous monstres (on whome scarcely for horror any yie dare loke) the foule vnhappy sorte of lepres, and other sore people, nedy, impotent, blinde, lame, and sike, that live onely by almesse, howe that theyre nombre is daily so sore encreased that all the almesse of all the weldisposed people of this youre realme is not half ynough for to susteine them, but that for verey constreint they die for hunger.[42]

As in the lollard petition, the poor beggars' predicament stems from the greed and negligence of the country's clergy, who are themselves *false* beggars: "the Bisshoppes, Abbottes, Priours, Deacons, Archedeacons, Suffraganes, Prestes, Monkes, Chanons, Freres, Pardoners, and Somners. And who is abill to nombre this idell rauinous sort whiche (setting all laboure a side) haue begged so importunatly that they haue gotten ynto theyre hondes more then the therd part of all youre Realme."[43] The *Supplication*'s claim that the clergy owns more than a third, perhaps half of the kingdom, precisely echoes the early fifteenth-century lollard disendowment bill and many other similar petitions.[44]

For Fish, like the lollards, this problem is traceable to the doctrine of purgatory and the practice of special prayers and alms. Hence Fish offers a radical revision of purgatorial logic: "They sey also that if there were a purgatory, and also if that the pope with his pardons for money may deliuer one soul thens: he may deliuer him aswel without money: if he may deliuer one, he may deliuer a thousand: if he may deliuer a thousand he may deliver theim all, and so destroy purgatory."[45] With purgatory at the root of the Catholic Church and its simoniac practices, hospitals on the traditional model cannot exist in Fish's scheme. His proposal goes much further than the lollard disendowment bill, which had carefully *not* advocated the dissolution of existing hospitals. Fish's "remedy" is radical. He argues that although the king's predecessors had richly endowed monasteries with land so that they might both support the poor and say intercessory masses daily, "they giue neuer one peny" and "they sey neuer one."[46] Hence he proposes, "if your grace will bilde a sure hospitall that never shall faile to releue vs all your poore bedemen, so take from theim all these thynges."[47] The notion of such "a sure hospitall" acknowledges that the *idea* of the hospital is worth saving: though hospitals are built, as the lollards had argued, on the "wicked" foundation of almsgiving, nevertheless as institutions of charity and intercession they should be preserved in some form.

Fish's remedy proposes that vicious priests be punished, defrocked, and, most important, deprived of misgotten alms. If such steps were to be taken, "Then shal aswel the nombre of our foresaid monstruous sort as of the baudes, hores, theues, and idell people decreace. Then shall the great yerely exaccions cease. Then shall not your swerde, power, crowne, dignite, and obedience of your people, be translated from you."[48] If applied correctly, the king's sovereign power, superior to the clerical estate, may rid the realm of undesirables ("baudes, hores," etc.) while maintaining the all-important "obedience" of his subjects.

Fish floats the idea that the laity might liberate hospitals from clerical greed while preserving something essential in their caring mission: "Then shall your comons encrease in richesse. Then shall the gospel be preached. Then shall none begge our almesse from us. Then shall we haue ynough and more then shall suffice vs, whiche shall be the best hospitall that euer was founded for vs. Then shall we daily pray to god for your most noble estate long to endure."[49] In the absence of clerical participation, he suggests that the hospital may persist as a rationally organized, charitable institution that contributes rather than detracts from the common profit, and in which, crucially, the king's own salvation remains paramount.

The Reformation Parliament of 1529–36, which met to consider a petition advocating partial disendowment of the Catholic Church and the temporary transfer of ecclesiastical jurisdiction to the Crown, coincided with the *Supplication*'s publication. The timing was auspicious: free copies of the *Supplication* were handed out in London on the very day that the Reformation Parliament convened.[50] The *Supplication*'s mention of clerical incontinence intersected with many Londoners' concerns about clerical vice.[51] As we shall see in chapter 6, in St. Bartholomew's refoundation documents, concern for sexual propriety looms large as the hospital strives to reinvent itself in a new form resistant to slander.

## COPLAND'S *HYE WAY TO THE SPYTTELL HOUS*: THE HOSPITAL IN CRISIS

In contrast to Fish's *Supplication*, which leverages a radical critique of purgatory to intervene into the provision of charity, Robert Copland's *Hye Way to the Spyttell Hous*, printed circa 1536, neither fully condemns nor fully reimagines the hospital. Instead, Copland's long, impassioned poem maps the hospital's contemporary predicament in a uniquely nuanced manner. This largely overlooked work, partially a translation and free adaptation of Balsac's *Le Droict Chemin de L'Ospital* (1509), complements Copeland's earlier translations from French, which testify to his interests in organizing physical, moral, and spiritual health.[52] Copland's *Secrete of Secretes*, a translation of the *Secretum Secretorum* from an abridged French version, appeared in 1528. His *The maner to lyue well deuoutly and salutaryly euery day for all persones of mean estate*, which Erler calls "a daily spiritual regimen for lay persons concerned both with the fulfillment of worldly obligations and with spiritual advancement," was printed several times appended to François Regnault's primers in the 1520s and 30s.[53] In the *Hye Way*, Copland suggests, in satirical verse that nevertheless actively searches for answers, how St. Bartholomew's might fit as a charitable institution into the increasingly poor, overrun, and religiously reformed world of London. Orme and Webster rightly contend that this work belongs in a separate category from contemporary critiques, such as Fish's *Supplication*, for the centrality of the hospital within it: "It survives in only two copies and uses hospitals as the starting-point of a discussion of society rather than a topic in their own right. It is original, nevertheless, in the extent of its interest in hospitals and valuable in showing how a contemporary viewed the strengths and weaknesses of hospitals on the eve of the Reformation."[54]

Although I agree with Orme and Webster's assessment of the work's interest and value, I depart from their view that in the *Hye Way* the hospital functions as a mere "starting-point." I contend that Copland's innovative work places the hospital—St. Bartholomew's to be precise—at its very center. His poem shows, in its original content, in its adaptations from the French source, and in its final section delineating beggars according to the seven deadly sins, how the institution's own history intersects awkwardly with the symptoms of contemporary London poverty.[55] Like Daly, who suggests that Copland found hospitals "worth salvaging for the valuable social services they rendered," Orme and Webster view Copland's portrayal of the hospital as largely "favourable."[56] On the one hand, they note that the poem's porter (a central figure) appears "at the gate where he should be; he is highly experienced in the ways of the world and skilled in distinguishing between the poor. Hospital sisters minister within, and those who die are charitably buried." Yet on the other hand, they note that the poem acknowledges the poor management of some hospitals, fails to mention the hospital clergy, and even suggests that some institutions actively welcome the unworthy poor.[57]

My analysis contributes a more complex sense of how Copland represents the hospital at this moment in its history. Copland's emphasis on deceptive performance and confusions of identity and social function marks his *Hye Way* as an early example of rogue literature, perhaps representing "a kind of origin to the genre."[58] Yet this is not a generalized "doctrinal complaint," but a complaint with a purpose related to the hospital itself.[59] In the *Hye Way* such confusions render it difficult to tell deserving from undeserving, to understand people's motives for coming to the hospital, or to discern what role the hospital should play in their lives and within the wider city. Rather than going unmentioned, the hospital clergy actually do appear in refracted, debased forms in the clerical figures who haunt the hospital's gates as paupers but are denied admission.

The first half of the *Hye Way* is original to Copland, not derived from the French source. From the start, the work discloses a specific knowledge of St. Bartholomew's history, from alluding to the founder Rahere—"To these poore folke / and god his soule pardon / That for theyre sake / made this foundacyon"—to listing the worthy poor as a group corresponding with traditional categories of patients received at St. Bartholomew's:[60]

Forsoth they that be at suche myschefe
That for theyre lyuyng can do no labour
And haue no frendes to do them socour
*As old people / seke / and impotent*
*Poore women in chyldbed haue here easement*
Weyke men sore wounded by great vyolence
And sore men eaten with pockes and pestylence
*And honest folke fallen in great pouerte*
*By myschaunce or other infyrmyte*
Way faryng men, and maymed souldyours
Haue theyr relyef in this poure hous of ours,
And all other which we seme good and playne
Haue here lodgyng for a nyght or twayne
*Bedred folke / and suche as can not craue*
*In these places / moost relyef they haue*
*And yf they hap / within our place to dye*
*Than are they buryed / well and honestly*
But not euery vnseke stoborne knaue
For than we shold ouer many haue.

(98–115; emphasis added)

Offering a traditional list of the "deserving poor," the porter's litany names categories of residents seen at St. Bartholomew's since Rahere's time: the poor and ill ("pauperes et infirmi"), pregnant women, travelers, the elderly, all of whom may receive proper burial there if necessary.[61] The current problem is confusion in the hospital's mission: Does it receive everyone who seeks relief there, or does it discriminate worthy from unworthy poor? The Porter gives an equivocal answer: "Forsoth yea / *we do all suche folke in take* / That do aske lodgyng for oure lordes sake / And in dede it is our custome and vse / *Sometyme to take in / and some to refuse*" (48–51; emphasis added). It seems strange that the Porter, who is literally the gatekeeper, cannot articulate a consistent policy on hospital admissions. I suggest a reason for this beyond simple incoherence. As an early example of rogue literature, the *Hye Way* links the newly amplified category of rogues and vagrants with a crisis in the administration of traditional charity at the hospital. As familiar identity categories begin to break down, and vagrants increasingly impersonate the deserving poor (a key element of their practice, as represented in rogue pamphlets), it becomes more difficult to discern the categories that had in earlier days, Copland implies, been more transparent.[62] Interrogating the implications of this social change for the hospital is a major preoccupation of the *Hye Way*, making it a central work for a literary history of the hospital.

Attempting to clarify his earlier comments, the Porter is at pains to explain which categories of supplicants are not welcomed at the "spytell house." Some categories of beggars are simply charlatans, including the "masterless men" and "nyghtingales of newgate" (jailbirds), familiar from other rogue literature. But the characters of "Rogers" (306–23), "Clewners" (324–44), and "Sapyent" (347–455) seem especially unusual and deserve further scrutiny. And although other critics have recognized the poem as "an independent and topical satire" on London poverty, and more globally as a searching critique of the failures of charity, intimating a "transnational, transhistorical critique of wealth," there has been little attention paid to the meaning of the *hospital* within the poem, beyond agreement that it depicts St. Bartholomew's, and that it suggests the hospital is generally doing a good job upholding its "ancient duty of ministering to the sick, infirm and needy."[63] I suggest that these strange figures point us to the poem's searching commentary on the past, present, and future civic role of the hospital. They become keys to Copland's larger project if we read the work with an understanding of the hospital's historical functions, as a place of intercession, clerical discipline, and medical care. Each of these portraits embodies a degraded version of the spiritual and medical practices that the institution had historically supported, indicating that it has ceased to perform them and that these individuals impiously abuse the trust of founders and benefactors, but without arguing that the traditional practices are in themselves unredeemable.

Copland uses the Roger, the Clewner, and the Sapyent to suggest that although there may have been right ways to live collectively and productively in the hospital, these figures are failing to embody them. At the same time, the *Hye Way* shows that the hospital's traditional practices have become untenable at this historical moment. As a site for spiritual and physical healing, the institution finds itself at a point of reckoning where it must change to survive the current crisis. The poem's incoherence, as it lurches between three parts, as to whether the hospital is discriminating or not with its charity, what kinds of people are welcome there, and what kind of institution it is—a prison, a school, a home?—speaks to an impasse in the institution's mission, one which Copland exposes not to condemn, but to reform.

Having evoked the hospital's history and the confusion of its mission, Copland hits his stride with descriptions of various unsavory groups who come to the hospital even though they do not deserve its charity. Having expressed ambiguity as to who is actually admitted to the hospital, the following section does little to clarify this question, instead multiplying lurid portraits of urban vice. Clearly, exposing the deceptions of rogues and vagabonds is part of the poem's purpose, as Copland shows how counterfeiting, mobility, and roguery intersect, to the institution's detriment.[64] At the same time, with these early portraits, the "Copland" speaker begins to show knowledge and sympathy for the spiritual aims of the hospital: in relation to the "maysterles men" who claim to have "serued the kyng," "Me thynk it is a *great soule heale* / To help them tyll they were pouruayd / Into some seruyce" (199–201; emphasis added). The hospital's mission is not just to provide lodging but to promote "soule heale" (spiritual health), making a particular concern for the hospital integral to the "doctrinal complaint" that the poem articulates. The ambiguity in his phrase "it is a great soule heale" suggests that spiritual health may travel in two directions, as a benefit experienced both by those who "help" (the hospital staff) and those who are helped by the charity, delivered at least temporarily from lives of destitution and vice. Although the speaker Copland's naïve belief that these masterless men truly did serve the king is disabused by the Porter's explanation that "they do were souldyers clothyng / And so beggyng deceuye folke ouer all / For they be vacabondes moost in generall" (205–7), nevertheless the motive of "soule heale" remains valid, confirmed by the Porter who agrees, "That is trouth" (204), before he goes on to reveal their deceptions. The traditional centrality of "soule heale" in the hospital milieu demands that readers attend to this value and its current fortunes.

The idea that the hospital is linked to a historical project of spiritual healing, one that has been submerged and betrayed, but not forgotten, undergirds the following portraits, which reference the historical ideals of "soule heale" (liturgical, spiritual, medical) even as they depict a crisis in the hospital's current practices. In describing these figures, Copland expresses an awareness of and perhaps a nostalgia for the old routines, even as he suggests that they can no longer be practiced amid the current crisis in legibility where the "deserving poor" are impersonated by "vagrants." Copland's description of the "Rogers," itinerant student beggar clerics, is the first to evoke and then pervert traditional hospital routines and priorities.

The label "Rogers" is of uncertain origin, apparently the first recorded use of the term to mean "a corrupt clerical-student beggar."[65] The first activity mentioned is their performance of prayers:

> But to our purpose / cometh not this way
> Of these Rogers? / that dayly syng and pray
> *With Aue regina / or De profundis*
> *Quem terra ponthus / and Stella maris*
> At euery dore there thy foot and frydge
> And say thay come fro Oxford and Cambrydge
> *And be poore scolers / and have no maner thyng*
> *Nor also frendes / to kepe them at lernyng*
> *And so do lewtre only for crust and crum.*
> With staffe in hand / and fyst in bosum.
>                       (306–14; emphasis added)

At first glance these unfortunate "rogers" seem to signal a widespread employment crisis in the clerical proletariat, one that had persisted well into the sixteenth century. Copland's passage distantly recalls the lament of *Piers Plowman*'s C text narrator, a university-educated cleric who has lost his patrons and vows to work where he can with the only tools he has, including "*pater-noster* and my prymer, *placebo* and *dirige*, / And my sauter som tyme and my seuene psalmes."[66] Both poets, though distant in time from each other, evoke the desperate poverty that would lead an unbeneficed cleric to sing liturgical devotions for anyone and everyone who could pay. These poor clerics have become virtually indistinguishable from beggars: Langland's clerical speaker is a beggar "withoute bagge or botel but my wombe one," while Copland's wandering "rogers" pathetically "lewtre only for crust and crum, / With staffe in hand / and fyst in bosum." Both wandering clerics palpably suffer the pains of hunger.

Whereas Langland's speaker cites "*placebo* and *dirige*," readings from the Office of the Dead that make up some of the standard "labouring psalms" performed by proletarian clerics,[67] Copland's lines more closely evoke the hospital context in their references not only to the Office of the Dead ("De profundis"), but more prominently to Marian devotions ("Aue regina," "Quem terra ponthus," and "Stella maris").[68] These Marian works were by no means unusual—they were familiar songs within hospitals, practices that we have repeatedly seen privileged in their literary remains. Devotion to the Virgin Mary was amply attested in the regulations, bequests, and surviving books of St. Leonard's and St. Bartholomew's: both houses possessed altars dedicated to Mary at which antiphons such as Ave Regina were performed daily. Copland thus evokes the commemoration of the dead and Marian devotions prominent in hospital liturgies: key practices that contributed to the "soulc hcalc" of brothers, patients, and dead patrons.

Copland's portrayal of the wandering "rogers" evokes a rupture in the clerical life cycle, recalling a range of "poor scolers" traditionally associated with the hospital. In the *Hye Way*, these figures perform prayers daily, but aimlessly, without a liturgical home or a clear purpose. Their status as wandering clerks seeking entrance to the hospital evokes both the "poor scholars" provided for by St. Bartholomew's hospital residents, such as Thomas Gyvendale and Beatrice Lurchon, and a debased version of the hospital brothers who received dispensation to study then returned to the house to resume duties of prayer and pastoral care. The fact that they "lewtre" (loiter), or stay in one place in order to beg, is striking in relation to the historical hospital: loitering (a characteristic mark of the vagabond) ironically mimics the stability required of hospital brothers, a lifetime commitment to a single spiritual home in contrast to a temporary place of convenience.

Again making a mockery of the proper Augustinian clerical life cycle, these figures who should be spiritually productive in their youth wrongly rcsort to the hospital before their time:

Such folkes of trouth cometh here dayly
*And ought of ryght this house for to vse*
*In theyre aege* / for they fully do refuse
The tyme of vertuous exercyse
Wherby they shold vnto honour aryse.
            (319–23; emphasis added)

Such people, university clerks (if they truly are) should not need to "use" the hospital until they are old: this would be the "ryght" way for them to live in the house. This image calls to mind the hospital's traditional function as a place for such clerks in their old age, a place of retirement, as for older Augustinian brothers, such as John Cok, who recorded the passing of time with his tremulous hand, and the numbers of secular retirees, male and female, we have encountered in this study.[69] The complaint that these Rogers make, that they "haue no maner thyng / Nor also frendes" (312–13), is repeated again by the Clewners, their superiors and "mayster Wardeyns" (326), who likewise complain, in order to gain entrance to the house, that "frends haue they none / To gyue them ony exhybycion" (334–45). Although he presents them as somewhat like a corrupt fraternity, a rogues' brotherhood akin to those depicted in later rogue texts,[70] the ideal implied is that of the *hospital* in its traditional capacity as a community of "frendes": clerical brothers, the "master" who oversees them, and a varied group of other residents, including women, children, and students.

For a contrast to this crisis of priestly fraternity, in which clerics violate their life cycles only to suffer abandonment by "frendes," one might look to the nearby "Pappey" hospital (the Fraternity of St. Charity of the Priests of London).[71] Copland's readers may well have known this institution. Like St. Bartholomew's, the Pappey was sited in the north of London along the city wall, to the east rather than the west. In keeping with broader fifteenth-century foundation patterns, this fraternity received a royal license in 1442 as an exclusive, self-regulating clerical institution. The Pappey gathered aged, feeble chantry priests under a priestly master and two wardens to offer "obsecraciones, oraciones, postulaciones et graciarum accciones" (supplications, prayers, intercessions and giving of thanks) for the king and heirs.[72] A mid-fifteenth-century observer approvingly described the house as follows: "Pappy Chyrche . . . ys a grete fraternyte of prestys and of othyr seqular men. And there ben founde of almys certayne prestys, bothe blynde and lame, that be empotent; and they have day masse and xiiij d. a weke, barber and launder, and one to dresse and provyde for hyr mete and drynke."[73] The house's officers (master and two wardens) were charged with supervising the ailing brethren, meeting their physical and spiritual needs and ensuring their good conduct.[74]

In order to constitute a coherent, self-regulating community, the fraternity's detailed regulations vested power in members to elect the master and wardens. Brethren and successors "sui Magistrum huiusmodi de seipsis tociens quociens expediens viderint eligere, perficere et ammovere possint" (have power to elect, appoint, and remove such master as often as they should think fit), and the fraternity is described as "vnum corpus in lege et communitas perpetua" (one body in law, and a perpetual community).[75] The Pappey's accounts indicate that the house continued to enlarge its property and accrue donations until its dissolution in 1548, when six brothers were recorded in residence.[76] Perhaps the founders' minute efforts to legislate communal self-regulation and supervision enabled the hospital to avoid the breakdowns in clerical hierarchy and community that Copland suggests had befallen St. Bartholomew's, where those claiming the title of "mayster Wardens" are exposed by the Porter not as duly elected leaders but as "deceuyers of people ouerall" (330).

Without financial support or a community, the Clewners are would-be chantry priests lacking the means to perform their liturgical duties properly. Their main task appears to be commemoration, the duty of a chaplain and one of the hospital's core functions:

> And how that they forth wold passe
> To theyr countrees / and syng theyr fyrst masse
> And there pray for theyr benefactours
> And serue god all tymes and houres
> And so they lewtre in such rogacyons
> Seuen or eyght yeres walkyng theyr stacyons
> And do but gull / and follow beggery
> Feynyng true doyng by hypocrysy.
>
> (336–44)

The Clewners desire to return to "theyr countrees" to perform intercessory prayer, but they cannot. This picture of what they wish they could do looks much like the idealized vision of the hospital: a life in which they daily "pray for theyr benefactours" and serve "god all tymes and houres." But like the Rogers they "lewtre" idly and temporarily rather than finding a permanent spiritual home. One could certainly argue, as most critics of the poem have assumed, that these are simply pictures of deceptive opportunists attempting to exploit the hospital's charity, and this would not be wrong. But I am suggesting that in evoking these particular rhythms of spiritual life, Copland gestures meaningfully to a culture of "soule heale" that was once robust, but in the current atmosphere of religious change, lack of funding, and profusion of destitutes, can no longer function as it had just ten or twenty years before.

The previous two characters portray the debasement of "soule heale," yet I see Copland's portrait of the Sapyent as commenting on the hospital's traditional commitment to healing (or at least comforting) the bodies of the poor and ill, particularly women and children. In the portrait of the horrifying mountebank who claims to be a healer yet does nothing to help an ailing child except extract money from his poor mother, we see a faint echo, more diffuse than in the earlier two portraits, of the hospital's historical medical role. Following the story of the Clewners, Copeland describes

> fals brybours, deceytfull and fraudelent,
> That among people call themselfs Sapyent
> These ryde about in many sondry wyse
> And in straunge aray / do themselves dysguyse
> Somtyme in maner of a physycyan
> And another tyme as a hethen man
> Countrefaytng theyre own tonge and speche.
>                               (346–51)

As Erler notes, per Henry VIII's statutes, it was illegal to practice medicine without a license from the diocese (1512) or, as of 1522, when physicians were exempted from clerical control, without permission from the London College of Physicians.[77] We do not have many records of physicians working at St. Bartholomew's prior to the refoundation, but Mirfield's *Breviarium* and *Florarium* testify to the hospital's medical mission and to the genuine learning (albeit more theoretical than practical) that underpinned medical knowledge as it circulated within the late medieval institution. Here we see an inversion of the traditional hospital's combination of practical care, usually undertaken by the nursing sisters, and the learned medical tradition as compiled by clerics like Mirfield. The mountebank combines the worst of both, claiming bogus knowledge to effect useless cures. In his manifest falseness, he embodies an affront to the medical ideals that Mirfield expresses in the *Florarium*: physicians should be straightforward Christians, where he is indeterminately "hethen," and they must never privilege making money, which he accepts despite feigning disinterest. The following passage also incorporates language strongly recalling another statute of 22 Henry VIII, containing specific provisions that bring together vagabondage and pretensions of false learning:

And maketh a maner of straunge countenauce
With admyracyons his falsnes to auaunce
And whan he cometh there as he wold be
Than wyll he feyne meruelyous grauyte
And so chaunceth his hostes or his hoost
To demaund, out of what straunge land or coost
Cometh this gentylman? forsothe hostesse
This man was borne in hethenesse
Sayth his seruaunt. And is a connyng man
For all the seuen scyences surely he can
And is sure in Physyk and Palmestry
In augury, sothsayeng, and vysenamy [physiognomy].

(356–67)

His staged performance, complete with servant-expositor, layers deception upon itself: having feigned incomprehension of English in order to
"auaunce" his appearance of foreignness, he must then "feyne meruelyous
grauyte" to act the learned physician, even as his long list of knowledges,
which combines the occult "sothsayeng" with the more reputable practice
of "vysenamy" suggests something unsavory about him.[78]

Such a character would violate a royal statute promulgated in 1531,
which penalized begging scholars lacking authorization from their universities and others feigning particular forms of learning in order to trick people.
Copland seems to be alluding to the statute's collocation of offenders in his
interlinked portraits of the Rogers, Clewners, Pardoners, and Sapyents, especially in his phrase "Physyk and Palmestry / In augury, sothsayeng, and
vysenamy." In addition to censoring unauthorized begging by scholars, the
royal order specified that

all Proctours & Pardoners goyng about in any contrey or contrayes
without suffycyent authoryte, & all other ydell personnes goynge aboute
in any contreys or abydyng in any Cytie Boroughe or Towne, *some of
them usyng dyers & subtyle craftye & unlawfull games & playes & some of
them feynyng themselfes to have knowledge in Physyke, Physnamye,
Palmestrye, or other craftye scyences wherby they beare the people in hande,
that they can tell theire destenyes & fortunes & suche other lyke fantasticall*

*ymagenacions to the greate deceypte of the Kynges Subjects,* shall upon ex-
amynacion had before two Justices of Peace . . . yf he by Provable
Wytnes be founde giltie of any suche deceytes be punysshed by whyp-
pyng at two dayes together.[79]

Tracking closely with the statute's language, Copland points to the character of the Sapyent as not only a dubious but an officially censured character. In his version, this figure is a criminal offending against the hospital's
medical traditions, combining the reputable science of "physyk" with the
less savory practices of "palmestry" and its occult companions "augury,
sothsayeng, and vysenamy."

Related and perhaps most damning in the hospital context is the false
Sapyent's greed, a characteristic that Mirfield had argued was misplaced in
the physician, who should be a good Christian. Such a man "deberet curare
infirmum christianum etiam gratis si infirmus pauper sit, quia plus debet
valere apud eum vita illius quam eius pecunia" (ought to cure a Christian patient without making even the slightest charge if the man is poor;
for the life of such a man ought to be of more value to the physician
than his money).[80] Our Sapyent makes two protestations of generosity, first
via his servant—"No money he taketh, but all for gods loue" (378); "He wyll
no money / hostesse I you promyt" (400)—leaving the "hostesse," mother
to the afflicted child, to say to his "felawe," who comes round the next day, "I
maruell that he wold / But of charyte, in such a meane houshold" (432–33).
Entreating the Sapyent's partner to "Help this poor chylde, of this sayd seke-
ness," she presses upon him the large amount of ".xx. shyllyngs for your
payne / And your exspence for a weke or twayne" (438–39). It seems that
they are finally paid double, for the Sapyent's "felawe" also demands payment "for the drogges / that occupy he shall / The whiche be dere / and very
precyous" (443–44). Having supplied worthless drugs and lived "a fourte-
nyght a borde" with the unfortunate family, the charlatans escape to "make
theyr avaunt / of theyr deceytes / and drynk adew taunt" with friends in a
typical alehouse scenario (456–57).

This figure's association with the hospital is ambiguous in Copland's
rendering. He avers at the end of the portrait: "the spytell is not for theyr
estate / Howbeit they come dayly by the gate" (460–61). Is he arguing that
this medical charlatan attempts to practice there, or that he seeks charity at
the hospital when his money has run out? Either way, his false care and
greed make a mockery of the hospital's healing mission, for he has egre-

giously preyed upon a mother and child, traditional figures of pity and care at St. Bartholomew's.

In borrowing from Balsac's *Droict Chemin de L'Ospital* in the second half of his poem, as Moore has shown, Copland expands its examples of misbehavior to a different purpose. Whereas Balsac's project was to delineate all the types of bad conduct that landed people in poverty and despair, leading them to a (generic) hospital, Copland emphasizes the *hospital* as the destination, giving the place priority and making it a subtly different kind of place depending on the type of seeker. In my view, Copland does something more than turn Balsac's "formless catalogue" into an "independent and topical satire."[81] He shows that the institution has adapted itself, or has been forced, in current circumstances, to take in the variety of poor whose "very nede" means that they cannot be refused. In the final section of the poem, where Copland matches needy and vicious folk to each of the seven deadly sins, the familiar catechetical framework drives home a similar point. There are no alternatives to the hospital; the institution must take in even the most hardened sinners in the knowledge that they are rogues, unredeemable as such characters tend to be.[82]

Copland makes several changes to the form and content of Balsac's work, reshaping it for his new purpose. Balsac's prose lists on its first page a huge variety of misgoverned folk, from "Gens qui ont petit et despendent beaucoup" (those who have little and spend much) to "Gens qui nont gueres biens and entretiennent grant estat" (those who have few goods and yet maintain a great estate) to "gens opiniastres et incorrigibles" (willful and incorrigible folk). All are destined to end up "a l'ospital" (at the hospital). Their failings send them to a single rather amorphous destination, the hospital whose "priuileges droitz et prerogatives" (privileges, rights and prerogatives) they are entitled to "enjoy" by virtue of their "oeuures et maniere de viure" (works and way of life), as the ironic prologue reads. In contrast, Copland's translation captures and sentences each of these subjects in stanzas, adapting the final line of each stanza to indicate the *hospital*'s response to the sins or needs of each debased guest. In varying these final lines to make the hospital ("our hous" in the Porter's repeated phrase), a reluctant haven for everyone from the poorly wedded, to the vain, to old folks who unwisely give everything to their children, Copland deepens the ambiguity of the earlier lines, suggesting that the hospital does have to shelter most of those who seek aid there, despite their unworthiness. Therein lies the problem: the hospital's welcome of all comers, a policy that needs reforming.

Despite the deceptiveness and criminality of its subjects, this section of the poem emphasizes even more strongly that these undesirables are rarely turned away from the hospital. Enhancing Balsac's brief descriptions to increase the detail of their sinfulness, the stanzas also frequently conclude by emphasizing the intensity of the subjects' need. The following two stanzas develop two lines from Balsac (corresponding to lines 512–13) to create a picture of dissolution that nevertheless results in genuine need:

> Yong heyres that enioy theyr herytage
> Rulyng themself / or they come to aege
> Occupyeng vnthryfty company
> Spendyng vp theyr patrymony
> Whyles they be yong, and vse dyssolute playes
> *Of very nede they must come these wayes*
> All such people as have lytell to spend
> Wastyng it, tyll it be at an end
> And whan they be seke / and haue nothyng
> Toward the spytell than they be coming.
> (506–15; emphasis added)

Here we see a stern criticism of the "yong heyres" who spend their entire inheritance before they "come to aege" (an intriguing echo of the earlier clerics who arrived at the hospital before they had reached "theyr aege"). Despite the fact they these young heirs are wastrels, spending their money on the most frivolous and ephemeral thing—"dissolute playes"—nevertheless "very nede" compels them to seek help at the hospital. The lens suddenly widens to include "all such people as have lytell to spend" who are forced to seek out the hospital when they "haue nothyng." Copland uses the verse deftly to reinforce the sense of inevitability and genuine need that he is describing: the "nothyng" that leads to their "comyng" to the hospital.

One may discern this inevitability a few lines later in another adaptation that not only details the subjects' dissolution but also highlights the hospital's obligation to help them:

Landlordes that do no reparacyons
But leue theyre landes in desolacyons
Theyr housyng vnkempt wynd and water tyght
Letyng the pryncypals rot down ryght
And suffreth theyr tenaunts to renne away
*The way to our hous we can them not denay.*

(528–33; emphasis added)

The first lines elaborate on the spare source, adding evocative details and alliteration to vivify the landlord's destructive negligence of a house.[83] But the last line, completely new to the *Hye Way*, is both emphatic and ambiguous. If we consider the pattern of all of these stanzas, "Landlordes," the subject of the stanza, seems to be the antecedent for "them," yet alongside this negligent victim appear "theyr tenaunts," made homeless by the landlord's incompetence. It would seem then that the Porter is acknowledging the hospital's duty to welcome all those needing shelter, thereby fulfilling one of the works of mercy, whether the homeless have caused their own desperate situation or are innocent victims. Either way, the line implies, the institution "can . . . not denay" its obligation to those lacking shelter (see fig. 5.1).

The final section of Copland's work, in which he relates the seven deadly sins to the hospital's clientele, might again be seen as a simple litany of the destitute and sinful, as in Balsac's text. Yet here in a slightly different mode Copland is working within a didactic idiom familiar to the particular institution of the hospital, a place of catechetical teaching and devotional reading in which priests and laity shared, as we saw in chapter 4. Here we see characters grouped according to their salient sin, in a slightly eccentric list that includes swearing.[84] These folks seem far from sympathetic: they are "full of iniquyte" and "so full of couetyse / That all the wordles good can them not suffyse / But by vsury / rapyne / and extorcyon / Do poulle the pore folke of theyr porcyon" (797–99). And yet, their inclusion in this section, organized according to their own sins, speaks again to the hospital's quandary: its obligation to offer charity to those who need it, despite their obvious sinfulness. The passage presents people whose sin has placed them in an impossible predicament, friendless and alone. The exchange of Copland and the Porter shows the paradoxical yet necessary obligation to care for such people:

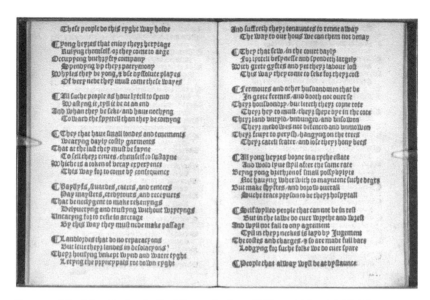

FIGURE 5.1   John Copland, *Hye Way to the Spyttell Hous.* © The British Library
Board, C.57.b.30, fol. C4. Reproduced with permission.

Copland.
How say ye by these folks full of yre
That brenne in wrath / hoter than fyre
And neuer be quyet / but chyde and brall
With wrath and anger fretyng hert and gall
Wayward / wode / furyous / and fell
For where they be / quyetnes cannot dwell
But always stryfe / mystrust / and greate dysease
And in no wyse non man can them please
Porter.
Hyther they come / and I will tell you why
None can lyue by them / well nor quyetly
But with eche one they fall out and make bate
Causyng people them for to hate
And wyll suffre them to dwell nowhere
But are fayne for to remayne here.

(847–60)

Copland's vivid description of the difficulty that anger presents to communal living evokes the impossibility of living with someone who is "Wayward / wode / furyous / and fell." In the face of anger, nobody can live in community. Yet paradoxically in generating "stryfe / mystrust / and greate dysease," anger drives sufferers to the hospital, that quintessential place of "dysease," a term that retains the psychological, physical, and emotional nuances that it possessed in late Middle English.[85] The hospital presents the only viable place for these people to come, for otherwise they are forced to "dwell nowhere." The hospital offers an unwilling refuge for the unwanted and the unacceptable, giving them a respite from erasure. There is nowhere else for these people to go, and it is of course ironic that the hospital *has* historically been a place for the intentional cultivation of community among laity, clergy, young and old. Copland is aware of this history and of London's need for an institution that will respond to urban poverty in its new complexity. A. E. B. Coldiron in her work on English translations from French, including the *Hye Way*, asks, "What does it mean to translate devotional verse—really a kind of applied doctrine—from France both before and after Henry VIII's break with Rome, when French religious discourses were also undergoing change?"[86] I suggest that by understanding the *Hye Way*'s evocation of the hospital's past, present, and future as a place of "soule heale," we may draw a line from the devotional literature of chapter 4 to this work, which attempts to serve a spiritual teaching function as well as a polemical one.

In this chapter, I have considered how a variety of writers envisioned the hospital as a problematic yet valuable, potentially salvageable place of spiritual and medical care. These voices bear vivid witness to the strains that economic and religious change placed upon the idea of the hospital as an urban charitable institution. In chapter 6, I will examine how our three hospitals used a range of textual and practical resources to respond to these developments, with results from disappearance to refoundation in variously reformed incarnations.

# SIX

# Dissolution, Disappearance, and Refoundation

## *Textual Strategies of Reconstitution*

In this final chapter, I consider the varied responses of our three hospitals to the civic and religious changes that gripped England from 1534 (King Henry VIII's breach with Rome) to 1553 (King Edward VI's death and the accession of Queen Mary). St. Leonard's, St. Bartholomew's, and St. Mark's were all subject to Henry's Act of Supremacy and subsequent appropriation of religious assets in the gradual process known euphemistically as the "Dissolution" of the religious houses. These institutions' responses to existential threat drew upon and reimagined the literary and cultural practices that they had cultivated over their long medieval histories, to very different ends. Beginning with St. Leonard's, I show that this venerable hospital remained culturally prominent in York, contributing to public religious ceremonial and civic welfare up to its surrender in 1539. Yet without strong support from the larger city, and in the politically perilous aftermath of the northern rebellions, St. Leonard's, with its rich endowments and desirable campus, became uniquely vulnerable to royal and ecclesiastical depredation, and ultimately disappearance, rather than the promised reformation. In contrast, St. Bartholomew's of London narrowly escaped dissolution to survive in a reformed secular reincarnation that depended upon the strategic use of texts: letters, regulations, and records. St. Bartholomew's new leaders answered both the reformed religious critique of purgatory and the secular desire to aid the poor, managing "a conscious abrogation of the hold of the past" and "a prioritization of resources towards meeting the needs of this world rather than the next."[1] Texts proved instrumental in that effort. Forging a third path toward reconstitution, after its surrender in 1540, St. Mark's Hospital, Bristol reemerged as a civic chapel, in a reduced yet visible pattern that may have enabled the creative recycling of older liturgical and spiritual texts by former hospital personnel.

Without rehearsing the convoluted history of the Dissolution, which has been well described elsewhere, I aim to consider how each hospital fared within the shifting landscape of reformation and refoundation after 1539.[2] For more than a century, English hospitals had been subject to critique on religious, political, and social grounds: it is impossible to disentangle these varying motivations in the story of their dissolutions. Henry VIII's break with Rome in 1534 over the matter of the royal divorce preceded the radicalization of his religious views, yet his desire for monastic assets and increasing hostility toward purgatory seem to have evolved in parallel.[3] When, after breaking with the papacy, Henry sought a valuation of church property in order to organize a new system of taxation, the religious houses presented a tempting source of revenue. In the *Valor Ecclesiasticus*, published in 1535, many hospitals were included (including St. Bartholomew's), if they were staffed with numerous clergy and resembled monasteries, but others were exempt if they dispensed alms at their founders' orders or if they did not have resident clergy (this latter category included many recent almshouse foundations).[4]

After a new parliamentary statute of 1536 authorized the Crown to dissolve religious houses with £200 income or less per year, a "creeping process" of individual surrenders rather than dissolution by statute led to the surrenders of St. Mark's, Bristol and of St. Leonard's, York in 1539.[5] We do not find a surrender document for St. Bartholomew's, which limped along with an uncertain future after 1539. Citizens soon realized that the disappearance of hospitals meant a loss of vital social services, and the reforming bishop Thomas Cranmer expressed grave disappointment that the wealth of dissolved institutions had not been put toward charitable purposes, such as "the founding . . . of grammar schools" or the "founding of hospitals, where poor and impotent people should have been sufficiently provided for."[6] Hence by 1539, Henry began to repurpose some of the buildings and wealth gained in the seizures. These efforts included turning dissolved properties to "better use" by maintaining old servants and reinvigorating almshouses and daily alms distribution, as well as founding new cathedrals and collegiate churches with poor relief as part of their mission.[7]

In addition to immediate practical losses of charity, the long-term spiritual implications of the hospital dissolutions were profound. Reconfiguring relations between the dead and the living amid the increasingly radical critique of purgatory presented a key challenge for hospitals as they reconstituted themselves in successive decades. Whereas St. Leonard's was never revived despite fitful attempts by York's citizenry, the reformation of St. Bartholomew's and St. Mark's into new civic forms depended upon textual means—civic letters, hospital orders, regulations, and liturgical practices. Another category of documents, records of the newly refounded St. Bartholomew's, testifies to the hospital's reformed self-understanding. As Paul Slack argues, since the early sixteenth century, "hospitals had been visualised as institutions which might not only express charitable instincts, relieve the poor, and protect public health, but in doing all those things bring about civic regulation and civic regeneration."[8] As I show, different kinds of "regulation" and "regeneration" unfolded and were interrogated in texts from St. Bartholomew's and St. Mark's. As part of this regenerative process, new hospital texts answered the literatures of complaint that we considered in chapter 5 and reflected (explicitly or not) on each institution's distinctive late medieval literary history.

### York's Hospital of St. Leonard:<br>Cultural Continuities and a Surprising Surrender

In the fifteenth century, St. Leonard's Hospital of York used its signature *Purification* pageant to broadcast the institution's long-standing devotion to Mary and advertise the house as a desirable spiritual home for widows. Although we do not know precisely when the pageant fell into abeyance, the hospital had certainly ceased to sponsor its drama some years before 1477, when the episode reentered the cycle to be produced by the Masons and Laborers. Despite the financial challenges of the later fifteenth century and the loss of its signature drama, St. Leonard's remained visible and viable well into the sixteenth century with a range of ongoing devotional, civic ceremonial, and educational functions. In this section, I consider evidence for these cultural continuities up until the hospital's surrender in December 1539. The surrender, by then-master Thomas Magnus, a noted pluralist and a member of the Council of the North, probably came as a surprise to many in York, yet it seems to have occasioned little civic outcry.

How could the north's largest, most venerable hospital surrender so readily despite its historic resilience? The surrender came after almost a decade of negotiations among Cardinal Wolsey, King Henry, and local ecclesiastics, rather than as a response to any significant reported malfeasance during the 1535 visitations of the northern religious houses.[9] St. Leonard's long-standing independence from civic control had at times proved a source of power, as when in the thirteenth century the hospital had resisted coming under the city's patronage.[10] But during Henry VIII's reign, St. Leonard's historic dependence on the monarch and relatively weak base of civic support made it vulnerable to the king's whims. By the late 1530s, Henry was avidly searching for sources of revenue in church properties and may also have hardened his attitude toward York's traditional religious houses after the 1536 Pilgrimage of Grace, a northern rebellion against his religious policies, which the city had supported. St. Leonard's, unlike other hospitals in York with stronger civic ties, would never be reconstituted.

### Devotion to the Virgin Mary and St. Leonard

Early in the sixteenth century, remaining in King Henry's good graces enabled the hospital to ride out some of the worst effects of financial exigency. In late 1515, the king granted St. Leonard's an exemption from its customary payment of tenths and subsidies. The king's letter patent of November 12 speaks fulsomely of his own traditional devotion, referring to "singularem deuocionem quam ad sanctam et indiuiduam Trinitatem gloriosissimamque virginem Mariam Dei genitricem et gloriosum Confessorem Sanctum Leonardum gerimus et habemus" (the singular devotion that I have and had to the holy and undivided Trinity, the most glorious Virgin Mary, mother of God, and the glorious confessor St. Leonard).[11] He makes the exemption from payments perpetual on the condition that the hospital's master, brothers, and their successors will pray "pro prospero statu nostro et precarissime consortis mee Katerine Anglie Regine dum vixerimus necnon pro animabus nostris et progenitorum nostrorum" (for our prosperous estate and that of my most dear consort, Katherine, Queen of England, so long as we live and also for our souls and those of our parents).[12]

   The king's letter implies that St. Leonard's retained its reputation for devotion to the Trinity, the Virgin Mary, and St. Leonard. The Marian piety that the hospital had once performed publicly with the *Purification* pageant continued to thrive within its precincts. We know from the hospital's 1294 ordinances, discussed in chapter 1, that devotions to Mary featured in the daily liturgy. The altar dedicated to her continued to receive gifts. For example, in 1505 Emmota Storm of Walmgate bequeathed "to oure lady grace of Saynt Leonerds a crosse of sylver and guylte."[13]

Lay residents of the hospital precinct also demonstrated continuing devotion to the Virgin Mary and St. Leonard during the first quarter of the sixteenth century. Just as the earlier wills from the hospital peculiarly reveal the presence of pious widows, the same register contains several sixteenth-century wills of men hailing from the nearby village of Newton-on-Ouse. Newton's lands had largely been in the possession of the hospital since their grant in the twelfth century, and the village's parish church was also controlled by the hospital.[14] Perhaps these precinct residents, who included several husbandmen, a weaver, a smith, and a laborer, had come to the hospital to work on its premises and then stayed for the rest of their lives. Most of these men were devotees of the guild of St. Mary in the Newton parish church: they wished to be buried in the church and left bequests to their guild in varying amounts. At the same time, some showed devotion to St. Leonard's, which must have served as another devotional hub over many years. A typical will is that of William Wrightson, husbandman, recorded in July 1522. Having asked for burial in the Newton parish church, Wrightson indicates, "I yif and will to the howse of Saynt Leonardes of York iij s iiij d. Also I will to our lady gild of Newton aforesaid ij d to be praid for."[15] A bit like Henry VIII on an extremely modest scale, Wrightson anticipated that his donations to St. Leonard's and the Virgin Mary would result in prayers toward his salvation. Many of these male testators left wives behind; one may imagine that these widows, already part of the precinct community, continued to live and worship in the hospital's orbit like the fifteenth-century widows who had preceded them.

### The Hospital, Civic Ceremony, and the Work of Charity

Although we might expect the hospital to have receded from public ceremonial responsibilities once it no longer sponsored its annual *Purification* pageant in the Corpus Christi cycle, St. Leonard's remained involved in provisions for York's yearly dramatic event, which continued to take place on the feast day even after King Edward's suppression of Corpus Christi in

1547.[16] The cycle was performed yearly with few exceptions until 1569, through the reigns of Henry, Edward, Mary, and Elizabeth.[17] In the later fifteenth and early sixteenth century, St. Leonard's continued to appear sporadically in civic records as contributing to the play's performance. An ongoing desire to publicize its mission in association with the play, but perhaps a downturn in fortunes, might explain why the hospital, sometimes with other groups and individuals, rented out the eighth pageant station at Stonegate landing (the station closest to its own campus). The hospital rented the station in 1454 together with the Augustinian friars and one Thomas Brignall, in 1468 (with unnamed others) and in 1499 (alone).[18] In 1499, perhaps owing to reduced circumstances, the hospital paid only two shillings four pence for the Stonegate station, the second cheapest rental that year.[19] In 1516, St. Leonard's paid for the rental of a hall (*aulo*) rather than a station. Richard Beadle notes of these rentals that "possibly this association with the Play substituted for the bringing forth of the pageant."[20]

By sponsoring a station or a hall (the latter's purpose is not clear), St. Leonard's publicized its own charitable activities to the play's spectators and contributed visibly to the larger annual urban devotional enterprise, which had itself long been understood by its producers as a work of charity. A 1399 petition describes the play as "en ouere de charitee pur le profitte de les ditz Comunes & de les Estraungers repairauncez a la dite Citee a lonor (..) dieu & nuresaunce de charitee" (a work of charity for the benefit of the said commons and of the strangers who have traveled to the said city for the honour of God and the promotion of charity).[21] Thus at the start of Henry VIII's reign, St. Leonard's remained visible as a promoter of charity on multiple fronts.

Even more venerable than its link to the Corpus Christi play was St. Leonard's privileged role in the Corpus Christi procession, a hierarchical public display on the day after Corpus Christi that shared a similar stated rationale: to promote "laudem dei, honestatem sacerdocii, edificacionem ac bonum exemplum tocius populi christiani maxime autem ad honore dei & ciuitatis Ebor" (the praise of God, the respectability of the priesthood, the edification and good example of all Christian people, but most of all for the honour of God and of the city of York).[22] Since at least 1426 the hospital had been the location where the Host was deposited mid-procession before its grand progress resumed: "Precedentibus numeroso lumine torchearum & magna multitudine sacerdotum in superpelicijs indutorum & subsequentibus maiore & ciuibus Ebor' cum alterius magna copia populi confluentis" (with the light of many torches and a great multitude of priests dressed in surplices preceding, and the mayor and citizens of York with a great abundance of other people flowing in following).[23] In the absence of evidence to the contrary, one may assume that St. Leonard's continued to play its long-standing role in the procession while the hospital remained in operation, at least until December 1539. The Mercers' records from 1539 indicate their participation in the procession, and presumably the hospital fulfilled its traditional role this year, perhaps for the last time.[24] We do not know whether or how the hospital's suppression altered the time-honored processional route, for extant records do not reveal any changes to the route after 1539.

Even after York's religious houses were surrendered one by one in 1538 and 1539, the city's House Books of the early 1540s register defiant adherence to such processional customs as remained.[25] In 1544 the city required the master and priests of the Corpus Christi Guild to process in their full finery: to "goo in the sayd procession in Coopes of the best that can be gottyn within the sayd Citie." Those whose houses lay along the route were to decorate gaily on pain of punishment:

> every howseholdr that dwellith in the hye way ther as the sayd procession procedith, shall hang before ther doores & forefrontes beddes & Coveryn-ges of beddes *of the best that thay can gytt and Strewe before there doores resshes and other suche flowers & Strewing as they thynke honest & clenly for the honour of god[d] & worship of this Citie* and this to be fyrmly kepte hereafter vpon pain of every man that doth the contrary this agrement shall forfait & pay to the Common Chamber of this Cite iij s. iiijd.[26]

The civic pressure exerted upon householders registers in the directive to display "the best" ornaments for the procession and in the insistent citation of the "honor and worship" that had justified the event from its earliest days. This emphatic, redundant order suggests that in these tense years between the suppression of the religious houses and the abrogation of Corpus Christi in 1547, the procession had taken on heightened significance as a performance of civic unity and traditional religion.

The 1535 *Valor Ecclesiasticus* assessment highlights one of the hospital's other major continuing contributions to "charity for the benefit of the said commons": the royally founded on-site grammar school, which had operated continuously since before 1300.[27] Along with St. Mary's Abbey, St. Leonard's had long housed the only other grammar school in the city until the appearance of several lay-founded schools in the early sixteenth century.[28] As such the hospital's school was indispensable to the city, and its loss at the surrender, along with the loss of St. Mary's school, was devastating to learning in York.[29] The venerable hospital school boasted several well-known masters. These included Thomas Ridley (d. 1448), whose will appears in the register of the hospital peculiar that I considered in chapter 1.[30] The late fifteenth-century schoolmaster William Burton was recorded in the York House Books for the dubious distinction of insulting King Richard III.[31] In 1535 the school supported twelve choristers "de elemosina dicti hospitalis" (from the alms of the hospital) who learned song and grammar there and also performed liturgical duties.[32] Although the school hardly seems to have been moribund, its student population was significantly smaller than in the fourteenth century.[33] This reduction may be due primarily to the hospital's (and city's) wider economic decline and loss of revenue. It may also be linked to the fact that Master Magnus, appointed in 1529, founded his own school the following year in his hometown of Newark, perhaps at the expense of St. Leonard's school.[34] The hospital's surrender brought an abrupt end to its previously uninterrupted tradition of grammar and song education.

### The Hospital's Surrender and Civic Responses

Although St. Leonard's continued to participate in public ceremony, support the poor, and educate young scholars, the city did little to sustain the hospital in its final years. Unlike some more recently founded hospitals that survived the Dissolution to be reconstituted in various forms, St. Leonard's did not enjoy a long tradition of civic support or the investment of a powerful local religious guild. The hospital found itself at the mercy of royal agents who controlled its leadership and ultimately its fate, granting the post of master to two royal favorites, Thomas Wynter and Thomas Magnus, between 1528 and 1539.[35] It is debatable whether the hospital was "out of virtuous religion, and the possessions in decay," as Thomas Donyngton ominously claimed in a 1527 letter to Archbishop Thomas Wolsey. He recommended that the house should be visited: "It would be a good deed to grant a commission to visit them."[36] The 1535 *Valor Ecclesiasticus* indicates a functioning institution with a total income of more than 500 pounds.[37] The house reportedly supported sixty poor.[38] This figure represented a major decline from the house's peak numbers in the thirteenth century, but it was still supporting far more "pauperes et infirmi" than any other northern hospital. These numbers did not include the transient poor that the house probably continued to support without recording an obligation to do so.[39]

The complex series of rebellions known locally as the Pilgrimage of Grace convulsed the north of England between October 1536 and February 1537. These uprisings stemmed from various grievances against Henry's religious policies, including the recently published Ten Articles, which praised salvation by faith over pious works, discouraged the worship of images, and cast doubt upon purgatory.[40] The risings were sparked by rumors that the king was contemplating a comprehensive crackdown on churches, including confiscation of church goods and amalgamation of parishes.[41] One Yorkshire rebel leader, gentryman Robert Aske, took particular exception to the parliamentary dissolution statute passed earlier in 1536, arguing against monastic dissolutions on liturgical/spiritual and material/charitable grounds. The transcript of his examination reports:

> to the statut of subpressions, *he dyd gruge ayenst the same & so did al the holl contrey, because the abbeys in the north partes gaf great almons to pour men and laudable seruyd God; in wich partes of lait dais they had but smal comfort by gostly teching.* And by occasion of the said suppression the devyn seruice of almightie God is much minished, great nombre of messes vnsaid, & the blissed consecration of the sacrament now not vsed & showed in thos places, to the distress of the faith, & speriuall comforth to man soull.[42]

Aske's complaint may not have been widely shared beyond his own faction, yet his charge articulates an understanding of the northern religious houses, including St. Leonard's, as embedded within the larger social fabric, serving interwoven religious and material functions.[43] Aske viewed the religious houses as bastions of orthodoxy whose suppression weakened traditional devotion and deprived the faithful of "speriuall comfort." In October 1536, the city of York gave safe harbor to the local rebels, led by Aske, for two months. Sir George Lawson, lay steward of St. Leonard's, offered his house for at least one meeting where Thomas Cromwell was denounced.[44]

Lawson's role in the rising was "equivocal," Palliser notes, for he was also a member of the Council of the North, charged with enforcing the regent's will upon the northern provinces. Like most challenges to Henry's authority, the Pilgrimage ended in defeat. Aske was hanged in chains in York, executed along with more than thirty other laymen and clerics.[45] Lawson went on to acquire a lease on the Augustinian Priory as soon as it was surrendered.[46]

From the start, the rhetoric of King Henry's dissolution effort had been one of "reform" rather than simply suppression. Yet as early as March 1536, Henry had offered the site of St. Leonard's Hospital to Sir Arthur Darcy, indicating that he was already contemplating its dissolution.[47] At the hospital's surrender in 1539, its future seemed unclear: it remained possible that the king intended to secularize and repurpose it. The hospital still had a relatively robust population: the surrender document lists the remaining officers (cellarer and receiver), three canons of long standing, two canons professed for more than three years; three "conductes" resident for more than two years; and four longtime sisters. Last come the "poore bedefolk called 'cremettes', as blind, lame, bedridden and very old bodies . . . and numbered of late 50 and now about 44."[48] Each was to be given a pension of 26s. 8d. "as long as they live," but it was not clear where they would live.[49] A week later, the king's commissioners reported that they had "altered" the place "after such order and fassion as we trust shall appeir to your lordship to be to the king's honour and contentacion," implying that St. Leonard's was being slated for survival in some form rather than dissolution.[50] The commissioners seem to have been uncertain of the king's plan, for when they indicated that the cremetts ("poore bedefolk") should receive their pensions for life "but no new to be chosen till the king's further pleasure," they implied the possibility of continuing support for poor residents.[51] Yet the king's pleasure did not tend in this direction, and the house's endowments began to be leased and granted away by 1541.[52] Some of the hospital canons eventually found other employment as chantry priests, but the fate of the other personnel and of the cremetts is unknown.[53]

By the time King Henry finally visited York in 1541, four years after the last rebels had been executed, the city was anxious to perform its fealty. Citizens did so with a grand entry that included abject apologies for having "greuously heynously and traitoryously offendyd your high invincible and moste Royall maiesty" and pleas for "your moste gracyous and charytable remissyon frank and ffree pardon."[54] In addition to other entertainments, including singing and allegorical floats, the final spectacle was a staging of the Mercer's *Last Judgment* pageant on its traditional wagon stage at Ousegate end. Patricia Badir notes that staging this pageant was risky: "It always gestures to an uncertain and precarious future as much as it apologizes for a past that stands at the king's judgment."[55] Badir also observes that the pageant evoked the powerful long-standing connections among the Corpus Christi feast and York's civic pride: the oft-repeated combination of "the honour of God and of the city of York" in which St. Leonard's too had visibly invested as recently as 1516.[56] The Mercers could still stage their pageant, with its Catholic associations, but members of York's religious houses, including St. Leonard's, with its own historic connection to performance, are noticeably absent from the records. Although the king's visit might have given the city council a chance to sue for the restoration of the religious houses, particularly hospitals, which traditionally cared for the poor in hard economic times, York's citizens did not take this opportunity. Perhaps the memory of steward George Lawson's ambiguous involvement in the rising was too fresh; perhaps the city was too preoccupied with its own difficult financial situation.[57]

Having always stood within yet apart from the city of York, occupying its own liberty, St. Leonard's was not in a strong position to seek civic support in its time of need. We might look for contrast to York's Trinity Hospital, supported by the powerful Mercers' Company, or to the Hospital of St. Thomas, patronized by the Corpus Christi Guild. At the Reformation, the Mercers had quietly de-emphasized their hospital's religious orientation.[58] St. Thomas's had in 1478 made the canny decision to establish joint governance by the guild and its own members, an arrangement that doubtless contributed to its survival after the Dissolution.[59] In a further strategy to secure its existence, after the 1547 dissolution of the Corpus Christi Guild, St. Thomas joined forces with the city in 1551, adopting the mayor as its primary lay patron and electing him master of the hospital. The hospital officials tell the story of their refoundation at the beginning of a new book of ordinances copied in 1551. Beset with "trobles and vexacions that he susteyned for the defence of the right of the said hospitall," the beleaguered master beseeched the "lorde maior and his brether aldermen of the Citie of Yorke to vowchesafe of ther favor and goodnes for to be brether with vs in the same hospitall, and that wolde bee the rediest waie to upholde the said house and maynteyne the poore folkes."[60] When the mayor declares that "it was a charytable dede to releif the poore, and said openly that he and his brethern was well contented to be brether with you in your said hospitall," the threatened institution is rescued from penury and obscurity. Its officers proceed to elect the mayor its master and his aldermen its wardens. The city's House Books record the hospital turning its leases over to the city, noting the hospital's intention to "electe and chose dyverse other newe brethern of the most honest and discret persones of this Citie for the good order, mayntenaunce and preservacion of the same hospitall and poore folke in the same according to the first foundacion."[61] Thus in the civic record and in the hospital's own book, St. Thomas's Hospital and the city become collaborators in the "preservacion" of a venerable charitable mission.

St. Leonard's Hospital did not receive any similar civic investment. The only substantial civic response to the hospital's closure came in relation to its traditional educational role. After the hospital closed its doors and shut its grammar school, as had St. Mary's Abbey, the city, in response to the dearth of grammar schools, founded a new grammar school on Ouse Bridge in 1555.[62] But little is heard in the civic record about St. Leonard's after its surrender, except for an isolated 1556 appeal for its restoration during the reign of Catholic Queen Mary and King Philip. The House Book records

> a supplicacon made to my Lord Cardynalle grace, in name of my lord Mayour and his bretheren thaldermen, for his graces helpe to the Kyng and Queenes maiesties to the restoryng and renewyng of the late hospitall of St. Leonards in York, whiche was new reddy and by the seyd presens was well allowed and aggreed that not only the seal of office shold be sett to, but also that they all wold subscribe the same with their owne hands.[63]

This record is isolated and enigmatic within the House Books. Even though it is made "in name" of the mayor, the "supplicacon" seeks the patronage not of the city, but of the Church and the monarchs, who were presumably more sympathetic than Henry VIII to the hospital's traditional mission. In contrast to the strategies of St. Thomas's Hospital, which welcomed substantial citizens and the mayor into its governance, here the mayor seems to hold St. Leonard's at arm's length, seeking patronage from outside. The terms "restoryng and renewyng" suggest a return to old traditions, much as the 1551 record had promised maintenance of St. Thomas's hospital "according to the first foundacion." Although those present evidently supported the petition, the identity and fate of this document are unknown. This last-ditch attempt to revive the hospital came too late. Despite a long history of performance, charity, and visibility within the city, St. Leonard's would never regain a foothold within York's changed religious landscape.

ST. BARTHOLOMEW'S AND REFOUNDATION:
TEXTUAL TRACES AND ACCOMMODATIONS

The long, winding story of St. Bartholomew's refoundation has been told in detail by historians of the institution.[64] Building on this work, I focus here on the distinctive literary history of this period. In the letters, petitions, and agreements of the citizens and the king (1538–46) we see coalescing the key ingredients for the reformed hospital: a response to the critique of dilapidation and immorality, a continued focus on "soule heale," both of patron and poor, and a new emphasis on the coordination of Crown and city to their mutual benefit. These efforts culminate in the 1552 *Ordre*, a (re)foundation document worthy of the original *Book of the Foundation*. In this work, London's "good citizens" defend the institution against "slander" in terms that privilege an ordered textuality, respect for the poor, and a balance of spiritual and medical concerns at a moment when concern for moral reformation had reached a fever pitch in London.

St. Bartholomew's dissolution and refoundation took place at a time of intense anxiety about illicit behavior in London, during which vagabondage, crime, and sex were linked and punished in newly harsh ways. Martin Ingram argues that London "became, in effect, a laboratory for the implementation of a far more radical and severe programme of moral reformation, and in the late 1540s and early 1550s, it witnessed a quite extraordinarily intense campaign against illicit sex."[65] The hospital's textualized refoundation in notorious Smithfield, still the site for public punishments, explicitly avoided such sins while "forging links between royal policy and London civic moralism."[66] We see these priorities emerge in the documents, culminating in the 1552 *Ordre*, even as the latter announces the hospital's independence from the king and its identity as a more thoroughly civic institution.

Although uncertainty remains to this day as to whether St. Bartholomew's was ever officially surrendered, after the 1536 Act of Dissolution the hospital's properties and rents became the king's property. Yet Moore notes, "The site was not sold, nor the buildings destroyed. Some of the inmates lingered where they were, unwilling or unable to move, and were supported by the casual alms of the charitable."[67] The hospital continued to function at a reduced level, and London's mayor, aldermen, and commonalty stepped in to petition for its preservation, together with St. Thomas's, St. Mary's Spital, and the New Abbey of Tower Hill, along with the four houses of friars (Augustinians, Black, Grey, and White Friars). The city's obsequious 1538 appeal absorbs and repurposes contemporary critiques of the hospital. It privileges ancient charitable ideals while adding an up-to-date condemnation of dissolute clergy and undeserving beggars and proposing a secular, medicalized model of care. Most strategic, the letter casts the king as a pious founder deserving spiritual merit in a traditional mode. The city's letter propitiates Henry as a righteous leader in command of religious reformation and civic benefit, calling the king "the self same person whom God hath constytuted and ordeignyd bothe to redresse and reforme all crymes offences and enormytyes beyng repugnant to hys doctryne or to the detryment of the common welth and hurte of poor people beyng your naturall subiects, and also to see and vigillantly to provyde for the reformacion of the same."[68] Thus, reformation of "doctryne" and of the "common welth" are folded into the same magnanimous sphere of action, with "poor people," those most vulnerable "naturall subiects," the ideal population to benefit from the "reformacion" that only Henry can provide. Countering the critiques of the hospital we saw in chapter 5 from Copland and Fish—that in supposedly striving to help the deserving poor it proved indiscriminate in its care—the citizens beg Henry to exert himself "for the ayde and comforte of the poore sykke blynde aged and impotent persones, beyng not hable to helpe themselffs nor havyng any place certeyn wheryn they may be lodged," thus directing his charity at the traditional worthy objects of the hospital (1). The London hospitals are, the letter maintains, ready and waiting to help such people, not "preestes chanons and monks carnally lyvyng as they of late have doon, nothyng regardyng the myserable people lyeng in the streete" (2). In alluding to clerical immorality, the citizens assure Henry that upon resuscitation, the hospitals will be run by *secular* governors, will include properly paid medical professionals, and will treat the truly needy rather than sheltering the undeserving: "all impotent persones not hable to labor shall be releved by reason of the sayd hospitalles and abbey, and all sturdy beggers not wyllyng to labour shall be punisshed" (2). In treating only the deserving and dispensing with "sturdy beggers," the hospital will again respond to the double need for Christian charity and civic reformation.

Even in a reformed climate, the petition suggests, hospitals may still function as sites for accumulating spiritual capital as they have in the past. If he agrees to the petition, Henry will receive the benefits of an old-fashioned hospital patron, and more: he "shall not alonely merit more toward God and your people than any of your most noble progenitors whiche have fownded so many abbeys but shall also have the name of the conservator protector and defender of the poore people, with their contynuall prayer for the helth welth and prosperytye of your Highness and the noble prynce your sonne" (2). Henry's new title of champion of the poor may win him more merit than his progenitors, since now he has the chance to heal contemporary social ills rather than simply secure intercession for himself.

Henry's belated 1544 response emphasizes restoration of the hospital's original function even as he positions himself as its founder.[69] Vaunting his inspiration by "divine mercy," the king expresses his desire "that the true works of piety and charity should not be abolished there but rather fully restored and renewed [*renouentur*] according to the primitive pattern of the genuine sincerity."[70] Using language similar to that of the York mayor's petition to "restore and renew" St. Leonard's, Henry appeals to the apostolic practices of charity and to the seven works of bodily mercy, casting himself as founder—"We determine to create erect found [*fundamus*] and establish [*stabilimus*] a certain hospital"—giving himself credit for this (re)new(ed) creation.[71] Yet the traditional function of prayerful intercession has disappeared, befitting the reformed circumstances and the king's hardening views on purgatory. To run the hospital, Henry proposes a master (a priest) and four additional priests: the vice-master, curate, hospitaller, and the visitor of Newgate. These suggestions may have been inspired by his father's hospital, the Savoy, which stipulated a master and four priests (vice-master, sacristan, confessor, and hospitaller).[72] Henry is preoccupied with restoring the hospital site with its ancient privileges, liberties, and free customs: in short, with his own role as "founder" and with the institution's legal viability.[73]

Although the City Corporation did not fully approve Henry's 1544 proposal and petitioned for the possession of St. Bartholomew's, the king issued a deed of covenant settling the matter in December 1546, a month before his death.[74] This document represents something of a compromise, more fully outlining a plan for the hospital's new form and sources of support. In addition to carving up the old ecclesiastical area of priory and hospital to constitute a new parish called Christchurch, which would eventually house Christchurch Hospital for children, the indenture hands over the former Grey Friars, St. Bartholomew's, and their rental incomes to support the reformed hospital. Reflecting the king's desire to "create erect found and establish" the institution, the house is to be called "The House of the Poore in West Smithfield, in the suburbs of the City of London, of King Henry the Eighth's Foundation."[75] This short-lived change bespeaks Henry's desire to remake the institution free of popish associations and to claim the hospital as his proprietary institution. In the seventeenth century, a stained-glass window was created to memorialize Henry's refoundation with appropriate splendor: it pictures the king enthroned, handing down the new charter to Thomas Vicary, the King's surgeon and a governor of the new hospital (see fig. 6.1).

The officers, rather than the governors, are defined carefully in Henry's covenant, along with their duties and wages: notably a matron to oversee the patients and twelve sisters to serve as nurses.[76] The officers of beadles invest the hospital with authority amid the hypervigilant neighborhood search culture into which the institution now reinserts itself: their job is to search for and bring in the sick people, "and to expulse and avoid such valiant and sturdy vagabonds and beggars as they shall find dayly within the said city and the suburbs of the same."[77] In addition to formally establishing the roles of physician and surgeon, the indenture also gives the hospital's overseers the right to tax citizens to support the hospital.[78] A lasting solution to the problem of funding came through the hospital's solicitation of the London livery companies for regular support: "Sixty-one of the companies 'willingly granted' relief to the poor in St. Bartholomew's, headed by the Mercer's Company giving £24, and the Grocers, Drapers, and Merchant Taylors each pledging £20."[79] Although the grants ceased to be compulsory after 1554, this system of regular investment bound members of the livery companies to the reformed hospital, as company members served as officers and cooperated closely from the start in defining the new hospital's identity, supervising its functions, and protecting its reputation.

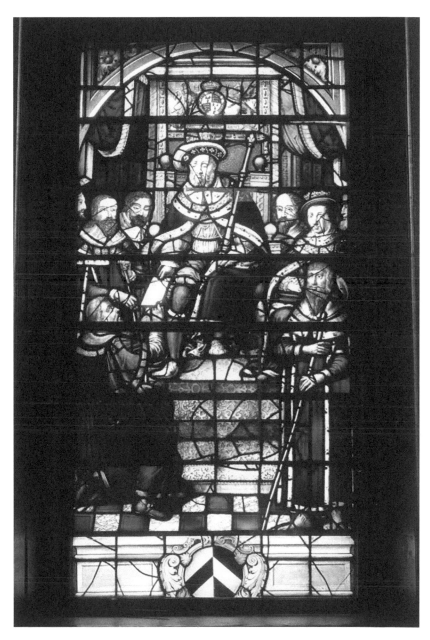

Figure 6.1. St. Bartholomew's Hospital, the "Charter Window." SBHX4/12. Reproduced with the kind permission of Barts Health NHS Trust Archives and Museums.

## The 1552 *Ordre of the Hospital*: A New Foundation Book

In 1552, the refounded hospital, overseen by the mayor and a cadre of lay and religious officers, published its own regulations (see fig. 6.2). This book bears some parallels to York St. Thomas's Hospital manuscript of 1551, with its fulsome narrative of refoundation followed by new ordinances, yet its printed form was evidently designed for a broader public.[80] Enshrining the new regulations in a text for a citywide readership, the hospital's leaders recount its travails and defend its refoundation with the hope of unveiling its good works to the public and raising money. A fundraising goal may well have been the main reason for publishing the *Ordre*: Daly argues that the work was "intended to sensitize a wide reading audience to the valuable tasks officers and staff regularly performed."[81] This multifaceted work creates a new textual beginning for the hospital. The *Ordre* features a preface, descriptions of all the officers' duties and wages, a liturgical Service for the Poor, and finally "a passe porte for the poore at their deliuerie" to be copied for each person leaving the hospital cured. Some aspects seem to draw upon the Savoy Hospital's statutes, yet the self-consciously public quality of the *Ordre* and its explicit concern to combat slander respond to the recent history of St. Bartholomew's Hospital and the political demands of the moment.

Historians of Reformation London have taken varied views of the *Ordre*, from sanguine to cynical. Susan Brigden argues that the work, particularly its services for the poor, manifests "the godly zeal which animated their foundation."[82] Slack, noting that the work is "articulate and sophisticated" compared to similar provincial documents, contends that in the *Ordre*, "crude incentives" such as directing the beadles to "throw vagrants in gaol and bring in any sick people loitering in the street . . . were papered over with the vocabulary of Christian humanism."[83] I focus on how this document endeavors strategically to reconstruct the hospital with an eye to the institution's past, present, and future. The *Ordre* is an ambitious work that attempts to encompass textually all the practices and people of the refounded institution. After considering its preface as a new statement of civic reformation in response to slander, I focus on the reconstitution of the hospital as a textual community in which documentation becomes essential to successful functioning. The *Ordre* attempts to recuperate what Copland had called "soule heale," delineating a regime to benefit residents and officers in a reciprocal dynamic that might also bring spiritual and civic reform into a new relation.

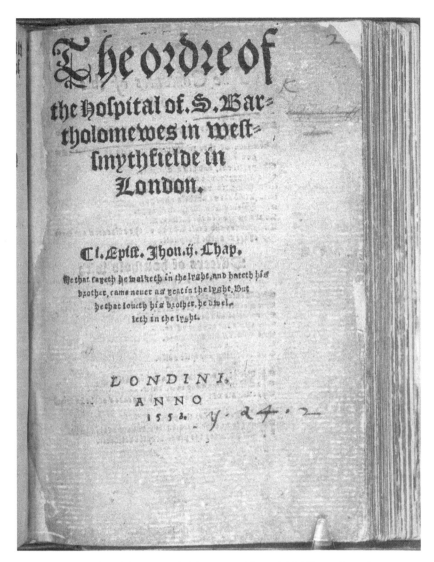

FIGURE 6.2. *Ordre of the Hospital*, title page. © The British Library Board, C.58.a.21.(2), folio A1r. Reproduced with permission.

*The Ordre of the Hospital of S. Bartholomewes in Westsmythfielde in London* was produced in 1552 by Richard Grafton, a reformist printer and member of the Grocer's Company. The *Ordre* appears to represent a collaboration between surgeon Thomas Vicary, a hospital governor and patient caretaker, and Richard Grafton, also a governor, who had served as treasurer in 1551. Vicary reportedly "devysed" the regulations for patient care, likely in consultation with the whole board. Grafton, a Protestant with evangelical leanings, probably supplied the preface and shaped the *Ordre*'s "clearly Edwardian" religious orientation and rhetoric.[84] Grafton had been instrumental in producing several controversial English Bibles, including the 1537 "Matthew" Bible and the Great Bible of 1539, followed in 1540 by a second edition with Thomas Cranmer's preface.[85] Grafton had been imprisoned three times: twice in 1541, for publishing material offensive to King Henry's religious regime and for offending against the Six Articles, and once in 1543 for printing "unlawfull" books.[86] Complementing his printing activities, Grafton was also an author. In 1543 he had published an edition of John Hardyng's fifteenth-century metrical *Chronicle* to which he added a prose extension up to the present day.[87] An experienced printer and administrator who had himself experienced persecution, Grafton was invested in reformed theology and in the refounded hospital's success.[88] The preface to the *Ordre* seems to be his work: it manifests a strongly proprietary interest, an understanding of the hospital's recent history, and a literary flair for appealing to a broad audience of pious, civic-minded readers.

From the start, the *Ordre of the Hospital of S. Bartholomewes* announces a return to the hospital's original name, an implicit rejection of Henry VIII's "House of the Poor" moniker. In renaming the hospital, the mayor and "good citizens" tacitly displace the king (now Edward VI) as patron in favor of a more fully civic regime, while hearkening back to the hospital's earlier combination of spiritual and medical purposes. The *Ordre*'s "Preface to the Reader" offers a strong riposte to the "slander" that the struggling new hospital, founded but poorly funded by King Henry "of famous memorie," had suffered since 1546 (see fig. 6.3). The Preface expresses defensiveness and guarded pride, responding to past satire and to the "prive backbiting" of the present, arguing for the success of the effort on the whole amid difficult financial and political circumstances. The Preface launches a strongly worded attack on the hospital's detractors: "The wickednes of reporte at thys daie good reader, is growen to suche rankenes that nothing almost is able to

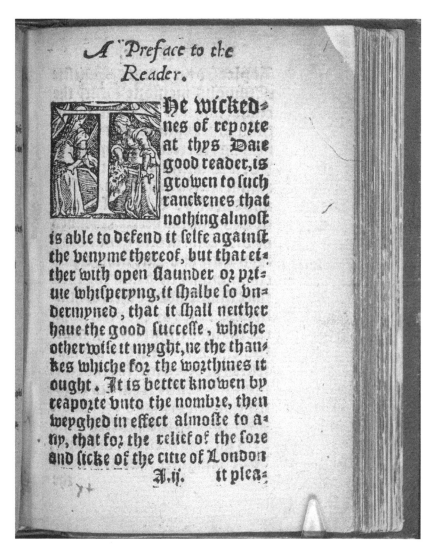

## A Preface to the Reader.

THe wickednes of reporte at thys Daie good reader, is growen to such ranckenes that nothing almost is able to defend it selfe against the venyme thereof, but that either with open flaunder or priuie whisperyng, it shalbe so vndermyned, that it shall neither haue the good successe, whiche otherwise it myght, ne the thankes whiche for the worthines it ought. It is better knowen by reaporte vnto the nombre, then weyghed in effect almoste to any, that for the relief of the sore and sicke of the citie of London

A.ij.          it plea=

FIGURE 6.3. *Ordre of the Hospital*, preface. © The British Library Board, C.58.a.21.(2), folio A2r. Reproduced with permission.

defend it selfe against the venyme therof, but that either with open slaunder or priuie whisperyng, it shalbe so vndermyned, that it shall neither haue the good successe, whiche other wise it myght, ne the thankes which for the worthines it ought."[89]

Without explicitly connecting the hospital to this "wickednes of reporte," the Preface encourages readers to make these connections and recognize them as unmerited.[90] The accompanying miniature features the Jewish heroine Judith in a modest widow's headcovering, decapitating the tyrant Holofernes.[91] Within Christianity, Judith had long signified steadfast chastity, and some English reformers shaped her specifically into an emblem of resistance to false religious authority. In a widely publicized Lenten sermon of 1549, Hugh Latimer had lauded Judith's refusal of Holofernes's sexual advances as an exemplary resolution "rather to sanctify God's name, to do God's will, than the will of the devil; therefore God gave her such a triumphant victory."[92] The appearance of this steadfast widow reinforces a message of godliness in the face of "wickednes of reporte," and a determination that the refounded hospital will eventually achieve a "good successe." Judith's chastity also makes her a fitting mascot for the refounded hospital's commitment to avoid sexual impropriety.

The subsequent narrative unfolds the story of Henry's (re)foundation: "for the relief of the sore and sicke of the citie of London it pleased the kinges Maiestie of famous memorie Henry the eight . . . to erecte an hospitall in West Smithfield, for the continual relief and help of an C sore and diseased" (A2v). Although the institution was underfunded, with decayed rents and dissolute residents, the citizens forged bravely ahead and "proceded with suche spied as they could to the redresse of all these decayes, disordres, and defaultes, and bestowed thereabout aboue their couanaunt of .v. hundred markes yerely . . . whereby (together with other their good endeuours) when they had wonne it to such poynct that it was fitt to receiue the nombre and to succour thesame with all necessaries requisite and in such case nedeful" (A4r–v). The passage shows palpable pride in the citizens' efforts despite difficult circumstances, with "decayes, disordres, and defaultes" adding an alliterative flourish. Next we hear strong resentment of the uncharitable citizens who attempted to undermine these efforts. Soon the slander started, as "certeyne busie bodies more ready to espie occasion how to blame other, then skilful how to redresse thynges" began to whisper privately and then "not contented priuately, one, and another, among their neighbours *to hynder the profette of the poore, and to slaunder the good citizeins occupied thereabout*, rounded into the eares of the preachers also, their tender consideracion" (A4v–5r; emphasis added). Privy slander becomes open accusation in the mouths of gullible preachers, and the good citizens "haue here receyued nothyng elles but for a commune benefight an open detraction and the pore . . . a larger hynderaunce" (A5v). In this account, slander becomes not only an affront to the hospital's caretakers in their endeavor to revive the institution, but, more grievously, it harms the poor, who should be the objects of civic care.

Thus the Preface links backbiting and slander to the detriment of civic charity toward the poor, the prime objective of the refoundation. "Slander" is a loaded term at this moment, one familiar to every reader. Defamation cases were the commonest sort brought in the Church courts of early sixteenth-century London; most citizens had probably experienced some sort of slander.[93] In this context, the term evokes malicious language intended to harm the institution's reputation, which it must now rebuild. In common law, "a slander was a personal injury equivalent to a physical assault or a trespass on land, a quantifiable damage to the reputation and livelihood of the plaintiff who brought the case and specified the damages to which he thought himself entitled."[94] The *Ordre* never identifies the "certeyne busie bodies," but its repeated evocation of slander argues for the hospital as unjustly libeled and deserving the Preface's strong defense. Grafton himself, imprisoned and released three times between 1541 and 1543 for his controversial printing, had certainly felt the sting of damage to personal reputation.

One of the Preface's main tasks is to establish slander as unmerited and contrary to the mission of the hospital. Abhorrence of slander runs through the whole document, and a formula against slander features in the charge to nearly every officer of the house: "if there shalbe any thyng done by any officer or other persone of this house, that shalbe unprofitable thereunto, or that may be occasion of any disorder, or shal engendre slaunder to thesame, that ye then declare it to some, one or two of the Gouernours of this house, and to non other persone, nor no further to meddle therein" (E1v).[95] Medieval visitation reports had expressed the need to avoid impropriety and the reputation for vice, for example in rules segregating men from women, but the explicit concern for slander is striking in the *Ordre*.[96]

Despite the obstacles of limited funds, decrepit buildings, derelict residents, and slander, the Preface seeks to instill admiration in its readers for what these "good citizeins" have wrought. Amid these impediments, in the years since its refoundation "there haue bene healed of the pocques, fystules, filthie blaynes and sores, to the nombre of .viii. hundrede, and thence saufe deliuered that other hauyng nede myghte entre in their roume" (A5v).[97] Moreover the hospital has cared for some "eyght skore and xii that have there forsaken this life . . . whiche elles myght have died, and stonke in the eyes and noses of the Citie" (A5v). (During this period St. Bartholomew's was allocated six suburban leper houses to care for pox victims at a distance from London proper, a significant help in this effort.)[98] Citing these hard numbers as proof of their success, against the weighty expenses that the hospital must bear, including wages and high prices, the *Ordre* notes its critics "might bothe *merueile* how so many are there relieued, and daily mainteyned, and with *repentaunce*, of that they have myssayde, endeuoure them selves with asmuch good reporte and prayse, to aduaunce both the died and the doers, to wipe away the slaunder, as they haue to hinder them" (A6r–v; emphasis added). Thus the *Ordre* offers its detractors the religious experiences of "merueile" and "repentaunce" as remedies to the harms they have caused. This passage revises the Priory's *Book of the Foundation*, which, as we saw in chapter 2, vaunted the miracles of the priory. Now that the hospital has survived the dissolution to which the priory succumbed, it may claim the mantle of "merueile" to make this sense of religious wonder part of its appeal to citizen generosity.

The *Ordre*'s claim that the hospital's healing should inspire "merueile" anticipates further attempts to recuperate what Robert Copland called "soule heale" in a reformed guise. Detailing the "charges" of governors and officers, the *Ordre* envisions the hospital's overseers and staff serving the spiritual needs of the poor and experiencing spiritual benefit in turn. This combination is encapsulated in the charge to the twelve governors, a combination of aldermen and commoners "elected by the Lorde Maior and his brethren" to run the hospital (B2r). These unpaid governors are exhorted to focus as exclusively as possible on the hospital, as if to a religious vocation. They are to "attende onely upon the nedeful doynges of this house, with suche a louyng and careful diligence, as shal become the faithfull ministers of God, whom ye chieflie in this vocation are appointed to serue, and to whom for your negligences or defaultes herein ye shall render an accompt" (B3r). Though these secular governors are not priests, they are charged with the sacred duty to treat "this house" as a religious institution once again, regarding the poor as embodiments of Christ. The text goes on to cite Christ's words (Matt. 25:40): "Whatsoeuer ye do to one of these nedy persones for my names sake, the same ye do vnto me. And contrary wyse if ye neglecte and despyse them, ye despise me" (B3v). Christ enters the *Ordre* as one of its authors, an appropriately apostolic, English source for the reformed hospital. But this speech could also evoke the Catholic connection between the deeds of mercy (Matt. 25:30) and the traditional tableau of the Last Judgment, a familiar subject for contemplation in the medieval hospital.[99] The governors' actions have eschatological consequences: if they succeed "so to comfort ordre and gouerne this house and the poore therof, that at the last daie, ye maie appere before the face of God, as trewe and faithfull Stewardes and disposers of all suche thynges as shal for the comfort and succour of them, (duryng the tyme of your office) be committed to your credite and charge" (B3v–4r).[100] If they fail at the daunting triple task of comforting, ordering, and governing, dire consequences are implied. By casting the lay governors of the house as latter-day secular masters, vested with spiritual responsibility if not technically with religious authority, the *Ordre* respiritualizes the hospital's mission within new civic parameters.[101]

Implying the traditional analogy between spiritual and physical health, the *Ordre* presses the parallels between the duties of the hospitaller, a priest charged with the welfare of poor residents, and of the surgeon, who tends their bodies but should also understand his role as spiritual. The role of hospitaller, referenced in Henry's 1546 indenture, has a predecessor in the Savoy Hospital, as one of the four priests (with vice-master, sacristan, and confessor) who assisted the master in running the hospital. The Savoy hospitaller tended to all matters related to the care of the poor, while the master and vice-master oversaw the entire house, the sacristan tended to religious possessions, and the confessor heard confessions.[102] Thus in the new model hospital, priestly authority was subdivided in line with traditional monastic roles. St. Bartholomew's office of hospitaller telescopes all of these duties into a single job description. The hospitaller must "visite the pore in their extremes and sickenesses, and to minister vnto them the moste wholsome and necessary doctrine of Gods comfortable worde, aswel by teachyng and preaching as also by ministering the sacrament of the holy Comunion" (D4r). Rather similarly, although the charge to the surgeons begins by exhorting these professionals to use the "vttermoste of your knowledge and connyng, to helpe to cure the greues and diseases of the poore of this hospitall" (E3v), it also privileges spiritual counsel on the doctor's part. Any time the surgeon visits a patient, he shall "geue vnto hym or her, faithfull and good counsaill, willing them to mynde to sinne no more and to be thankefull vnto almighty GOD for whose sake they are here comforted of men" (E4v). Thus, even as the institution becomes medicalized, emphasizing the professional knowledge of its surgeons, the *Ordre* stresses the traditional complementarity between medical and spiritual care, evoking a circuit of spiritual benefit that runs between the poor and their caregivers.

We know that books and records had long been central to the life of St. Bartholomew's Hospital. The house's revised statutes draw upon traditional modes of monastic record-keeping while making active documentation an explicit priority.[103] A self-consciously textualized organization of practice, detailing expenses, receipts, minutes, and patient information, works to benefit the poor by naming them, positively rather than punitively, as in the legal system, where naming had become central to persecuting "rogues."[104] The *Ordre* suggests, hopefully, that records may become a means to recognize the humanity of the poor: they are individuals with names, possessions to be returned when they leave the house, and passports to ensure their safe travels back home.

With the aid of careful record-keeping, the *Ordre* maintains, the poor will be cared for more efficiently and fairly. Notably, the work contains an "order for the saufekepyng of the euidences and writinges apperteining to the hospitall" to be kept in "one fayre and substanciall chest" (C4v): the chest is to have three locks, one for the president, one for the treasurer, "and a commoner appointed by the whole house, to haue the thirde" (C5r).[105] Just as the *Ordre* encompasses textually the work of the refounded institution, the chest will hold all the documents involved in this work.

Each officer's job description textualizes the duties of the traditional religious obedientiaries. The treasurers, central officers for "saufekepyng" and stabilizing the new house's precarious finances, are to work closely with the renter, who supervises the hospital's properties, and give a detailed written report every year: "Ye shal also yerely the .xx. day of October (within this hospitall) yelde and geue up in wrytynge vnto the President and gouernors of thesame a true and a perfect accompte of your whole charge, duryng the yere of your treasorourship" (B5v). The almoner, who cares comprehensively for the poor, making sure that "euery man do his dutie therein accordyng to hys charge" and that "there be peace and quietnes mainteyned" (B7v) and keeping track of patients healed and discharged, keeps "one entier and perfect inuentarie" of the house's possessions (C1r). He is supported by a phalanx of officers who must keep careful records. The "Auditour" focuses exclusively on keeping records:

Unto youre audite muste be brought these sortes of Bookes, *first the hospitall booke,* beyng in the custody of the Hospiteler, to whiche also ye shall loke that euery page or totall somme therof be *subscribed with two of the handes of the almoners.* And this booke shal ye conferre with *the Stewardes boke,* who first maketh the prouisions. Ye must also haue *the Scrutiners booke,* to examine the accompte of the Treasourer for money deliuered vnto hym. . . . Also the *booke of Surueye* to conferre the Bylles brought in by the Treasourer with the alowaunces of reparacions. . . . Also ye shall demaunde of the Renter, *his rental* for that yere, not forgetting alwaies to charge hym with the arrerages that remain the yere before. . . . And lastly to haue speciall regarde, if any somme of money haue bene paid by the Treasourer, by any decre or general order of this house, to loke in the *Journal for the same. And thus in the whole affayres of this house, shall ye perfectly be instructed.* (C3v–4v; emphasis added.)

This passage creates a remarkable picture of the house's textualized system of regulation, "instructing" the auditors to run the hospital's operations by superintending other officers in relation to their texts, ensuring they are consistent with each other. The *Ordre* describes a cooperative system of review and consultation that, via the scrutiny of records, will reveal any discrepancies, dishonesty, or vice and eradicate them.

The nature and purview of each book are specified in subsequent sections of the *Ordre*; all are deemed necessary, but it is the "Journal" that contains a "Calender [index], and it shal alwaies be brought further at suche tymes as the President and moste parte of the Gouernours shall sit within this hospitall, for the generall affaires of the same" (D3v–4r). This book is to record any "orders and decrees, as from tyme to tyme shall by the sayde Gouernours or greatest part of them, be decreed and ordeined." Every time an item is entered, it must be added to the Calendar within five days, giving a sense of how heavily the governors relied upon the journal: "that aswel when you are absent, as present the gouernours may without difficultie be satisfied of that they seke for therein" (D4r).

The final step in the poor resident's journey, if not burial in the hospital grounds, is delivery with the instrument of the "passeport to be deliuered to the poore" (see fig. 6.4). This text was a form letter addressed "To all Maiours, Bailiefes, Constables, +c" that could be tailored for each departing patient. It certified that she or he,

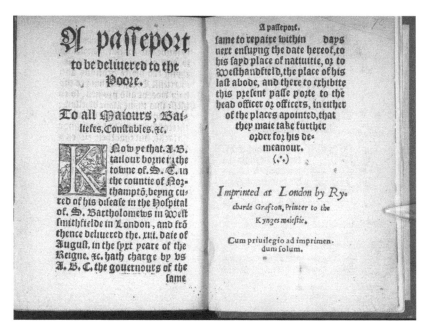

FIGURE 6.4. *Ordre of the Hospital,* passport for the poor. © The British Library Board, C.58.a.21.(2), folio I7v. Reproduced with permission.

beyng cured of his disease in the Hospital of S. Bartholomewes in West Smithfielde in London, and from thence deliuered on the .xiii. daie of August, in the syxt yere of the Reigne +c. hath charge by vs ABC the gouernours of the same to repaire within dayes next ensuyng the date hereof, his said place of natiuitie or to Westhandfield, the place of his last abode and there to exhibite this present passe porte to the head officer or officers, in either of the places apointed, that they maie take further order for his demeanour. (I7v–8r)

Once cured, and after submitting to this last measure of textual regulation, the hospital resident receives the "charge by vs" (the governors) to "repaire" either to place of birth or most recent residence, in orders that dovetail with contemporary poor law regulations. (This passport references the similar document that the accused vagabond would be issued after being duly punished.)[106] At this point, the patient is no longer protected by the hospital's textual system and must fend for him- or herself.

## MATRON, NURSES, AND SINGLE WOMEN
### IN THE REFOUNDED HOSPITAL

The refounded hospital's public textual representation of itself coexists with surviving records (the "Journal" or Governors' Minutes for 1549–61, and the Account Book for 1547–61).[107] Picking up some of the questions that I addressed in chapter 2 about the treatment of pregnant and laboring women at the later medieval St. Bartholomew's, I suggest that in the charged atmosphere of the early 1550s, the leaders of the reformed hospital demonstrate both charity and anxiety toward childbearing women, an ambivalence constantly informed by the fear of slander.

Describing the situation that the good citizens faced as they set about resuscitating the hospital, the *Ordre*'s Preface alludes to "thre or foure harlottes, then lieng in childbed" who remained in the derelict institution just prior to its refoundation, "so far had the godly meanyng of the gracious kyng bene abused at those days" (A3v–4r). This verbal picture offers a stark contrast to the chaste widow Judith included a few pages earlier. Within the *Ordre*, the matron and nursing sisters become key players in the effort to avoid slander. In the refounded St. Bartholomew's, the role of the nurse became "more fully recognized and delineated," and the *Ordre* implies that the nurses' newly textualized role will help to contain and redeem female sexuality.[108] Even as the term "nurse" was used in the period as a euphemism for whore or bawd, the valorization of nursing becomes linked to a rejection of unchaste women from the hospital, precisely for the purpose of avoiding scandal.[109] But as the hospital closes its doors to pregnant and postpartum women (and sends away residents, including poor and sisters, who become pregnant), it continues to care for them indirectly by paying local women to shelter them. A range of other women are connected, occasionally or regularly, to the house: some are paid to care for pregnant women, others for selling goods to the house. A network of local women becomes visible in these records, reminding us of Monserrat Cabré's argument that for the medieval period, "women's health actions form a continuum that runs from the ordinary to the occupational, from gratuitous therapeutic attention to paid acts of health care."[110] The hospital was one point on this continuum of care, which extended into the wider neighborhood.

The hospitaller was administratively responsible for the care of the poor, and the matron managed patients at a hands-on level. As the *Ordre* decrees, after their initial examination, the hospitaller "shall committ the same poore to the matron of this house, to be placed accordingly as the case shal require" (D5r).[111] And though all of the officers are charged with avoiding slander, the matron, as head of the sisters and the patients and responsible for monitoring their interactions, plays the leading role in this effort. She receives new patients as they are admitted to the hospital, and the bulk of her charges as "chief gouerneresse and worthy Matrone" (E1r) involve supervision of the sisters, who must "declare and shewe your selves gentle diligent and obedient to the Matrone of this house who is appointed and aucthorised to be your chief gouerneresse and ruler" (E2r). Here the matron takes on an abbess-like role, and with their new textual rule, the sisters replace the religious brothers and sisters of the old hospital. However, as Margaret Pelling notes, the matron was allowed to be married, unlike the nurses under her supervision: "She thus stood in a relation to them similar to that of a mistress of servants."[112] The first matron of the refounded hospital was Rose Fisher, "a redoubtable figure" nearly lured away from her post by competing offers from other hospitals.[113]

The *Ordre* constructs a system in which the matron supervises the sisters' work and ensures their immunity from slander. On the one hand she should check that they "do their dutie vnto the poore, aswel in makyng of their beddes, and keping their wardes, as also in wasshyng and purgyng their vnclene clothes and other thinges" (D8r).[114] On the other hand, just as important is her control over the sisters' movements at all times. The sisters must stay in the women's ward at night unless they need to leave to tend to a dying person, "And yet at suche a speciall tyme it shall not be laufull for euery Sister to go furth to any person or persones . . . but *onely for suche as you shall thinke verteous, Godly, and discrete*" (D8v; emphasis added). The matron's close supervision of the sisters enables her to know which are "verteuous" and which likely to err (an assumption about female weakness that is built into the text). This condition upon the sisters' care of the poor in the interest of avoiding slander seems a newly explicit priority: the Savoy statutes included strict rules about segregating male and female staff, but nurses were exhorted to visit the poor speedily at all times, lest an unattended patient should die.[115]

The assumption that women's inherent foolishness endangers their chastity is implicit in the charges to the sisters. The *Ordre* exhorts the sisters in their care of patients to "Vse unto them good and honest talke, suche as may comforte and amend them, and utterly to aduoyde al lyght, wanton, and foolishe wordes, gestures and maners, vysyng your selues vnto theim with all sobriete and discretion. And aboue all thynges se that ye auoyde, abhorre and detest skoldyng, and dronkennesse, as moste pestilent and filthie vices" (E2v–3r). Even as the *Ordre* constructs the sisters as potential amenders of patients, it transmits anxiety about their possible reversion to "lyght, wanton, and foolishe wordes," not to mention the possibility that the same lapses of judgment might allow them to welcome inappropriate visitors or "any lyght persone to haunt or vse unto you" (E3r). The matron is charged with controlling the sisters' movements in a context just as porous and dangerous to female chastity as the original hospital site, that Smithfield fens, which, the *Book of the Foundation* suggested, was both literally "uncleene . . . and as a maryce dunge and fenny" and morally questionable, haunted by the presence of prostitutes. The *Ordre* attempts to enforce a distinction between the contained, chaste sisters and young poor women very like them who might well be patients.

The refounded house's documentary records afford sporadic but meaningful insights into how leaders drew distinctions between respectable poor patients and unmarried poor pregnant women, who were by 1552 considered beyond the bounds of respectability and the hospital's purview. Linda A. Pollock argues that in early modern England, "the pregnant, unwed woman was a visible rent in the moral fabric of society and all the more unwelcome for that."[116] In contrast to the medieval hospital's documented mandate to care for pregnant and postpartum women until their purification, and the care offered in Mirfield's *Breviarium,* the hospital records of the early 1550s indicate that the hospital too found such women "unwelcome" and took steps to expel them. However, in doing so the hospital arranged for the care of childbearing women at a distance. Whereas the Account Books tend to focus on the expulsion of such women amid the danger to institutional reputation, the Journal discloses a more concerted effort to support them from afar. Further records indicate ad hoc efforts to care for vulnerable people no longer admitted to the hospital: the dying elderly and children, categories of poor who did not fall within the new mandate to treat only "sicke poore" adults. These efforts run parallel to the parish-based relief of local "impotent poor" that was mandated during the same period.[117]

In the context of payments to miscellaneous people outside the hospital, we find the institution policing the distinction between respectable and

scandalous female poor. Notable for its connection to the *Ordre*'s preoccupations is this Account Book record from 1551–52: "Item to a woman for to
take in a woman that travelde with chylde at the gate of this house *bycause
we wolde not haue this house slaundred with no suche persons*. xs."[118] The hospital asserts its abiding fear of "slaunder" by turning away a woman in the
throes of childbirth. The laboring woman has been rejected, but not without recourse: another anonymous woman is paid ten shillings to take her in.
Perhaps she was a neighbor who had previously taken in women rejected by
the hospital. The payment was included among the list of "rewardes," occasional payments distinct from regular "wages" and "casuall paymentes" in
the record book.[119] Similarly, but with less exposition, the Accounts record
that in 1552–53 the hospital paid fifteen shillings eight pence for "keping of
ii poore women in chyldbed."[120] The expense is listed under the "casuall and
foreyn paymentes," between a payment for "wynding shetes" for the dead
and the "redymyng of certen pewter of a poore woman's" from the hospitaller. There is not enough information in the record to know whether these
two women were rejected or expelled from the house, but the record without comment may imply that the "kepyng" of laboring and postpartum
women had become a mundane expense for the hospital.

Just as the first record above gave a scene of rejection and the motives
behind it, sometimes the Account Books give more detailed information
about the circumstances of pregnant women's expulsions. A record under
"casuall paymentes" from 1554–55 records payment of 14s 8d "to Alice Hall
a woman for keping of a pore woman that was sent out for that she was
withe chyld as by dyuers bylls apperyth."[121] Here the name of the carer appears, suggesting that Alice Hall was a regular casual employee.[122] If we take
the ambiguous term "dyuers bylls" in its common sense of public statements or petitions, written or otherwise, it may be that the hospital sent
this pregnant woman away in response to some sort of pressure.

The Governors' Minutes (the "Journal" named in the *Ordre*) also testifies to more formalized decisions on the "kepyng" of pregnant and postpartum women. On the same leaf of the Journal are two detailed records
from 1552, the second dated January 27.[123] The marginal note to the first
one reads, "For the kepyng of a woman with chylde": "This day yt is agreed
that Master Vycar[y][124] shall pay unto a woman in Cok Lane that hathe the
kepyng of a woman that was fownd with chyld after she was admyttyd to
the hospitall wekely xd tyll she be delyueryd, and then xijd by the weke tyll
she be churched, whereof xd ys alridy delyueryd vnto the woman." Rather

than emphasizing the woman's abrupt expulsion from the house, the record describes discovery and procedure: the woman in question was "fownd with chyld after she was admyttyd to the hospitall." A set amount is established for her care, with a two-pence supplement after the birth. The reference to churching recalls the medieval hospital's custom of housing women until after this ritual. This concern may be an attempt to preserve something of that spiritual solicitude for the woman's welfare, to frame this "kepyng" not merely as a matter of convenience, but an act consistent with the refounded hospital's claim to care for "the herboure and succour of the dere members of Christes body" (*Ordre*, E1v).

A related record on that page offers a similar payment to a different woman, already delivered of her child, residing very nearby: "This day yt was orderyd that the woman that was delyueryd of childe wythin the close shall haue xii d by the weke tyll she be churchid and that Master Vycary and the matrone shall take order for the childe." The woman presumably was not resident in the hospital, but she "was delyueryd of childe wythin the close," and hence the governors perhaps felt that they should take responsibility for her support until her churching. Maybe she had previously been a hospital resident.[125] And though the house no longer took in orphaned children, the note that "Master Vycary and the matrone shall take order for the childe" suggests that the officers remained concerned for the welfare of vulnerable children as they had since the foundation.

As this care for the newborn child shows, despite its narrower charitable mandate and its abiding fear of slander, St. Bartholomew's continued to make accommodations for the vulnerable. Children fell through the cracks of civic charity, at least before the foundation of Christchurch hospital, and various payments indicate the hospital's support of neighborhood women who cared for poor and afflicted children. In 1552–53, among the hospital's lists of payments, including a legacy to the matron and sisters, is found a twelve-pence payment "to a woman for takyng in a poore chylde."[126] In the following year the hospital paid four shillings "to a poore woman for helyng of a boyes head," and made another payment of the same amount to the same woman "in ernest to amend a nother skald head."[127] The repeated payments suggest that the unnamed poor woman served as a valued adjunct to the hospital's care of the poor and sick. Despite the *Ordre*'s seemingly clear-cut categories and exclusions, in practice the institution remained flexible enough to superintend a range of charitable care in the neighborhood, subsidizing poor neighbors who performed vital functions that the hospital no longer could.

## St. Bartholomew's, St. Mark's,
### and the Reformation of Civic Piety

Although much had changed in the post-Dissolution hospital, the leaders of the refounded St. Bartholomew's, keen to disavow past derelictions and create a respectable, efficient institution, expressed continuity with the past in their insistence upon the hospital's spiritual role. Despite their rejection of pregnant women and refusal to support childbirth on-site, the hospital's governors remained attentive to the importance of rites, such as churching, that marked the passage of sacred time. If we turn to the religious service at the end of the 1552 *Ordre*, we see how liturgical regulation and practice become integral to its plan for the well-ordered hospital. The hospital's simplified twice-daily liturgies parallel those in Cranmer's 1549 Book of Common Prayer, which contains only two services. The *Ordre* likewise contains two services, both quite long.[128] The obligatory services are central to the house's daily discipline, as the initial instructions show:

> At the Houre of eyght of the clocke in the mornyng, and .iiij. of the clock at the afternoone, throughout the whole yeare, there shal a bel be rong the space of halfe a quarter of an houre, and immediately upon the seassyng of the bell, the poore liyng in their beddes that cannot aryse, & kneling on their knees, that can aryse in euery warde, as their beddes stande, they shal by course as many as can rede, begyn these praiers folowyng. And after that the partie whose course it shalbe, hath begon, all the rest in the warde shal folow and aunswere, vpon paine to be dismissed out of the house. (F6r–v)

All are required to participate in the service to the extent possible, even those unable to rise from their beds. The "service for the poor" enlists the poor in praying for their own salvation as well as for their leaders and the king. This ritual recalls the requirements enjoined upon the residents of the new fifteenth-century almshouses. At the same time, the *Ordre*'s emphasis on the patients' performance of the prayers, and the texts themselves, anticipate the demands by testators in this period and the 1560s that the poor, beneficiaries of charity, embody proper religious conduct and belief in order to merit that charity. By the late 1560s, testators who funded hospitals, almshouses, and schools were demanding that the "deserving" poor show not just "moral probity" but "adherence to the true religion."[129] Testamentary evidence of this period shows slight changes in "the context and rationale of established [charitable] customs" rather than a wholesale reinvention of practice. Now rather than the donor hoping to reduce his or her time in purgatory, it was the poor who were enjoined "to demonstrate their worthiness by leading lives of exemplary piety and ultimately by following the correct form of religion."[130] As early as 1552, the rule-abiding poor of St. Bartholomew's Hospital were already on their way to embodying the "true religion" of this transitional moment.

In some respects the twice-daily service reflects the wider liturgical changes of the Book of Common Prayer, offering a simplified sequence of psalms and readings and identical litany and suffrages at the end (to be performed three times a week).[131] Yet unlike the Book of Common Prayer with its varying calendar of psalms and readings for each day of the year, the Service for the Poor was unchanging, requiring the poor and their ministers to perform identical rites without fail or "to be dismissed out of the house." Its sequence of psalms and lessons reflects upon the poor, miserable condition of the residents, echoing the *Ordre* itself. As an extension of the *Ordre*, the service functions to propitiate God and discipline the bodies and spirits of the ill. Psalm 51 (*Miserere*), featured in the morning after the "anthem of the poore," speaks to the need for purgation and health, recalling the language of the sisters' charge: "Thou shalt purge me with Isop, and I shalbe cleane; thou shalt wash me, and I shalbe whiter than snowe" (G2v). The literal purging of the patients' clothing and washing of their bodies is imagined in a spiritual key. The following lesson exhorts them to control their flesh, recalling the older catechetical function of texts in John Cok's Latin manuscript, updated to apply not to canon-brothers or elderly elite residents but to the poor themselves, plucked from the teeming streets of London. The text warns, "The dedes of the fleshe are these, aduoutrie, fornication, vnclenness, wantones, worshypyng of ymages, witchecrafte, hatred, variaunce, zeale, wrathe, strief, sedicious sectes, enuieng, murther, dronkenesse, glotony, and such lyke" (G4r). This list, with its particular attention to the sexual and violent sins of "rogues" as well as to the dangers of idolatry and religious dissent, speaks to the hospital's abhorrence of slander and to its twinned mission of physical and spiritual reformation.

We may discern some of the same emphases in the evening service, likewise unchanging from day to day. The lesson from Romans 6 emphasizes the possibility of new life through Christ's resurrection, an apt remonstrance for the poor and ill, who will, the governors hope, be physically cured and spiritually reformed during their time at the hospital: "consider ye also, that ye are ded as touchynge sinne, but are aliue vnto God, through Jesus Christ our lord. Let not sinne therefore reigne in youre mortall body, that you should thereunto obey by the lustes of it. Neither geue you your membres as instrumentes of vnrighteousnes vnto sinne, but geue ouer your selues vnto God, as they that of deathe are lyue" (H5r–v). The process of reforming the body, from death to life, sin to purity, is emblematized in the very words that the poor hear every day of their time in the hospital.

Like St. Bartholomew's of London, St. Mark's of Bristol experienced a combination of rupture and continuity in its religious life during the Reformation. In 1552, the year St. Bartholomew's *Ordre* was printed, Edward's revised Book of Common Prayer was issued, and all churches across the nation were required to obtain it. W. R. Barker notes, "Accordingly the following entry is made the same year:—Item, for a book of the new order of the last setting forth, for the Gaunts."[132] By this time, the hospital had been dissolved and given over by King Henry to the mayor and city council to become a civic chapel.[133] Repurposing the hospital's church as a civic institution under corporation control removed the hospital from the nexus of charity and poor relief into which St. Bartholomew's had been reinserted, yet it returned St. Mark's to visible participation within a reformed religious system. In my epilogue, I piece together the early Reformation history of this new chapel, whose curate, John Ellis, was a former hospital brother. I suggest that despite radical changes in liturgical fashions, up to 1552 (and perhaps beyond), the chapel's rites for the dead may have retained some of the associations with purgatory and intercession that the medieval institution had cultivated.

As early as 1533, Bristol had become a flashpoint for religious controversy. At Easter, Hugh Latimer, a supporter of the royal divorce, preached a series of radical sermons that brought him to national attention. Latimer's sermons, which inveighed against pilgrimages, purgatory, and prayers to saints, were pivotal to the early Reformation, triggering Cranmer's edict in 1534 prohibiting preaching about purgatory, saints, priestly marriage, justification by faith, pilgrimages, or miracles, "considering these things have caused dissension amongst the subjects of this realm already."[134] With this edict, "the existence of purgatory, a given of late medieval religion, had been relegated to the status of a contentious opinion."[135] At the same time that reformist positions such as the doctrine of justification by faith and an emphasis on vernacular scripture were circulating in Bristol, traditionalist preachers such as Roger Edgworth fought back publicly, defending the pope's authority, the traditional role of the clergy, and the Mass.[136] The opinions and beliefs of Bristol's laity are difficult to gauge given the lack of documentation. Most Bristolians may not have supported radical reform. Martha Skeeters emphasizes the division of lay loyalties among numerous religious institutions and the fragmentation of the Bristol clergy itself under the pressure of competing religious views. She suggests that the fissures among laity and clergy may have "undermined the *status quo*; clerical squabbling undoubtedly created apathy or even anticlericalism among many lacking strong doctrinal convictions."[137] Compared to the London citizens' loud defense of local hospitals, the response of Bristol's laity to the dissolutions of its religious houses was muted, with little resistance on record.[138] It is possible that given the changing attitudes toward the poor in the 1530s, support for religious houses and their traditionally indiscriminate charity had begun to wane in some quarters.[139] David Harris Sacks has connected local religious disaffection to the foundering cloth trade and a diminishing spirit of guild unity.[140]

Yet during this period, we find scattered evidence of continued loyalties to local hospitals: this is true in the case of St. Mark's, where lay worshipers testified to its centrality in their spiritual lives. After Master Colman and the few remaining brothers had signed on to the Act of Supremacy in 1534, Jane Guildford, resident widow, became concerned about the house's fate and her ability to worship there. As Mary Erler has described, Guildford had lived and worshiped in the hospital, received counsel from Master John Colman, and sponsored the construction of the lavish Poyntz chapel. In her 1535 letter to Thomas Cromwell, the king's officer, she voices anxiety about maintaining her lodging and access to the church, if not the chapel:

> A suit I have now unto you, by reason of certain injunctions that I understand are given to the master of the Gaunts in Bristol, that no woman shall come within the precincts of the same, where I have a lodging most meetest, as I have chosen, *for a poor widow to serve God now in my old days.* And I trust both for myself and for my women, like as we have been hitherto, to be of such governance with your licence to

the same, that no inconvenience shall ensue thereof. And where hereto
before I have used from my house to go the next way to the church, for
my ease, through the cloister of the same house to a chapel that I have
within the quire of the same, I shall be content from henceforth, if it
shall so seem convenient to you, to forbear that, and to resort to the
common place, like as other do, of the same church.[141]

Seeking a relaxation in some new "injunctions" that followed the 1534 agreement, a "reforming sweep" that prohibited women from monastic precincts,
Guildford sues to maintain her physical and spiritual home in the hospital.[142] She casts herself as a "poor widow," not quite a vowess but one dedicated to the hospital, as we have seen other widows were. Her language also
strongly recalls that of the widow Anna in the York *Purification*, who states,
"Here in this holy playce, I say, / Is my full purpose to abyde, / To serve my
God bothe nyght and day." Guildford is willing to give up access to her private family chapel in order to maintain a connection to the hospital, and
she also asks that Cromwell "license the master of the house [Colman] to
go abroad to see for the common weal of the same [the hospital]," suggesting that by 1535 Colman was seeing his own freedom curtailed and the
hospital's fortunes imperiled.

Although the hospital evidently still hosted local worshipers such as
Guildford, such support was not sufficient to hold off its dissolution. In
1539, the hospital, along with St. Augustine's Abbey, was formally surrendered to the king. The following entry appears in the Bristol mayor's *Kalendar*: "this year the Abbott and Conuent of Seynt Augustynes of Bristowe sur-
rendred that monastry vnto the kynges moost noble graces handes. And
so in like wise the maister and his brothers of Gauntez, with theire assentz
made."[143] Whereas St. Augustine's Abbey was eventually turned into a cathedral church, St. Mark's Hospital was to take on a civic function as a chapel,
but without further formal service to the poor.[144] In 1541 it was turned over
to the city for a large fee. Moved, King Henry states, "as much by the sincere
affection that we feel for our town of Bristol as by the sum of a thousand
pounds sterling," he grants the hospital's site and the manors, including all
properties and rents, to the mayor and the commonalty of Bristol.[145] Earlier
civic records show that the town had worked hard to win Henry's affection,
currying his favor with lavish gifts in 1535 and offering fulsome praise of his
newborn son, Edward, in 1537.[146] This attention evidently paid off in the

transfer of power to civic leaders; the antiquarian Barrett's characterization of the deal is telling: "[the hospital] was granted the 33rd of Henry the 8th. 1540, from the crown to the mayor, burgesses, and commonalty of Bristol *for public uses, who are now in the place of the master and cobrethren of the hospital of St. Mark.*"[147] In arrangements reminiscent of those at London's St. Bartholomew's and York's Hospital of St. Thomas, the mayor and aldermen slip into secularized versions of the traditional hospital leadership roles. Although it does not appear in the sixteenth-century document, Barrett's phrase "public uses" is suggestive, for with this transfer the hospital chapel, which would later become the Lord Mayor's Chapel, now became available to any worshiper wishing to attend services there. Unlike the hospital, a private institution, home to the "special prayers" of intercession detested by lollards and Protestant reformers alike, both the space and the liturgy of the former hospital chapel were now open to all.

Changes to the chapel at the Dissolution indicate that the hospital was quickly relieved of its valuables. In 1540 the city paid for "certeyne baskettes to pake the churche plate that was caryede to London" and for "maylynge corde for the same" and "brede and ale for the caryers."[148] Canvas was procured for wrapping the "charters to be caryed to London." It is not clear which charters these were, but the action suggests the Crown appropriating the house's documentary record for itself.[149] As Barker notes, in 1541 charges appear for the expenses of Easter week, which were largely subsidized by the city corporation.[150] These included physical changes in the chapel, such as the addition of pews ("the setting of forms"), enabling worshipers to congregate comfortably. In contrast, Barker notes, at this time "the Monastery (St. Augustine's) is referred to as 'still void.'"[151] This observation suggests that post Dissolution, the former hospital may have received lay worshipers previously attracted to St. Augustine's, with which it had long sparred for the devotion of local people. Though in a reduced form, St. Mark's, like St. Bartholomew's, was on its way to becoming a site for the expression of reformed civic piety and charity.

# Epilogue

*Rites for the Dead and the End of Purgatory,*
*1540–1552*

At the Dissolution, a St. Mark's Hospital brother, John Ellis, was appointed curate of the new chapel for a pension of 8 pounds.[1] Ellis continued to receive the pension until his death in 1558.[2] The Dissolution documents sometimes call St. Mark's a "parish," and a plan may have existed when it was signed over to the city corporation to constitute it as a parish church. Yet it never became one, for it was situated within the parish of St. Augustine the Less. "The character of the Chapel thus transferred to the Corporation was peculiar, it being neither strictly parochial nor strictly private," notes Barker. "It is clear that in addition to its Conventual use [abrogated as of 1540], it was regarded as a place of worship for the Gaunts' Precincts."[3] The new chapel was not a parish church, but a religious home for people of the district who attended services voluntarily. Ellis served as curate of the repurposed chapel from 1540 to 1558, through the reigns of Henry, Edward, and Mary. Like some other ex-religious just after the Dissolution, such as the London Franciscans whom Erler has studied, Ellis remained closely connected to his original house.[4] The chapel would have been used for daily liturgies as well as baptisms, marriages and funerals, but we have no records of these from Ellis's period.[5] If we consider funerals specifically, the rites for the dead were the most fraught part of the liturgy during the Reformation, subject to radical changes yet also strongly defended by traditionalists. We may well wonder how Ellis administered the chapel through these repeated changes.

I conclude this book by speculating about how Ellis might have administered these rites in the turbulent years 1540–52. The scanty records note Ellis's appointment in 1540, his obligation to perform a traditional funeral for another former hospital brother, Richard Fechett, in 1546, and the corporation's 1552 purchase of "a book of the new order of the last setting forth, for the Gaunts" (the new Edwardian prayer book). Building up a picture from these three records, I suggest that Ellis's practices probably reflected continuity between the chapel's emergence from the dissolved hospital and the moment that the radical liturgical alterations of 1552 were imposed. Rites for the dead are central for considering how the chapel might have negotiated its new liturgical function in relation to the hospital's traditional work of commemoration amid the ongoing debate over purgatory. Another key source for this investigation survives in Bodleian MS Lyell 38, Master Colman's Latin manuscript. The book features Rolle's *Expositio super novem lectiones mortuorum* (hereafter *Super novem*), commentaries on the Job readings that lay at the heart of the Sarum Dirige service.[6] How might the spiritual influences of Sarum, Rolle, and Colman have informed Ellis's practice during these tumultuous years, when purgatory became controversial, then officially nonexistent?

The years just before and after the Dissolution saw several iterations of the English prayer book, in 1534, 1535, and 1539.[7] We do not know whether Ellis was enjoined to use the latest English version of the prayer book, Bishop Hilsey's 1539 *Manual of Prayers*, when he took up his post, or whether he continued to employ the old service books. The extensive medieval Latin rites had included a procession accompanied by suffrages, a commendation service, and the Dirige rite featuring ten separate psalms, the seven penitential psalms, plus the nine interlinked readings from Job with responsories. The Sarum Dirige stressed the Christian's repentance for sin, the experience of life as continual suffering, and a lengthy confrontation with death, bolstered by a faith in God's stabilizing power and a diffuse anticipation of resurrection, as articulated in the first "Dirige" (Job 19:25–26), the responsory for the first lection: "For I know that my Redeemer liveth, and in the last day I shall rise out of the earth. And I shall be clothed again with my skin, and in my flesh I will see my God." The 1539 English Dirige kept a similar shape, retaining the psalms and nine lessons. Yet even though it included Sarum's lengthy readings from Job 14, this Dirige replaced six of the Job readings with texts from Augustine and the New Testament, changing the emphasis somewhat.[8]

The reformed service, even in retaining the psalms' expression of penance and faith turned palpably from death to resurrection, at times criticizing an undue focus on death. The new service marshals Augustine in the fourth lesson to impugn "the pompe of the Dirige" as contributing more to "the comforte of the lyue, then the helpe of the deade," citing the "mynistery of angels" who attended the burial of Lazarus, resurrected at Christ's hands.[9] The resurrection theme is expanded in the New Testament readings, notably lection seven, drawing upon 1 Corinthians 15: "Behold I saye vnto you a mystery, we shall not al slepe, but we shall all be chaunged. . . . But whan thys corruptyble shall put on incorrupcion, and this mortall shall put on immortalite, then shall the worde be fulfylled: Death is swalowed vp in victory."[10] In this lection, the focus is shifted from Job's painful encounter with death (Job 17:1–3; 11–15) to the anticipation of the Resurrection and its fulfillment of the Word, another key reformed preoccupation.

Evidence from 1546, the year former hospital brother Richard Fechett requested an ultratraditional funeral, suggests that Ellis was probably still using the old service. Ellis figures prominently in Fechett's will, which discloses a long standing friendship between the two priests and assumes the continuation of traditional liturgical practices at the chapel.[11] Fechett (sometimes recorded as "Fletcher") was pensioned in 1539, but unlike the three other remaining priests, he seems not to have taken up another post.[12] He asks to be buried "within the Quyer of parish ( ) Saint Maikes church" and gives six shillings and eightpence to cover the expenses.[13] His first bequest is to the church: "a peir of vestementes of blewe tyssen an alter clothe of dioper with a masse booke."[14] Showing orthodox Catholic devotion, he invests curate Ellis with gifts and spiritual responsibilities: "I geve and bequethe to Sir John Ellis curate of that churche iij s. iiijd. in money and oon of my best Surplices at the discrecion of my executor to be delyvered to hym for a remembraunce to praye for my Soule and all my Frendes and Christen soules."[15] Fechett was a bookish priest, bequeathing not only the mass book to St. Mark's, but also giving "Sir John Robyns prist my goostly Father" his "best and v bookes which is the whole wurkes of Vincent [of Beauvais?] and a nother book called Sermones discipuli *a dirige booke of vellom* with a Claspe of Silver & gilte."[16] He gives another mass book to a friend, Edward Prym, of "the parishe church of St. Mathos otherwise called the Churche of Clyfton within the Countie of Gloucester," asking him "*to kepe dyryge and masse* and to make a drynking to that companye of that parish after diryge vs."[17] In addition to contributing to the fabric of St. Mark's (money for repairs of the church and the water pipes), he shows a traditional concern for the neighborhood poor, with twenty shillings to be given at his burial, his month's mind, and his year's mind. Moreover he asks for the traditional "tryntall of masses to be kepte to the some of xjs. *Item my mynde and will is to have a dirage and masse the daie of my buryall with xx*$^{ti}$ *pristes* which costes shall amount to the some of xvjs. at the monethes mynde lykwyse xvjs."[18] Fechett is focused on gifting liturgical books and on the proper execution of the Dirige and mass for the benefit of his soul. A "dirige booke of vellom" was presumably the Sarum version (the new one being on paper). It seems likely that he wished Ellis to perform this traditional service.

Whether in 1546 Ellis used the Latin Sarum version or the 1539 English *Manual of Prayers* to perform his former hospital brother's funeral, he would have been able to marshal his traditional knowledge and his study of Rolle's *Super novem* to inform Fechett's funeral services. I suspect that Ellis would not have skimped on references to the misery of death, the passage through purgatory, or the need for intercession by the community, all of which were emphasized in Rolle. These were priorities for Fechett that Ellis also would have understood. The Sarum Dirige included Job 14:1–6 and 13–16 as lections five and six, and the 1539 liturgy includes Job 14:1–5 and 7–16 as lessons two and three. Hence most of the same content would have been shared:

(1) Man born of a woman, living for a short time, is filled with many miseries. (2) Who cometh forth like a flower, and is destroyed, and fleeth as a shadow, and never continueth in the same state. (3) And dost thou think it meet to open thy eyes upon such an one, and to bring into judgment with thee? (4) Who can make him clean that is conceived of unclean seed? It is not thee who only art? (5) The days of man are short and the number of his months is with thee: thou hast appointed his bounds which cannot be passed. (6) Depart a little from him, that he may rest, until his wished for day come, as that of the hireling. (7) A tree hath hope: if it be cut, it groweth green again, and the boughs thereof sprout. . . . (13) Who will grant me this, that thou mayst protect me in hell, and hide me till thy wrath pass, and appoint me a time when thou wilt remember me? (14) Shall man that is dead, thinkest thou, live again? all the days in which I am now in warfare, I expect until my change come. (15) Thou shalt call me, and I will answer thee: to the work of thy hands thou shalt reach out thy right hand. (16) Thou indeed hast numbered my steps, but spare my sins.

If we consider some of the passages that Colman marked with his characteristic pointing hand and brackets, we may appreciate the emphasis that this lection had received in the hospital, where these readings perhaps served as guides for the canons' reflections on sinfulness, brotherhood, and purgatory.

Commenting on Job 14:1, Rolle expounds on the connection between suffering and sin: "multe sunt miserie quibus repletur miser homo. Et non habet miseriam nisi propter peccatum. Quot sunt peccata tocius vite; tot miscriarum habebit tormenta" (Miserable man is full of miseries, and the sole cause of misery is sin. As many sins as there are in his life, so many miseries he will have).[19] He later enumerates these pains in detail: "miseriam vestis, miseriam caliditatis, miseriam frigoris, miseriam sitis, miseriam famis, miseriam putredinis, miseriam fetoris" (misery of clothing, misery of heat, misery of cold, misery of thirst, misery of hunger, misery of corruption, misery of stench).[20] A pointing hand and an abbreviated marginal note signifying "miseria propter peccatum" mark the start of this chapter, visually drawing brothers' attention to the range of life's sufferings and the sinfulness causing them.[21] Rolle's emphasis on a continuum of pains during life and the degradation of the body after death keeps the focus on suffering. These expositions and annotations were originally intended for the brothers' own contemplation, like the *Emendatio vitae* text, with its emphasis on an ascetic break from the world and an avoidance of fleshly temptations. Rolle's reflections upon the Job text might also have served Ellis when performing his duties in the new setting, perhaps embellishing the readings with a sermon or counseling worshipers on the fear of death.

Rolle's commentary on Job 14:2, "quasi flos egreditur et conteritur et fugit velut umbra et numquam in eodem statu permanet," would be as fitting in 1546 as earlier, with its emphasis on the sinner's solitary confrontation with Christ and desperate propitiation for mercy. Of this verse Rolle notes, "Pensate fratres mei condiciones vestre fragilitatis, et nolite polliceri vobis vitam longam. Vigilate in preceptis dei et parati estote in omni tempore; quia nescitis diem neque horam qua Dominus noster uenturus sit" (Think, my brothers, of the conditions of your frailty, and do not wish for a long life. Be vigilant in God's precepts and be ready at any time; for you know neither the day nor the hour when our Lord shall come).[22] The fleeting quality of life pushes Rolle to emphasize readiness and constant adherence to holy precepts. For hospital brothers, these would have included the vows and practices of the religious community. But as we saw in chapter 4's *manus meditationis* at the end of John Cok's Latin book, MS Additional 10392, such warnings of death as imminent but mysterious would also have relevance for lay readers or auditors in the hospital. We can imagine the appropriateness of this commentary not only for memorializing Richard Fechett, once Ellis's spiritual brother, but also for other worshipers as "brothers." These are no longer brothers in the hospital or in fraternity with the institution, but brothers (and sisters) worshiping in the new civic chapel.

Given the confusion attending life and the long anticipation of death that the Job texts emphasize, purgatory had offered Rolle a useful image for the majority of people who remained uncertain of their ends even as they hoped for bliss. The status of purgatory was under heated debate in 1546, a year before it was categorically denounced by Cranmer in the new Book of Homilies and the Royal Visitation Injunctions.[23] Like Fechett, seemingly untroubled by religious controversy or the winds of reform, some worshipers at the chapel may have remained confident of purgatory's existence. Commenting on Job 14:5, "Constituisti terminos eius qui praeterire non poterunt" (thou hast appointed his bounds which cannot be passed), Rolle remarks on the vigilance that this boundedness must engender. Colman placed a maniculum just above this passage: "Nos quippe terminum nescimus, finem nostrum penitus ignoramus. Et ideo magi cauere debemus, quia magnum periculum nobis iminet" (Naturally we cannot know our end; we remain ignorant of our death).[24] Those who dwell "in celo" (in heaven) are "securi . . . scientes quod termini glorie non videbunt" (secure . . . knowing that they will never see the end of glory). In contrast, those who are punished in hell will know no end of suffering. Yet those in purgatory

> in medio sunt, inter infernum et celum, quia quamquam torqueantur in flamma, habent tamen terminum constitutum quando liberabuntur a pena. Unde et securiores sunt de gloria celi. . . . Sciunt enim post illam punicionem se perducendos ad paradisum. Nos vero eciam quamuis in tribulacionibus hic uiuimus. . . . Et cum huiusmodi sit homo in carne manens, uel in purgatorio existens.

> ———

> They are in the middle between hell and heaven, for although they are twisted in flames, nevertheless they have an end ordained when they will be liberated from pains. Then they are more secure of the glory of heaven. . . . They know that after their punishment they will be led to paradise. Truly, we are living here in tribulation. . . . And in this way man must remain in the flesh, or in purgatory.[25]

For Rolle, purgatory not only represented a hopeful middle state from which sinners would eventually be liberated, but it also provided a metaphor for the uncertainty and pain of earthly life. In this passage, purgatory becomes a way to speak about life after death and to analyze the difficulties of earthly life. Purgatory is conceptually central to Rolle's exposition of Job, just as it had been central in practical terms to the life of the medieval hospital. Although its existence was under debate, and although the chapel could no longer officially perform intercession, purgatory would have remained powerful as a teaching tool and a sympathetic expression of the common "tribulation" shared by all Christians.

By 1552, when the corporation purchased "a book of the new order of the last setting forth," Ellis was still presiding over the chapel, but much had changed in theology and politics. Marshall has argued that "the Edwardian campaign against purgatory represents a moment of rupture, perhaps the most abrupt and traumatic of all the cultural apertures opened up in sixteenth-century England."[26] The 1549 Injunctions had forbidden the mention of purgatory, and the 1549 prayer book had removed all references to the third place.[27] The year 1549 represented a liturgical tipping point: despite some lags in acquiring the new prayer book, its purchase was widely enforced as the old service books were systematically purged from churches.[28] The 1549 service retained psalms 116, 139, and 146 and an address to the corpse, which suggested some continuing relationship between the dead and the living. However, the version of 1552 would have been nearly unrecognizable to Ellis, offering an even starker text than that of three years earlier.[29] It fully replaced intercession with resurrection, opening with certainty in Christ as its vehicle: "I am the resurrection and the life (sayth the Lord): he that beleveth in me, though he were dead, yet shall he live" (John 11:25).[30] Now Job was enlisted not to bemoan at length the sin and sufferings of life and death, but instead to broadcast redemption. After the reading from John, we find Job 19:25–27, once the responsory for the first Sarum lection. Here, removed from the context of death and suffering, the spoken text gestures only to the promised redemption: "I knowe that my redeemer lyveth, and that I shall ryse out of the yearth in the last daye, and shalbe covered again with my skinne, and shall see God in my flesh: yea and I my selfe shall beholde hym, not with other but with these same iyes."[31] A second reading from Job 1 (repeated in 1 Timothy 6:7), not found in any previous Dirige service, asserts not only the fleeting nature of life but also utter human incapacity to affect one's fate, encapsulating the reformed conviction of justification by faith.

Finally, Job 14, the centerpiece of the Sarum lections and subject of Rolle's extensive commentary, is truncated to include just the first two verses, on the shortness of life and suddenness of death, proceeding without visual separation into a Lutheran hymn: "In the myddest of lyfe we be in death, of whom may we seke for succour but of thee, o Lorde, which for our synnes justly art moved."[32] Derived from a ninth-century work by Notker of Gall, this hymn in its new context emphasizes that God alone can deliver souls from pain, as the hymn continues: "But spare us Lord most holy, o God moste mighty, o holy and mercifull saviour, thou most worthy judge eternal, suffre us not at our last houre for any paines of death, to fal from the."[33] Although the Christian community still speaks as a collective "we," within the further reformed setting, gone are the allusions to the process of death and its pains, to the consoling presence of God evoked in the psalms, to the community surrounding the dying person, or to the possibility of passage through purgatory toward heaven.

The congregation is still exhorted to pray together, but now that intercessory prayers and the possibility of purgatory had been excised from burial and postburial practices, those surrounding the corpse were in theory obligated to take sole responsibility for their misdeeds as they confronted God without reliance upon purgatory as a middle ground between heaven and hell. Ellis was instructed to use this version of the prayer book, but we cannot know if he actually did. Recorded orthodox responses to the 1552 funeral service were strongly negative. Robert Parkyn, a conservative Yorkshire curate, sardonically noted the absence of "diriges or other devoutt prayers to be songe or saide for suche as was departtide this transitorie worlde, for thai nedyde none (saide the boyke). Why? By cawsse ther sowlles was immediattlye in blisse and joy after the departtynge from the bodies, and therfor thay nedyde no prayer."[34] Parkyn was clearly devoted to the traditional Dirige service: the first text that he collected in his commonplace book was Rolle's *Super novem*.[35]

Curate John Ellis may have felt similar. Perhaps he did not use the new prayer book. But even if he were using the 1552 version and wished to embellish the service, Rolle's exhaustive emphasis on misery and its link to sin remained extremely fitting, even in the midst of a profoundly changed liturgy. As curate of St. Mark's Chapel, Ellis would have been officially prohibited from invoking purgatory, yet his spiritual charges might have lived in a quite purgatorial state on earth, doubtless quite "ignorant of [their] death" and of their resurrection, perhaps fearing it more given the religious changes witnessed during their lifetimes.

When Mary ascended the throne in 1553, liturgical customs were again turned upside down, with the repeal of Edward's prayer book and the return of the Sarum service decreed in 1554. There is no record of St. Mark's Chapel restoring the original liturgy, but we have seen, with Richard Fechett's bequests of mass books and Dirige books in 1546, that such volumes remained in circulation. Evidence from elsewhere in the country suggests that by 1555 many congregations had returned to traditional liturgies, including the "dyryge and masse" that Fechett had requested.[36] The Bristol corporation's Audit Books of that year record a payment "for making of [an] Altar in the Church," and in 1557 they record "a processional for the Gaunts church at St. Mark's fair."[37] Practices were beginning to resume as before the breach with Rome, yet even proponents of Reformation continuity like Duffy argue that after two decades of wrenching changes, something fundamental in the "continuity" between living and dead had been lost forever.[38] However, some of Master Colman's books survived to testify to the hospital's literary legacy and lasting influence. As the hospital became an independent chapel, still referred to by Bristolians as "the Gaunts," its liturgical services, held in the space ringed by medieval tombs, may have changed radically or little during the intervening decades. We cannot know. The continued presence of a former hospital brother, a disciple of Colman and Rolle who was closely linked to the old ways, testified to the city's continued investment in a place to link the living with the dead, on terms that may have been rather flexible. Although I will not speculate about Ellis's practice in his final years (1553–58), a restoration of the Sarum service in the space of the former hospital chapel may have met with guarded relief from the aged ex-brother. He would not live to see the next iteration of reform during Elizabeth's reign.

In contrast to the afterlife of St. Bartholomew's, London, which recombined worship, charity, and medical care in the "new" hospital, the coda to St. Mark's dissolution speaks to the separation, in Bristol, of reformed worship from civic charity. Even as St. Mark's Chapel continued to operate as a public place of worship, the mayor's "Kalendar" records that in 1586 a local benefactor, John Carr, esquire, endowed a new charitable venture: "an hospitall w[i]thin the Cittie for the bringinge up of poore fatherless children according to the order of the hospitall of Christchurch in St Bartholomewes in London."[39] The institution was to operate on the site where the

Gaunts house had once stood. It was chartered by Queen Elizabeth in 1590 and approved by an act of Parliament in 1597.[40] The hospital's charitable purpose was reimagined as an institution for the nurture of poor orphans and children, inspired by reformed London models. It was not quite a public place—a fee was required for entry—but as a civic initiative enabled by the Dissolution and by local charity, its development paralleled the emergence of St. Mark's as a chapel. The new Bristol hospital became a secular place of care, training, and avoidance of the roguery widely feared in this period. Thus the medieval hospital's legacy was bifurcated into the reformed chapel and the new secular hospital.

We have records of these new and refounded institutions but little evidence of the kinds of literary practices that had flourished in later medieval English hospitals, such as the performance of drama or the copying of poetry and devotional texts. An exception is Thomas Vicary's *Anatomie of Man*, a medical treatise that emerged from St. Bartholomew's in the mid-sixteenth century, connecting the hospital's learned traditions with its reconception and future as a scientific institution. Yet this brief work, which Vicary modestly describes as containing "certayne Lessons and smal Chapters a parte of the Anatomie, but touching a part of euery member particulerly," was largely derivative of Galen and medieval medical authorities and less comprehensive than Mirfield's *Breviarium Bartholomei*.[41] The mixed religious, charitable, and medical mission of our three medieval hospitals made them sites for a unique complex of literary practices, yet the institutions' imbrication in Catholic culture, particularly intercession for the dead, made full continuity with the past impossible. Yet in the near term, as we have seen with St. Bartholomew's and St. Mark's, textual strategies of reconstitution and reuse may have enabled some traditional ideals and practices to persist, even under the watchful eyes of the new secular overseers. In some ways, England's hospitals suffered the narrowing of scope and imagination that James Simpson has associated with the institutions and literature of England's "cultural revolution."[42] Many simply did not survive. Yet each of the three hospitals considered here persisted in some ever-shifting configuration of text, practice, and space. Whether in the revised lines of the York *Purification* pageant, the off-site care of destitute mothers at the new St. Bartholomew's Hospital, or the partially altered rites for the dead in the Bristol Mayor's Chapel, older literary traditions continued to intersect with reformed practices, reshaping the care and the "soule heale" that these hospitals had long performed.

# NOTES

## Introduction

1. Rawcliffe, *Medicine for the Soul*; Rubin, *Charity and Community.*

2. Coletti, "Social Contexts." Also see Coletti, *Mary Magdalene and the Drama of Saints*, 39–43.

3. Notably, Erler, "Widows in Retirement"; Kumler, "*Imitatio rerum.*"

4. Rawcliffe, "Written in the Book of Life," 131.

5. Rawcliffe, "Christ the Physician," 83.

6. Geltner, "Social Deviancy," 34.

7. Gilchrist, "Christian Bodies and Souls," 116.

8. Rubin, "Imagining Medieval Hospitals," 15.

9. See Watson, "Origins," 79, for a list of common terms denoting hospitals. Phrases such as "*domum hospitalem, domum infirmorum, domum leprosorum . . .* pair the notation of the house . . . with a description of aid or support" (ibid.).

10. Orme and Webster, *English Hospital*, 18. On the development of hospitals within early monasteries, see Crislip, *From Monastery to Hospital.*

11. See Gilchrist, *Sacred Heritage*, 74–75, on monastic infirmaries and regimes of health.

12. Watson, "Origins," 87. She notes that the model of the hospital as a community under a religious rule is taken from French and Belgian models that do not fit most early English foundation patterns (81).

13. Also see Watson, *On Hospitals*, 108–13, on the critical importance of fulfilling the donor's wishes in the foundation and management of a hospital.

14. Watson, "Origins," 91.

15. Ibid., 89.

16. Watson cautions against assimilating English hospitals to Continental models, but comparative work can illuminate important parallels and differences. See Horden, "A Discipline of Relevance." Also see the geographically diverse collections in Horden, *Hospitals and Healing*, and Horden, *Cultures of Healing.* On hospitals in the medieval Levant and Egypt, see Ragab, *Medieval Islamic Hospital.*

17. European hospitals, always distinct from monasteries, had such a variety of forms and leaders that even the farthest-reaching canon law (*Quia contigit*,

from the Council of Vienne, 1311/12), acknowledged that they were not necessarily always "ecclesiastical" institutions. Watson notes that "*xenodochia*/hospitals did not fundamentally belong to the church" (Watson, *On Hospitals*, 308–9).

18. Rawcliffe, "Medicine for the Soul," 329–30. Quoted passage from the statutes of Ewelme almshouse (see chapter 5 for more on this foundation). Watson aptly characterizes each "charitable foundation" as "a living testament to an act of *caritas*" (Watson, *On Hospitals*, 312).

19. Adam Davis notes that a precursor for the foundation of hospitals in thirteenth-century Champagne was the valorization of "charitable service through the performance of the corporal works of mercy," which in turn stemmed from the "larger apostolic movement of the twelfth and thirteenth centuries" (Davis, *Medieval Economy of Salvation*, 48–49).

20. The most significant legal restrictions on hospitals related to "the possession of a chapel and burial ground, which might compromise the rights of the local parish church" (Orme and Webster, *English Hospital*, 37–39). Hospitals often clashed with parish priests over such rights, as did St. Mark's in the fifteenth century.

21. See Rawcliffe, "Word from Our Sponsor," 168–69. On lay spiritual affiliation with hospitals, also see Rawcliffe, "Communities of the Living and of the Dead."

22. Kealey, *Medieval Medicus*, 97.

23. For the canons of St. John's Hospital, Cambridge, see the rule printed in Rubin, *Community and Charity*, 300–301; for lay obligations at Ewelme, see Richmond, "Victorian Values."

24. Davis, *Medieval Economy of Salvation*, 275.

25. Augustine, *Enarr. in Ps.* 48.1.11 (*PL* 36:551), cited in Arbesmann, "Concept of 'Christus Medicus,'" (15). John Henderson remarks on the importance of the *Christus medicus* idea and the frequent presence of Christ's image in early hospitals (Henderson, *The Renaissance Hospital*, 113–17).

26. Tanner, ed., *Decrees of the Ecumenical Councils*, 1:245. Catherine Batt notes that this image was anticipated by Alain de Lille's *Liber Poenitentialis*, in which Alain makes the analogy between a medical doctor seeking a correct diagnosis and a priest ministering to the spiritually ill (Henry of Grosmont, *Livre de Seyntz Medicines*, 35; and Alain de Lille, *Liber Poenitentialis*, 2:15–16). A devotional work expressing penitential anguish and hope for healing, Henry's *Book of Holy Medicines* seems related in spirit to the hospital of the Annunciation of St. Mary in the Newarke, Leicester, which his father founded in 1330 and which he reconsecrated (Henry of Grosmont, *Livre de Seyntz Medicines*, 39–40).

27. Citrome, *Surgeon in Medieval English Literature*, 5.

28. McCann, *Soul-Health*, 82–85. On the latter, he cites (at 84) Augustine, *In Epistolam Joannis ad Parthos*, tract 9.4: "Timor Dei sic vulnerat, quomodo medici ferramentum; putredinem tollit, et quasi videtur vulnus augere" (The fear of God wounds like the knife of the physician: it takes away the festering, and seems to enlarge as it were, the wound). Translation from Arbesmann, "Concept of 'Christus Medicus,'" 22n102.

29. McCann, *Soul-Health*, 5.

30. See, e.g., Gilchrist, "Christian Bodies and Souls," 108–10, and Rubin, "Development and Change," 51, on the sparse surviving records of medical care in hospitals.

31. Park, *Secrets of Women*, 10.

32. Medical works are relatively rarely attested in extant English hospital library lists. Ramsey and Willoughby list a few anonymous medical works (a "Liber medicine" and "Liber de physica") recorded in library lists from Rome's Hospital of the Holy Trinity and St. Thomas and Writtle's Hospital of All Saints, respectively. See Ramsey and Willoughby, *Hospitals, Towns, and the Professions*, 535.

33. Gilchrist, *Sacred Heritage*, 106.

34. Cullum, *Cremetts and Corrodies*, 3. Female carers might be characterized as "nurses" or provide nursing care without being formally recognized. See Ritchey, *Acts of Care*, 80–94, on health care by nuns and semireligious women in hospitals of the Low Countries.

35. Rawcliffe, "Christ the Physician," 89.

36. Gilchrist, "Christian Bodies and Souls," 103. Gilchrist notes the gradual development of hospitals, such as the Domus Dei of Bury St. Edmunds, which acquired a chapel and cemetery when it moved to a larger site.

37. On St. Bartholomew's, see ibid., 112, and on water supplied to St. Mark's, see Burgess, *Right Ordering of Souls*, 77. Also see Davis, *Medieval Economy of Salvation*, 265–66, on water and hygiene in Champenois hospitals.

38. Hall, "York's Medieval Infrastructure," 80.

39. Watson, "City as Charter," 238.

40. Ibid., 262.

41. Orme and Webster, *English Hospital*, 41.

42. Watson, "City as Charter," 262.

43. Geltner, "Social Deviancy," 31.

44. Davis, *Medieval Economy of Salvation*, 189, also notes the "mixed" nature of hospital populations as one of their distinctive institutional characteristics.

45. Text of the longer version (*Praeceptum*) from *La Règle de Saint Augustin*, 1:418. Translation by Robert Russell, OSA, at http://faculty.georgetown.edu/jod/augustine/ruleaug.html (italics in translation).

46. Dickinson, *Origins*, 196.

47. On St. Leonard's, see Cullum, "Hospitals and Charitable Provision," 146–47.

48. These regulations are printed in Dugdale, *Monasticon Anglicanum*, vol. 6, pt. 2: 610. My translations here and below except where otherwise noted.

49. See Cullum, "Hospitals and Charitable Provision," 156, and details in chapter 3 herein.

50. This phrase was coined by W. A. Pantin (*English Church*, 28) to describe the large group of fourteenth-century unbeneficed clergy, including chaplains, who worked for a salary rather than holding a benefice. Kerby-Fulton contends that "the unbeneficed contributed disproportionately to the resurgence of Middle English literature, which also, often, contains poetry recording or representing their plight" (Kerby-Fulton, *Clerical Proletariat*, 2).

51. In her conclusion, Kerby-Fulton details the "tendencies" of clerical proletarian writers, including, in summary: "*disgruntlement with both church and state*"; writing in which "the border . . . *between the secular and religious is blurred*"; "*strong voices of compassion for the poor*"; "*encouragement and counsel to women*"; possession of "'*the means of production*' *via book production supplies*"; "*marvelously complex poetic speakers*"; "*multilingualism and even literacy* itself"; "*a sense that, against all odds, intellectual or ecclesiastical material can be the stuff of great poetry*" (Kerby-Fulton, *Clerical Proletariat*, 300–304; italics in original).

52. See, for instance, my discussion of John Shirley in chapter 3.

53. Carlin, "Medieval English Hospitals," 32.

54. For the Ospedale di Santa Maria Nuova, see the statutes translated in Park and Henderson, "First Hospital among Christians," 180–83.

55. TNA, C270/20, membrane 1. When citing from medieval manuscripts, I have retained original spellings and silently modernized capitalization and punctuation. We also find detailed rules for the matron and nursing sisters in the statutes for London's Savoy Hospital, founded by King Henry VII. These were written circa 1515.

56. TNA, C270/20, membrane 1.

57. Cullum, "Hospitals and Charitable Provision," 168–69.

58. Gilchrist, *Sacred Heritage*, 89.

59. For St. Leonard's, York, see Cullum, "Hospitals and Charitable Provision," 166. See chapters 1 and 3, below, on the evidence of testators' regard for sisters at St. Leonard's and St. Bartholomew's.

60. Rawcliffe, "Hospital Nurses," 57.

61. *Rotuli Parliamentorum*, 4:19.

62. See Roffey, "Medieval Leper Hospitals," 215–16.

63. Rubin, *Charity and Community*, 301.

64. From the 1295 ordinances as recorded in Dugdale, *Monasticon Anglicanum*, vol. 6, pt. 2: 610.

65. On corrodies at St. Bartholomew's, see Rawcliffe, "Hospitals of Later Medieval London," 3–4.

66. Married retirees are to be distinguished from the married couples who sometimes pledged themselves to work at Continental hospitals and were required to observe chastity; on such couples, see Watson, *On Hospitals*, 267.

67. Rawcliffe, "Eighth Comfortable Work," 387. See Kerling, *Cartulary*, 105 (item 1059).

68. Dickinson, *Origins*, 137. For example: "Hospitals were generally committed to follow the most flexible of the monastic rules, that of St. Augustine (Gilchrist, "Christian Bodies and Souls," 103). Rubin, "Development and Change," 49, also uses this term.

69. In one fascinating example, Sethina Watson discusses three thirteenth-century hospitals founded by aristocratic women, two of which (North Creake and Lechlade) eventually adopted the Augustinian Rule under their founders' guidance. See Watson, "A Mother's Past."

70. Le Grand, *Statuts*, v.

71. Verheijen, *La Règle de Saint Augustin*, 1:148; translation by Russell, as in note 45, above. The sentence "Ante omnia . . . nobis data" opens the short version of the Rule (*Ordo monasterium* or *Regula Secunda*), and many medieval versions of the *Praeceptum* (*Regula Tertia*) begin with this sentence, then proceed with the longer version, as in Oxford St. John's College MS 173, John Colman's book, which I consider in chapter 4.

72. By the 1060s, regular canons across Europe were adopting some version of the Rule in order to ground their vision of a full common life in a text distinct from the monastic rules. Dickinson cites a letter by Alexander II of 1067, noting that the community of St. Denys, Rheims, was living "*sub regula beati Augustini*" (Dickinson, *Origins*, 54). As Jean Becquet notes, in contrast to the Benedictines, for which the rule was "essential," for the Augustinian canons in the eleventh and twelfth centuries, the Rule was still a "secondary" element; see Becquet, "Chanoines réguliers," 364.

73. See Davis, *Medieval Economy of Salvation*, 22–24, on the importance of the regular canons within the Champenois hospital movement of the twelfth and thirteenth centuries.

74. See Dickinson, *Origins*, 172, on the paucity of early Augustinian customaries in England.

75. Saak, *High Way to Heaven*, 182. On the other hand, the influential Augustinian hermit Jordan of Quedlinburg (or Saxony) cast the hermits in Augustine's model, as "the imitators of our Father Augustine" (ibid., 283).

76. Ibid., 365.

77. Ibid., 366.

78. Bynum, "Spirituality of Regular Canons," 36.

79. Ibid., quotations from 43 and 46.

80. See Reinke, "'Austin's Labour,'" 165. The *Expositio* is attributed to Hugh of St. Victor, but its authorship is disputed. The General Chapter of 1308 required that every house should hold a copy of the rule and the *Expositio* and read them daily. Most English Augustinian hospitals, including the three I consider, were independent houses under diocesan control, not that of the General Chapter.

81. His phrase is "surtout peut-être, le goût de l'étude"; Pouzet, "Quelques aspects," 174.

82. Forde, "Educational Organization," 22.

83. This phrase from ibid., 23.

84. See Roger, "Blakberd's Treasure," 93, on John Bokyngham of St. Bartholomew's Hospital, who was granted papal permission to study "theology and other lawful faculties" for seven years in the early fifteenth century.

85. Forde notes that Barnwell priory's *Observances* "imply that canons could copy their own books and also borrow from the common *armarium* with the Precentor's permission" (Forde, "Educational Organization," 25).

86. Pouzet, "Book Production outside Commercial Contexts," 232.

87. For St. Leonard's, see Moran, *Growth of English Schooling*, 74–75. For St. Bartholomew's, see Caroline Barron, "People of the Parish," 357.

88. Saak, *High Way to Heaven*, 475.

89. Ibid., 544.

90. Cullum, "Hospitals and Charitable Provision," 68, citing from British Library, MS Cotton Nero D. III, fol. 5r.

91. Carpenter, *Cartulary of St. Leonard's Hospital*, 1:xl.

92. Ibid., 1:xlii.

93. Cullum, "Hospitals and Charitable Provision," 87; also see ibid., 97.

94. Ibid., 158.

95. Ibid., 164–65.

96. Cullum, *Cremetts and Corrodies*, 28. The 1364 visitation (TNA C270/20, membrane 3) ordered that the "Barnhous" under the infirmary be prepared for children who would be cared for by one of the sisters.

97. TNA C270/20, membrane 1. Also see Cullum, *Cremetts and Corrodies*, 7–8.

98. Cullum, "Hospitals and Charitable Provision," 49.

99. As Watson "Origins," 93, notes, St. Bartholomew's did not follow the prevalent English foundation model of "sited alms"; it was inspired by a hospital that Rahere had visited in Rome.

100. See Kealey, *Medieval Medicus*, 85–106, on the "blaze" of Anglo-Norman hospital foundations, with discussion of St. Bartholomew's at 98–101.

101. Moore, *History of St. Bartholomew's Hospital*, 1:39–42. Also see Reddan, "Hospital of St. Bartholomew, Smithfield."

102. Moore, *History of St. Bartholomew's Hospital*, 1:52.

103. Daly, "The Hospitals of London," 30. This statute was reaffirmed in 1437 (see *Calendar of Patent Rolls, 1436–41*, 48).

104. Daly, "Hospitals of London," 29, referencing the 1316 visitations copied in LMA DL/A/A/004/MS09531/001, fol. 39v.

105. See Moore, *History of St. Bartholomew's Hospital*, 1:584–90, for the ordinances in translation. They are copied in the Hospital Cartulary (SBHB/HC /2/1, fols. 61–62), and catalogued in Kerling, *Cartulary*, 19 (item 48). By 1379–81, we find information about the hospital's staff from city records on taxation of clergy. They record three brothers, two chaplains, and three sisters paying taxes (McHardy, *Church in London*, 2).

106. Ross, *Cartulary*, xii–xiii.

107. Ibid., xiii.

108. Ross, *Cartulary*, xv. See Watson, "A Mother's Past," 242n143.

109. For the charter text, see Ross, *Cartulary*, 7–8 (translation) and 268 (Latin).

110. Ibid., xv–xvi.

111. From the Charter of Robert de Gournay, dated between November 1230 and August 1232 (see Ross, *Cartulary*, 2–3, for translation, and 266–67 for Latin).

112. Ross, *Cartulary*, 2. Ross notes that the number twenty-seven may have been falsified by the compiler of the cartulary, since earlier copies of this same charter indicate that one hundred poor were to be fed daily (ibid.).

113. Ross, *Cartulary*, 7 (English) and 268 (Latin).

114. Ibid., xvii.

115. See Ralph, *Great White Book*, 60.

116. See Barker, *Mayor's Chapel*, 51.

117. Orme and Webster, *English Hospital*, 127.

118. E.g., Martha Carlin argues for the general decline and mismanagement of English hospitals over this period, with a few exceptions, including St. Bartholomew's, London (Carlin, "English Medieval Hospitals," 34–35). Noting a low point, Reddan finds that "the tone of a house must have been deplorable when, as in 1375, the master, Richard de Sutton, was publicly defamed for incontinence with one of the sisters" (Reddan, "Hospital of St. Bartholomew," 152). Rubin suggests that fourteenth-century economic and demographic changes resulted in altered, more "suspicious" views of charitable institutions and led to greater discrimination in the provision of charity (Rubin, "Development and Change," 53).

Rawcliffe emphasizes the ways in which different hospitals adapted to the times, in which a "considerably smaller and generally fitter" English populace began to require different forms of poor relief (Rawcliffe, "Eighth Comfortable Work," 378).

119. Rawcliffe, "Eighth Comfortable Work," 383.

120. Ibid., 384.

121. Barron, "People of the Parish," 369–70; Roger, "Blakberd's Treasure," 95–96.


O N E .  St. Leonard's Hospital, Civic Drama, and Women's Devotion

1. Coletti, "Social Contexts," 297. As Coletti notes, the phrase "theater of devotion" comes from the pathbreaking Gibson, *Theater of Devotion.*

2. Most York pageants were sponsored by artisan companies, but some had mercantile sponsors, including the Vintners (*The Marriage at Cana*), the Drapers (*The Death of the Virgin*), and the Mercers (*Doomsday*). In 1999, Theresa Coletti remarked on the turn in locally oriented drama scholarship toward recognizing "the dynamic character of both the archive and the dramatic event," noting a critical emphasis on "theater performing cultural work in and for communities, institutions, and individuals; mediating political tensions between and within social groups; creating and contesting urban identities; drawing the boundaries, even inscribing the significance, of urban dramatic space itself" (Coletti, "Genealogy, Sexuality," 26). Coletti's dynamic and complex vision of urban drama has strongly influenced my own methodology.

3. For an exposition of the first theory, see Goldberg, "From Tableaux to Text." Goldberg characterizes these "two differing camps" (275). Also see Goldberg, "Craft Guilds, the Corpus Christi Play and Civic Government." For the latter view, see Swanson, *Medieval Artisans*, 120. For a close connection between the guilds' "internal structure" and their pageants, see Johnston, "Cycle Drama in the Sixteenth Century," 9. For the terms "irregular evolution" and "big bang," see Dobson, "Craft Guilds and City," 101.

4. Goldberg notes that "conventional craft guilds were not alone responsible for all the individual pageants" in the dramatic cycles of Beverley and York (Goldberg, "Performing the Word of God," 149–50).

5. My work may thus complement Goldberg's speculative argument for the greater participation of women workers during the cycle's early days, before women were "displaced" from the cycle during a later fifteenth-century period when artisan guilds increasingly discriminated against women. See Goldberg, "From Tableaux to Text," 262. Several recent monographs have focused on women's participation and representation in late medieval drama. On the cycle

plays, see Normington, *Gender and Medieval Drama*, and on the Digby Mary Magdalene and the East Anglian devotional context, see Coletti, *Mary Magdalene*. Also see Kathleen Ashley's important work on gendered representation and reception of drama in Ashley, "Sponsorship, Reflexivity, and Resistance."

6. I discuss the *Ordo paginarum* in detail in the next section. Few medieval records survive from St. Leonard's. For a summary of the remaining materials, see Carpenter, *Cartulary*, xliii–xlvii. Extant records include two of three original cartulary volumes (BL MS Cotton Nero D. III and Bodleian MS Rawlinson B. 455); a coroner's roll for the hospital liberty 1386–89 (PRO, JUST 2/243); a bundle of extents and other documents that traveled to Lichfield (Lichfield RO, D 30/12/106-115) and to York (York Minster Library, MS 2/6 b–e). From this last, section b contains the hospital receiver's accounts (June–September 1409), lists of debtors (September 1404–September 1405 and September 1408–June 1409); section c contains selected accounts from 1343–86; section d contains later accounts from 1461–62; e contains a register of wills belonging to the hospital's peculiar jurisdiction (1410–1533). Other documents in e include selected presentations, inquests, and proceedings; a summons from 1452; and a grant of sanctuary from 1518.

7. The Masons had previously sponsored *Herod and the Magi* together with the Goldsmiths. For detailed discussion of their earlier coproduction and the later reassignment, see Rice and Pappano, *Civic Cycles*, 83–116. On the controversies leading to the reassignment, also see Evans, "When a Body Meets a Body."

8. On the state of the text, see Beadle, *York Plays*, 2:141–43. The York Register (London, British Library, MS Additional 35290) is the sole copy of the entire cycle. For an introduction, see Beadle and Meredith, *The York Play: A Facsimile*, ix–xlviii.

9. Twycross, "*Ordo paginarum* Revisited," 112.

10. Ibid., 105.

11. Ibid., 110.

12. Twycross, "Forget the 4:30 am Start," 106 (emphasis in original).

13. Niebrzydowski, *Bonoure and Buxum*,167.

14. *REED: York*, 1:19; 2:705.

15. Twycross, "*Ordo paginarum* Revisited," 111. Goldberg, "From Tableaux to Text," 258–59, emphasizes the "intensely visual nature" of the descriptions, downplaying their "possible textual nature," while acknowledging that some "descriptions do imply speech." He suggests the representations were "more tableau at this date."

16. For this record, ordering the joining together of the Painters' and Stainers' pageant with that of the Pinners and Latoners so that people might better hear the "oracula" (words) of the players, and in which one guild takes over the

other's "materiam loquelarum" (matter of the speeches), see *REED: York*, 1:37–38, and 2:723 for translation.

17. Twycross, "*Ordo paginarum* Revisited," 119.

18. Quoted phrase from ibid.

19. *REED: York*, 1:25, and 2:710 for translation. Twycross, "*Ordo paginarum* Revisited," 124, notes this dating and argues that Burton slightly revised the descriptions of the *Ordo* list "so that they would become much more like descriptions of plays, like, in fact, his Second List."

20. The Vulgate Bible, Douai–Rheims translation, is cited throughout.

21. Schorr, "Iconographic Development," 17.

22. For the development of the feasts, see Schorr, "Iconographic Development," 17–19. She notes, "Pope Sergius I is said to have instituted a procession with candles on the Feast of the Purification. His famous contemporary, the Venerable Bede, refers to the substitution of Mary's procession for the pagan rites in February and describes how the people and priests went through the church singing hymns and carrying candles" (18).

23. Lee, "'Women Ben Purifyid,'" 49.

24. Young, *Drama of the Medieval Church*, 2:250.

25. The first prayer addresses God and speaks of Christ being presented in the Temple: "Domine, Sancte Pater ... benedicere, et sanctificare digneris ignem istum, quem nos indigni suscipimus per invocationem Unigeniti Filii tui Domini nostri Jesu Christi, quem hodie praesentatum in templo justum Simeonem diu expectantem in ulnas suscepisse novimus" (Lord, Holy Father, deign to bless and sanctify this fire, which we, unworthy, carry in respect of your Son, the Unbegotten Lord Jesus Christ, whom today, we know, was presented in the Temple and was received by the just man Simeon, having waited for a long time) (Henderson, *Missale ad usum insignis Ecclesiae Eboracensis*, 2:17). Translations are mine unless otherwise noted.

26. Cf. Luke 2.32: "A light to the revelation of the Gentiles, and the glory of thy people Israel." The antiphon, to be sung at the altar of the Virgin, praises her as "caelestis porta" (gate of heaven) and claims, "ipsa enim portat regem gloriae" (she indeed bears the king of glory) (Henderson, *Missale*, 2:18).

27. Record cited in Young, *Drama of the Medieval Church*, 2:252. On this record in relation to the custom of churching, see Gibson, "Blessing from Sun and Moon," 20.

28. In the fifteenth century, the King's Lynn Corpus Christi procession featured an image of the Virgin Mary "in gesine" (in childbed) taken from the Gesyn chapel of St. Margaret's Church (Marks, *Image and Devotion*, 147).

29. Based on the evidence of local records, the cycle dramas staged in Newcastle and Norwich seem not to have featured *Purification* episodes. For

lists of pageants performed in Newcastle, see Anderson, *Records of Early English Drama: Newcastle-Upon-Tyne*, xi–xv; for Norwich, see Lancashire, *Dramatic Texts and Records*, 237–38. The Newcastle Shipwright's play of *Noah's Ark* and the Norwich Grocers' play of the *Fall of Man* are edited in Davis, *Non-Cycle Plays*, 25–31, 8–18, respectively. According to an early sixteenth-century pageant list, Beverley's cycle contained a *Symeon* episode, but no text survives; see Wyatt, "Play Titles without Play Texts," 70. The Towneley (Wakefield) pageants will not figure in my analysis, because their auspices are uncertain, and the surviving *Purification* episode is incomplete; see Palmer, "Recycling 'The Wakefield Cycle.'"

30. Gibson, *Theater of Devotion*, 137. For N-Town's possible association with regional religious guilds, see Sugano, *N-Town Plays*, 3–4, 7–12. Within the N-Town compilation, the *Purification* was added at a relatively late point and is followed by the date 1468 (ibid., 7).

31. Coletti, "Genealogy, Sexuality," 26.

32. For explorations of the connections between dramatic representations and religious group identities, see Gibson, *Theater of Devotion*, and Coletti, "Genealogy, Sexuality." On artisan groups and dramatic production, see Fitzgerald, *Drama of Masculinity*, and Rice and Pappano, *Civic Cycles*.

33. *Killing of the Children*, lines 9–15, in Baker, Murphy, and Hall, eds., *Late Medieval Religious Plays*, 96.

34. *The Purification*, in Sugano, *N-Town Plays*, lines 123–26. All quotations from the N-Town *Purification* will be taken from this edition, with lines cited parenthetically hereafter. In her early work on the N-Town plays, Gail McMurray Gibson posited a monastic provenance, yet she noted a possible connection between the *Purification* and the Bury St. Edmunds Candlemas guild; see Gibson, "Bury St. Edmunds," 65–66. She connects the epithets "salver of seknes" and "lanterne of lyght" to Candelmas. Gibson has recently accepted Sugano's arguments for N-Town as "compilation" rather than "cycle"; see Gibson, "Manuscript as Sacred Object," 521n4.

35. Matthew Sergi's new study brilliantly widens our critical conception of the Chester cycle's artisanal origins, production, and revision, using the model of "community-based performance" to argue for the Chester cycle as "a performance tradition characterized by massive, participatory urban engagement" (Sergi, *Practical Cues*, 114).

36. Alakas, "Seniority and Mastery," 17.

37. *The Weavers' Pageant*, in King and Davidson, *Coventry Corpus Christi Plays*, lines 461–66. All quotations from the Weaver's pageant will be taken from this edition, with lines cited parenthetically hereafter.

38. Alakas, "Seniority and Mastery," 23–24.

39. One York pageant whose production was originally shared between religious and secular groups is the *Second Trial before Pilate*, attributed to the Tilemakers. The pageant was sponsored and produced by the York Minster vicars choral, who owned two tileworks in the city, Kerby-Fulton notes: "The vicars regard the play as their own, referring in 1420 to expenses for the play in their accounts as "pro ludo nostro" (Kerby-Fulton, *Clerical Proletariat*, 233). In a new reading of the pageant, she argues that the vocational concerns, discourses, and grievances of the vicars choral appear prominent in the text (ibid., 233–43). For discussion of this pageant's complex production history, see Beadle, *York Plays*, 2:288–96.

40. See Fitzgerald, *Drama of Masculinity*, 95–144, on the centrality of "male homosocial communities" to the York cycle.

41. Beadle, "Nicholas Lancaster," 33.

42. For the decree, see *REED: York*, 1:112–13 and 2:777–78.

43. Beadle, "Nicholas Lancaster," 51. He concludes, "It would not be surprising to discover that the York Corpus Christi Play, as it happens to have come down to us in the form of British Library Additional MS 35290, was, at this stage in its long career, becoming an enterprise with a Ricardian aspect" (52).

44. On the Masons' and Laborers' sponsorship of the *Purification*, see Rice and Pappano, *Civic Cycles*, 106–16.

45. See discussion in Beadle, *York Plays*, 2:146.

46. Ibid., 2:141.

47. Christie, "Bridging the Jurisdictional Divide," 73.

48. Ibid.

49. King, *York Mystery Cycle*, 128.

50. *The Purification*, in Beadle, *York Plays*, 1:130. All quotations from the York *Purification* will be taken from this edition, with lines cited parenthetically hereafter.

51. Simeon's speech bemoaning his old age is only twenty lines long in the Coventry Weavers' play (lines 197–217).

52. For similar diction, see the York Shipwrights' *The Building of the Ark*, where Noah, having earlier complained about the weakness of his old body, is rejuvenated by his contact with God: "Full wayke I was and all vnwelde, / My werynes is wente away" (Beadle, *York Plays*, 1:43, lines 93–94). Beadle also notes that this is "a formulaic expression, echoed in relation to older men who are granted a special grace in later pageants," including Joseph and Simeon (ibid., 2:47). Revisers of the *Purification* probably drew upon these other pageants for inspiration. On the aged male body in the Coventry Weaver's play, see Alakas, "Politics of Ageism," 19–20.

53. Based on these lines, Sergi remarks upon Simeon's representation as a "very old priest" (Sergi, *Practical Cues*, 177). The Chester *Purification* shares a

common source with the *Purification* episodes of York, Coventry, and Towneley, as shown by W. W. Gregg, " 'Christ and the Doctors' and the York Play." Chester's version also incorporates considerable content from the *Stanzaic Life of Christ*, and splices in the episode of *Christ and the Doctors* (probably derived from York's version). The latter addition, in which Christ expounds the Ten Commandments, strongly increases the pageant's focus on the transmission of masculine knowledge. On the incorporation of earlier material into the Chester *Purification*, see Sergi, "Un-dating the Chester Plays," 83–84. For an extended discussion of how the Chester *Purification* incorporates *Stanzaic Life of Christ* material, see Sergi, *Practical Cues*, 171–82.

54. The term "decrepitude" is from Alakas, "Politics of Ageism," 20.

55. Beadle, *York Plays*, 2:137. Also see Christie, "Bridging the Jurisdictional Divide," 59.

56. Christie, "Bridging the Jurisdictional Divide," 74.

57. Cited in Cullum, "Hospitals and Charitable Provision," 191.

58. The procession was probably established by 1366, when we find a local rector leaving a bequest "ad sustentacionem solempnitatis corporis Christi in Civitate Ebor singulis annis" (to the solemnity of Corpus Christi celebrated each year in the city of York) (see *REED: York*, 1:2; 2:688 for translation). A record of 1426 describes the processional route (ibid., 1:42–43). See *REED: York*, 1:3, for the 1376 reference to pageant wagons that has long been considered the first mention of the play. However, Twycross, "*Ordo paginarum* Revisited," 113, notes that this date has been written over an erasure by a later hand and may thus be, "to say the least, unsafe." Procession and play were separated, with the play performed on Corpus Christi and the procession the day after, sometime between 1468 and 1476. On the relation between procession and play and possible reasons for this rearrangement, see Rice and Pappano, *Civic Cycles*, 48–52.

59. Beadle, *York Plays*, 2:138. Another connection between St. Leonard's and wider civic religious celebration is recorded in the *Ordinale* of St. Mary's Abbey, which indicates a procession to the hospital on Rogation Tuesday; see *Ordinale and Customary*, 319.

60. The 1385 record indicates, "to two minstrels on the feast of the Purification of the Virgin Mary in the presence of the warden and the brothers" (*Item ij ministrallis in festo Purificationis Marie virginis in presencia Custodis & ffratrum*) (*REED: York*, 1:2–4, and 2:688, 690 for translations). See *REED: York*, 1:92, for the hospital's payments to minstrels on the Feast of St. Leonard in 1461.

61. The others were St. Egidio and St. Lucia, as noted in the hospital's early sixteenth-century ordinances. See Park and Henderson, "First Hospital," 179.

62. King, "*Civitas* versus *Templum*," 92. See Rice and Pappano, *Civic Cycles*, 24–28, for discussion of actors in the York and Chester cycles.

63. The Chester Assumption is mentioned in the Early Banns of 1539–40; see Baldwin, Clopper, and Mills, *Records of Early English Drama: Cheshire Including Chester*, 1:85. For evidence of women performing in English royal and private households, parish settings, and civic productions, see Stokes, "Women and Mimesis" (182–83 on civic performance). On the Reformation-era narrowing of opportunities for women to perform, see Stokes, "Women and Performance." I thank Matthew Sergi for helpful suggestions about women performers.

64. Stokes, "Women and Performance," 27. In the context of his larger argument for the Chester cycle as a massive civic collaboration, Sergi argues that evidence such as the Wives' *Assumption* play and the relatively large numbers of "unattached women" appearing in other Chester pageants may point to a "local collaborative traditional of female inclusion" that was eventually suppressed by "extramural misogyny" in the later sixteenth century (Sergi, *Practical Cues*, 151).

65. The work of Kate Matthews on contemporary French convent drama is also relevant here. The Easter plays of Origny-Sainte-Benoîte, performed by nuns, combined Latin with vernacular French and were played in the abbey church for an audience that included lay spectators. Matthews suggests that the women's performance may have worked to "heighten the role that emotion and female spirituality play in the Easter story" even as it functioned to "display the wealth and status of the Abbey"; see Matthews, "Textual Spaces/Playing Places," 75 and 79 for quotations.

66. Christie, "Bridging the Jurisdictional Divide," 65, posits a thematic connection between the aged Temple-dwellers Simeon and Anna and the hospital's care of the elderly. Beadle, *York Plays*, 2:138, also suggests this possibility.

67. Rawcliffe, "Medicine for the Soul," 323.

68. These ordinances are printed in Dugdale, *Monasticon Anglicanum*, vol. 6, pt. 2: 610.

69. See the discussion of the Lady Mass in Sumpter, "Lady Chapels," 41.

70. When the hours are to be sung, the chaplains and boy choristers should enter the church "ad ostium versus porticum beatae Virginis" (at the door across from the porch of the blessed Virgin). Dugdale, *Monasticon Anglicanum*, vol. 6, pt. 2: 610.

71. Ibid.

72. Cullum, "Hospitals and Charitable Provision," 299.

73. This is certainly not to claim that St. Leonard's devotion to the Virgin was unique. See the rather similar liturgical customs at the Pontefract almshouse, described in Cullum, "Hospitals and Charitable Provision," 356.

74. For discussion of prayers, relics, and amulets, see L'Estrange, *Holy Motherhood*, 55–68. On amulets, shrines, girdles, and other aids to childbirth,

also see French, "Material Culture of Childbirth." Orme and Webster, *English Hospital*, 50, mention St. Leonard as a patron of "nursing mothers."

75. Knowles and Hadcock, *Medieval Religious Houses*, 313–38, record more than fifty English hospitals originally dedicated to St. Leonard or St. Leonard together with another saint. However, Orme and Webster warn that these earlier figures may "underestimate the number of hospitals in the earliest periods" and "overestimate the number after 1350, when some early hospitals changed into chantries and chapels" (Orme and Webster, *English Hospital*, 11).

76. The *Vita S. Leonardi, Acta Sanctorum*, November, 3:153, reads, "Postquam autem haec omnia gesta sunt, remansit sanctus Leonardus in eodem loco, quem ei rex praebuerat, videlicet in ipsa nemoris solitudine; ubi etiam construxit oratorium in honore sanctae Dei genetricis Mariae" (After all these things had occurred, St. Leonard stayed in the same place, which the king had offered to him, namely, in the solitude of that forest, where he built an oratory in honor of St. Mary mother of God).

77. St. Leonard was also invoked in childbirth. A prayer for safe childbirth, attributed to the saint, is featured in Anne of Brittany's prayer book (L'Estrange, *Holy Motherhood*, 260–62).

78. These vows are outlined in the 1364 visitation record; see TNA, MS C 270/20 (membrane 1).

79. French, "Maidens' Lights," 403.

80. For example, goldsmith Alan de Alnwyck gave pittances to the brothers and sisters in 1374; John Yhole, who died in 1390, donated money to buy clothing for the seven poor men and women and was buried at St. Leonard's. See Cullum, "Hospitals and Charitable Provision," 249, 257.

81. Ibid., 173.

82. See *Calendar of the Patent Rolls: Henry IV*, 1:131.

83. King, "*Civitas* versus *Templum*," 86, notes that in this period most mayors preferred bequests to maisons-dieu rather than to the hospital.

84. Cullum, "Hospitals and Charitable Provision," 322.

85. Ibid., 323–25.

86. Cullum, "'For Pore Peple Harberles,'" 47. Also see Cullum, "'And Hir Name,'" 183, for evidence of women's bequests from 1389 to 1398.

87. See Cullum, "'For Pore Peple Harberles,'" 48.

88. Cullum, "'And Hir Name,'" 199.

89. Cullum, "Hospitals and Charitable Provision," 445.

90. For a rare case where a hospital (St. Mark's, Bristol) claimed the right to purification and its associated fee, see Ross, *Cartulary*, 48.

91. Johnston, "The *York Cycle* and the Libraries," 356.

92. Ibid., 367.

93. The library list, from Trinity College Dublin MS 359, has been edited in Humphries, *Friars' Libraries*: for glossed texts of Leviticus, see items 10 (12) and 27 (14); for Luke, see items 41 (16) and 55 (18); for Hugh of St. Victor's "de virginitate beate Marie," see item 93 (29); and for Anselm's "de laude," see item 142 (42).

94. See ibid., item 145 (43).

95. For the former view, see Coster, "Purity, Profanation, and Puritanism." For the latter view, see Cressy, *Birth, Marriage, and Death*, 197–230.

96. Lee, "'Women Ben Purifyid,'" 40.

97. For the York *Ordo ad purificandum mulierem*, which begins with the psalm *Ad te levavi*, see Henderson, *Manuale et processionale*, 23.

98. The festive mood would of course be greatly muted if the baby had died. In the case of miscarriage, stillbirth, or infant death, the mother still required churching. I thank Shannon McSheffrey for pointing this out to me.

99. Gibson, "Blessing from Sun and Moon," 149.

100. Ibid., 143.

101. This point about the churching ceremony is noted by Coletti, "Genealogy, Sexuality," 45. For discussion of this custom, see Duffy, "Holy Maydens," 196. Also see Marks, *Image and Devotion*, 184–85, on churching bequests.

102. Beadle, *York Plays*, 2:144, continues, "Her purpose was to carry (as here) a basket containing the birds to be offered in sacrifice, and she sometimes bore, on the Virgin's behalf, the single candle customarily brought by women to their churching after childbirth."

103. See Swann, "'By Expresse Experiment,'" 2–4, for discussion of these sources.

104. Ryan, "Playing the Midwife's Part," 440–43, with cited passage on 443.

105. Ibid., 444.

106. The 1415 description reads, "Maria cum . . . Ioseph, obstetrix, puer natus iacens in presepio, inter bouen & azinum & angelus loquens pastoribus & ludentibus in pagina sequente" (Mary, with . . . Joseph, the midwife, the newborn boy lying in a manger between the cow and the ass, the angel speaking to the shepherds and the players in the following pageant) (*REED: York*, 1:18, and 2:704 for translation). Ryan, "Playing the Midwife's Part," 441, has noted the early presence of the midwife and her disappearance. The midwife in the early *Nativity* is also noted in Swann, "'By Expresse Experiment,'" 5. Woolf, *English Mystery Plays*, 195, remarks that the *ancilla* featured in the *Magi* pageant, following the *Nativity*, may have originated as the *obstetrix* who featured in the early *Nativity* pageant.

107. Ryan, "Playing the Midwife's Part," 439.

108. Ibid., 446.

109. Brown, *Stained Glass*, 54, notes that this window dates from ca. 1340 and was "reused" ca. 1370 for the new Lady Chapel. The panel is the third in a narrative sequence including "small scenes of the Adoration of the Magi, Massacre of the Innocents, Presentation in the Temple, Flight into Egypt and the Annunciation of the Virgin's Death." See ibid., 54–55, for images of these windows.

110. For a discussion of the wimple as mark of the married woman from the twelfth century onward, see Gabriela Signori, "Veil, Hat, or Hair?," 31.

111. Marks illustrates his point with a Purification image from a late fifteenth-century book of hours made for the Bray family (Stonyhurst College Library, MS 60, fol. 26v). See Marks, *Image and Devotion*, 164, 166 fig. 117. I thank Kathryn Smith for directing me to this reference.

112. Rieder, *On the Purification*, 127.

113. Niebrzydowski, "Secular Women," 139; see 136 for parallels between stages of the churching ritual and of *Purification* dramas.

114. Niebrzydowski, *Bonoure and Buxum*, 167.

115. Simeon's sons, Leucius and Karinus, relate their experiences in the apocryphal *Gospel of Nicodemus*. See Elliott, *Apocryphal New Testament*, 190–204; for the mention of the white robes, see 196.

116. Beadle, *York Plays*, 2:144, notes that including Simeon's sons in drama is "highly unusual." He uses the term "prefigurative" at 145, noting their connection to Simeon's "prophetic role" in the York pageant.

117. Niebrzydowski, *Bonoure and Buxum*, 166, also flags Mary's line, "As other women doith in feer," as notable.

118. See Lee, "Men's Recollections." Some banquets featured minstrels (ibid., 231).

119. *Killing of the Children*, lines 565–66. Gibson, "Blessing from Sun and Moon," 140–41, notes the connection between this moment in the Digby play and the festive Candelmas procession.

120. The first phrase appears in the manuscript, suggesting a large group of girls, but the list of "pleyers" at the end of the text only accounts for "a virgyn" (see *Killing of the Children*, 111 and 115). The editor suggests that the virgins "would perhaps have been village girls collected for the occasion" (lxiii).

121. Coletti, "Genealogy, Sexuality," 30.

122. Mirk, *John Mirk's Festial*, 1:55 (emphasis added).

123. Ibid., 1:56.

124. Waller, *Virgin Mary*, 70, argues of women spectators to late medieval English Marian drama: "They would recognize both their own and the Virgin's sexuality, not just through the abstractions of theology but in the play space . . . physically present in the bodies of the actors from the community."

125. See Solberg, *Virgin Whore*, for a brilliant analysis of Mary's complex sexuality in late medieval English drama, particularly the N-Town cycle.

126. For example, in 1406 Master John Parker, a medical doctor, bequeathed twenty shillings to be shared among the sisters (see Raine and Clay, *Testamenta Eboracensia*, 1:342). Noted in Cullum, "Hospitals and Charitable Provision," 166.

127. See Cullum, "'And Hir Name,'" 201, for a table of liveries and corrodies recorded from 1392 to 1409.

128. Cullum, "St Leonard's York," 16.

129. Cullum, "Hospitals and Charitable Provision," 178–79. Also see Cullum, "Vowesses and Lay Female Piety."

130. Cullum, "'And Hir Name,'" 197.

131. The document is York, York Minster Library, MS M 2/6/e. For a printed index, see "Index of Wills from St. Leonard's Hospital." See Cullum, "Hospitals and Charitable Provision," 94–95, on the hospital's independent legal jurisdiction. Individuals whose wills were proved in the peculiar would have resided within the precinct.

132. On the need for caution in using probate evidence, see Goldberg, *Women, Work*, 366.

133. York Minster Library, MS M 2/6/e, fols. 36r (1459) and 36v (1464), respectively.

134. For example, Matilda Wighton, a litster's widow, asked to be buried in the church of St. John the Evangelist in York alongside her husband (see York Minster Library, MS M 2/6/e, fol. 36v).

135. Ibid., fol. 30v.

136. Ibid., fol. 36r.

137. Ibid., fol. 36v. I am grateful to Shannon McSheffrey for generous help transcribing and translating this document.

138. Ibid., fol. 36v. Wighton distributed her charity widely in York, also leaving money for distribution to the poor dwelling in places such as leper houses, maisons-dieu, prisons, and almshouses.

139. Roger, "Blakberd's Treasure," quotations at 100.

140. Erler, "Widows in Retirement," 70.

141. See Cullum, "'And Hir Name,'" 199, on women living in churchyards.

142. *MED*, s.v. "conversacioun," no. 1: "holi ~, life devoted to the ideals of Christianity."

143. Widows often kept vigil over the dead or prepared bodies for funerals; see Cullum, "'And Hir Name,'" 198. An image in the Hastings Hours depicts Elisabeth of Hungary as a widow distributing alms from a hospital (BL MS Additional 54782, fol. 64v).

144. Neither of the artisan pageants accords her a prophetic role: in the Chester *Purification,* Anna has the final words of the play and references her life of "penance and prayer" (195), yet she does not play a prophetic role. Male prophets take the stage to start the Coventry Weavers' play, leaving no room for Anna to prophesy.

145. Henderson, *Missale,* 2:18.

146. Collier, *Poetry and Drama,* 226, argues that from the moment Christ is offered to the Prisbeter by Mary and Joseph, "the silent Christ child is the focus of the action as the 'blyssyd babb' is celebrated in the sustained, exultant hymns and prayers of the Prisbeter, Anna, and Simeon."

147. For discussion of the term "beylde" in this pageant, see Rice and Pappano, *The Civic Cycles,* 114–16.

148. Beadle, *York Plays,* 2:148.

149. See the *Nativity,* line 111, where Joseph says, "Hayle my lorde, lemer of light."

150. As they prepare to offer Christ, Joseph says, "He is the lambe of God verray / That muste hus fend frome all our fray, / *Borne of thy wombe, all for our pay /* And for oure chere" (lines 263–69; emphasis added).

151. Henderson, *Missale,* 2:21.

152. As Solberg argues of the N-Town plays, "Mary steals the show: the arc of Jesus' lifetime nestles inside the larger dramatic frame of the Virgin's progress from her Immaculate Conception to her death and Assumption" (see Solberg, "Madonna, Whore," 191).

153. Gibson, "Bury St. Edmunds," 66, and quotation from 86. Gibson notes that the play's language "might well have been drawn from the common stock of Latin meditation and liturgical celebration of the Virgin Mary" (87). See, for example, the celebration of Mary as "star ever ruddy, ever bright" (*stella semper rutilans, semper clara*) in the sequence for vespers at the Feast of the Purification: *Breviarium,* fascicle 3, *Proprium sanctorum,* 146.

154. I am grateful to Margaret Aziza Pappano for help in formulating this conclusion.

TWO. Corruption and Purification at St. Bartholomew's Hospital, London

1. Orme and Webster, *English Hospital,* 109–10.

2. Carole Rawcliffe also notes that St. Bartholomew's had "special facilities for the unmarried mother" (Rawcliffe, "Hospitals of Later Medieval London," 2). Among hospitals outside of London, Holy Trinity, Salisbury was founded

with concern for "orphans, widows and 'lying-in women' above all others" (Rawcliffe, *Medicine and Society*, 204). St. John the Evangelist at Blyth was refounded in 1446 expressly to help unmarried women (Orme and Webster, *English Hospital*, 109–10).

3. For Edward's decree, see Dugdale, *Monasticon Anglicanum*, 6:296. It renders the hospital tax exempt in consideration, in part, of its care for "mulieres pregnantes quousque de puerperio surrexerint: necnon ad omnes pueros de eisdem mulieribus genitos, usque septennium, si dictae mulieres infra hospitale praedictum decesserint" (pregnant women until they arise from childbirth, and also all children born of these women, until age seven, if their mothers shall have died within the said hospital). Henry's decree grants the hospital master and brethren a license to acquire land in mortmain "in consideration of their great charges in receiving the poor, feeble, and infirm, keeping women in childbirth until their purification and sometimes feeding their infants until weaned" (*Calendar of Patent Rolls 15 Henry VI*, 3:48).

4. The English translation is very literal and often awkward, as Ralph Hanna, "Augustinian Canons," 41n38, notes.

5. The manuscript can be traced through ownership notes to the priory, and it was probably produced there (*Book of the Foundation*, x).

6. The extant Latin text is a transcript of the earlier work, which was probably composed between 1174 and 1189 (ibid., xi).

7. Varnam, "*The Book of the Foundation*," 58. Her essay analyzes the *Book*'s account of the church's construction "in order to explore the notion of the sacred which is produced through the interaction of the physical structure with its textual re-imagining" (ibid.).

8. Karras, *Common Women*, 3.

9. Roger, "Blakberd's Treasure," 85–86.

10. Moore, *History of St Bartholomew's Hospital*, 1:15–16.

11. Kerling, "Foundation," 147. Varnam also remarks on the *Book*'s promotion of the priory at the hospital's expense ("*The Book of the Foundation*," 72).

12. *Book of the Foundation*, 2. Subsequent page numbers will be cited in the main text. I cite from this edition with occasional silent emendations from the manuscript.

13. See Luke 8:2 for Mary Magdalen's exorcism and Matthew 16:18–19 for Christ's charge to Peter and promise to give him "the keys of the kingdom of heaven."

14. BL MS Cotton Vespasian B. IX, fol. 1v.

15. *MED*, fonnish, adj., "Unwise or innocent (person); erroneous (opinion); sinful (love)."

16. BL MS Egerton 1995, fols. 85r–v. See Gairdner, *Historical Collections*, i–x, for discussion of the manuscript. The list of churches resembles several other such lists in contemporary manuscripts, but this particular description does not appear elsewhere (viii).

17. *MED*, worship/e, n., 1(e) "reputation, repute; a person's good name, respectability; a woman's honor, perceived virtue, her reputation for chastity, modesty, etc."

18. Taylor, *Textual Situations*, 154. Taylor also cites the *Book*'s "clensynge" passage in connection to Smithfield's reputation for vice and uncleanness (154–55).

19. BL MS Cotton Vespasian B. IX, fol. 7r. Christopher Bonfield cites this passage as an example of an urban hospital being "surrounded by moral refuse and the miasma of sin," in Bonfield, "The *Regimen Sanitatis*," 192.

20. These physiological assumptions are discussed in Cadden, *Meanings of Sex Differences*, 169–201.

21. On miasma and contagion, see Rawcliffe, *Medicine and Society*, 42–43.

22. Caciola, *Discerning Spirits*, 144 and 145.

23. Karras, *Common Women*, 23. She notes the presence of a brothel in East Smithfield run by a married couple who were known to cater to foreign visitors (78).

24. Taylor, *Textual Situations*, 173.

25. Bovey, "Communion and Community," 76. I thank Kathryn Smith for directing me to this essay.

26. Ibid., 77. Taylor also remarks on the appropriateness of the illustrations to the Augustinian setting: "The Augustinian canons were known for their broad intellectual interests and their urban mission, which included preaching. A canon might be assumed to know the punchier legends for use in popular sermons and how to meld romance and piety in his own storytelling" (Taylor, *Textual Situations*, 190).

27. Bovey is interested in the ways that these two visual narratives privilege the Eucharist and the intervention of priests. She notes that the Thaïs story in particular had a connection to the Augustinian Order (Bovey, "Communion and Community," 66). Also see Taylor's discussion of the Mary of Egypt sequence (Taylor, *Textual Situations*, 183–87).

28. Bovey, "Communion and Community," 69.

29. The recorded miracles divide fairly evenly among men and women. For a table delineating "selected neuropsychiatric cases" from the *Book*, see Wilmer and Scammon, "Neuropsychiatric Patients," 9–10. The authors, both physicians, attribute cures to the hospital rather than to the priory, despite the *Book*'s emphases.

30. See chapter 15 ("Of a woman i-helyd").

31. On menstruation as a key site for pollution anxiety, see Elliott, *Fallen Bodies*, 2–6. Whereas earlier medieval medical authorities treated menstruation in fairly neutral terms, by about 1300 menstruation began to be treated in increasingly negative terms as male physicians came to monopolize the learned treatment of women's "secrets" (Green, "Flowers, Poisons," 58–59). Also see Cadden, *Nothing Natural*, 123–28.

32. Jennifer Kosmin calls virginal and pregnant bodies "the two bodies most critical to the social and cultural landscape of early modern Europe," despite the general lack of male medical knowledge about them. One could say the same of medieval England. See Kosmin, "Midwifery Anatomized," 84.

33. In the miracle accounts, the hospital is rarely mentioned. We find a passing mention of poor men lying in the hospital (chapter 24). Adwyne the carpenter, stricken with "contracte" sinews, is brought to the hospital, but the *Book* makes it clear that he is supported by the "almes of the same chirche" and healed "by the vertu of the Apostle" (29).

34. The Latin description of her seduction reads, "a quodam lenone ab utilitate iusti laboris ad uoluptatem seducta est sordidi criminis . . . incompa[ra]bili thesauro depredata est" (MS Vespasian B. IX, fols. 36v–37r).

35. Karras, *Common Women*, 3.

36. Ibid., 19. Young girls in domestic service were often forced into prostitution: "Such employment relieved the immediate economic pressure that drove some women into prostitution but did not protect them against being coerced into the sex trade when an employer forced his servant to work as a prostitute or to have sex with him" (ibid., 55).

37. Ibid., 63.

38. Ibid.

39. Caciola, *Discerning Spirits*, 157.

40. Ibid.

41. Among few changes to the Latin version, the Middle English translator adds this term elsewhere in the text as part of a litany of ailments: "bisy in this place was hadde of recouerynge men yn to helth of them that langwisshid / of drye men, *of contracte men* / of blynde men / dome men / and deif men" (*Book of the Foundation*, 31; emphasis added). What the *Book* calls "contraction," Wilmer and Scammon identify as "hysterical paralysis" (Wilmer and Scammon, "Neuropsychiatric Patients," 10).

42. This useful term is from Orlemanski, *Symptomatic Subjects*, 139. Considering the power of illness within exemplary narratives, she argues, "Exemplary illness is a long-standing technique of narrative meaning-making, which generates its significance in historically and discursively specific contexts" (ibid.).

43. His name appears as "Johannes de Mirfeld" (Mirfeld is a Yorkshire name) in Latin and has variously been translated "Mirfield" and "Mirfeld." I use "Mirfield," the more common spelling in recent scholarship.

44. Hartley and Aldridge, *Johannes de Mirfeld*, 4–5.

45. Ibid., 24–25. For brief mention of Mirfield and his two works, also see Bullough, "A Note on Medical Care," 76. Bullough suggests that Mirfield "probably gained some medical knowledge from his experience at St. Bartholomew's," despite his profession of ignorance about medicine in the *Breviarium* preface (ibid.).

46. Mirfield's chapter is largely taken from the pseudo-Aristotelian *Secretum Secretorum*, a translation of which was owned by John Shirley, a resident of the hospital at the end of his life. See Hartley and Aldridge, *Johannes de Mirfeld*, 122–59, for an edition and translation of the chapter, from which I cite below. The *Florarium*'s treatment of health regimen was perhaps appreciated by St. Mary Elsyng, Cripplegate, a hospital for sick clergy, which according to a 1448 inventory possessed a copy of the *Florarium* (see Rawcliffe, "Eighth Comfortable Work," 390).

47. Getz, "John Mirfield and the *Breviarium*," 25.

48. Getz, *Medicine in the English Middle Ages*, 52–53.

49. See Green, "From 'Diseases of Women,'" 23, for the phrases "natural-philosophical speculation" and "medical practicality." Green traces the gradual movement from a focus on "relieving women of their suffering" in the earlier medieval texts to "facilitating conception and birth," as the phrase "secrets of women" came to describe the hidden processes of generation (ibid).

50. Hartley and Aldridge, *Johannes de Mirfeld*, 46–47.

51. Ibid., 48–49.

52. Latin text from ibid., 48 and 50; translation from 51.

53. Riddle, "Theory and Practice," 170–74. Also see Bonfield, "*Regimen Sanitatis*," 46–49, on the disconnect between learned tradition (grounded in *scientia*) and the practical tradition (based on *experimenta*).

54. Riddle, "Theory and Practice," 162.

55. Hartley and Aldridge, *Johannes de Mirfeld*, 50–51.

56. In drug formulae, a medical writer might copy in one recipe "from various sources all the drugs he can find for a specific ailment . . . many of these documents were not used in medical practice because they could not be used. Medical theory in pharmacy was becoming less related to practice" (Riddle, "Theory and Practice," 175).

57. Hartley and Aldridge, *Johannes de Mirfeld*, 52–53.

58. Gottfried, *Doctors and Medicine in Medieval England*, 223.

59. Hartley and Aldridge, *Johannes de Mirfeld*, 48–49.

60. The grant was to last five years, and the two other hospitals included St. Thomas in Southwark and St. Mary without Bishopsgate (Rawcliffe, "Hospitals of Later Medieval London," 7).

61. Rawcliffe, "Hospital Nurses," 52 and note 44.

62. *Sickness of Women*, 462.

63. Cabré, "Women or Healers?," 23.

64. Ibid., 24.

65. "Que circa prouidus lector simplicitati compilatoris parcat corrigendo. Et discat potius deliberat ratione emendare" (Let the prudent reader spare the simpleness of the compiler by correcting the book, and let him learn to amend its faults with mature deliberation) (Hartley and Aldridge, *Johannes de Mirfeld*, 48–49).

66. An extract from the work, on the "signs of death," appears in London, Lambeth Palace MS 444. (This extract is printed and translated in Hartley and Aldridge, 54–73.) Book 15, the *Regimen sanitatis* (just the opening section), is excerpted in several manuscripts: London, BL MS Sloane 3149 and MS Additional 27582; Oxford, Bodleian Library MS Digby 29, MS Digby 31, and MS Bodley 58. Bodleian MS Bodley 682 contains excerpts from the *Breviarium*'s gynecological section at fols. 172r–196r.

67. Biddle, Lambrick, and Myres, "Early History of Abingdon," 56.

68. See Mowat, ed., Sinonoma. (The Sinonoma does not appear in the Harley MS 3 copy of the *Breviarium*.)

69. See ibid., 70 and 9.

70. Ibid., 31, 16.

71. Bonfield, "First Instrument of Medicine," 105.

72. Tony Hunt notes that many lists of drug substitutes traveled under the name *Quid pro quo*; see Hunt, *Popular Medicine*, 19. I have compared Pembroke's *Quid pro quo* to two versions of the alphabetical *Quid pro quo* appended to the *Antidotarium* of Nicholaus of Salernitanus, which became the standard when printed in 1471. The Pembroke version shares many common entries, but it is not identical to the list in BL Harley MS 2378 (a fifteenth-century English medical manuscript), fols. 110v–113r, or to the printed version (Venice: N. Jenson, 1471).

73. Getz, "John Mirfield and the *Breviarium*," 25. Bartlett bequeathed the book to All Soul's College, from which it came to Pembroke College.

74. Bakewell, "Bartlot, Richard," in *ODNB*.

75. See Roberts, "Dee, John," in *ODNB*. Dee purchased the volume in 1573, from the widow of William Carye, a London clothworker. On Harley MS 3, see Watson, "Christopher and William Carye," 137. The Harley MS has another manuscript of the *Breviarium* as its flyleaves, indicating the existence of another copy, but the rest has not been found.

76. Green, *Trotula*, 48–54.

77. Green, *Making Women's Medicine*, 30n3 (emphasis added).

78. The 1544 Strasbourg edition featured only two of the nine Salernitan recipes for vaginal constriction, perhaps because the editor Kraut "felt uncomfortable with the topic" (Green, *Trotula*, 59–60).

79. Green, *Making Women's Medicine*, 110.

80. BL Egerton MS 1995, fol. 86v. Whittington, known for his charitable activity, founded his own almshouse and several other ventures, including the Guildhall Library. See Imray, *Charity of Richard Whittington*, and Appleford, *Learning to Die*, 55–73, on Whittington's piety and many bequests.

81. Martha Carlin notes that this is the only reference to this bequest by Whittington. It does not appear in his will (Carlin, *Medieval Southwark*, 81). Whittington also donated to St. Bartholomew's, but not to the single women specifically.

82. See Karras, *Common Women*, 48–49, on the difficulty of surviving outside marriage; 81 on the potential legal problems associated with marriage to former prostitutes. Martin Ingram notes that pregnancy was also a bar to working in the Southwark stews (Ingram, *Carnal Knowledge*, 163).

83. Post, "Fifteenth-Century Customary," 424. Post's essay includes an edition of the Middle English regulations. Karras prints a translation as an appendix to Karras, "Regulation of Brothels" (see 427–33).

84. These same regulations prohibited pregnant women from working in the brothel (see Post, "Fifteenth-Century Customary," 424).

85. Though in very different circumstances, we find one record of a wealthy thirteenth-century widow placing her two boys in the hospital's custody for care and education until they came of age. See Moore, *History of St. Bartholomew's Hospital*, 1:440.

86. This was literally so in the Southwark regulations, which repeatedly use the term "single women" to refer to prostitutes (noted in Karras, "Regulation of Brothels," 425, and see the text of the regulations, 427–33).

87. See chapter 6, below, for discussion of the hospital's changing attitudes in the sixteenth century toward the support of women in childbirth and afterward.

88. Mirfield's text is unedited except for the sections included in Hartley and Aldridge, *Johannes de Mirfeld*. I cite from Oxford, Pembroke College MS 2, in which the gynecological section begins on fol. 142v.

89. In Fiona Harris Stoertz's survey of medieval English religious and medical texts related to childbirth, recipes for removing a dead fetus outnumber those for hastening a live birth (Stoertz, "Suffering and Survival," 107).

90. Oxford, Pembroke College MS 2, fol. 143ra.

91. Latin text from *Compendium medicine Gilberti Anglici*, 300ra-vb.

92. Green, *Trotula*, 144–45.

93. Ibid., 42.

94. Monica Green notes that this term "might mean literal buck's horn, or the plant, buck's horn plantain" (email communication March 27, 2018).

95. I am very grateful to Monica Green for her generous help with correcting my transcription and for translating the passage. I have slightly adapted this translation from the one that she kindly provided.

96. Trease and Hodson, "Inventory of John Hexham," 79–80.

97. See Mowat, ed. *Sinonoma*, 29, 16, 22, 17, 11, 9, 15, respectively.

98. Translation in Green, *Making Women's Medicine*, 83. Latin cited from Gilbertus, *Compendium medicine*, fol. 300ra.

99. Gilbertus, *Compendium medicine*, fol. 300ra.

100. Gilbertus also includes discussion of the possibility of feigning chastity through modest appearance and speech. Whereas the indicators of virginity are "pudor et verecundia cum casto incessu loquele gestus" (modesty and shame, with a chaste walk, speech, and gesture), some women "docte effrenos motus didicerunt castigare et falsitatem sub specie veritatis palliare" (have learned by a clever motion to correct and hide falseness under the appearance of truth) (Gilbertus, *Compendium medicine*, fol. 300ra).

101. See Pembroke MS 2, fol. 153ra. See Gilbertus, *Compendium medicine*, fol. 300rb, for a similar recipe.

102. See Gilbertus, *Compendium medicine*, fol. 300va, and Green, *Trotula*, 146–47.

103. Green, *Trotula*, 146–47.

104. Green, *Making Women's Medicine*, 110. Hartley and Aldridge suggest that Mirfield's comment that charms and incantations might not be effective in helping with difficult childbirth, and his inclusion of contraceptive recipes, might have "led to his rejection the first time he applied for ordination" (Hartley and Aldridge, *Johannes de Mirfeld*, 44).

105. In BL Harley MS 3, a key to reading the ciphers is included, suggesting a more concerted effort to assist in interpreting them.

106. Green, *Trotula*, 96–97.

107. Pembroke MS 2, fol. 153ra.

108. See Green, *Trotula*, 96–98, for the stone and weasel recipes.

109. Pembroke MS 2, fol. 153ra.

110. S. J. Lang's study of London surgeon John Bradmore's *Philomena* considers his borrowings from Mirfield on elements of surgery. See Lang, "*Philomena*," esp. chap. 3 and appendix 3.

111. I thank Monica Green for bringing this volume to my attention and for providing a typescript list of the section's contents. For a description, see https://medieval.bodleian.ox.ac.uk/catalog/manuscript_1674.

112. See Green, "Development of the Trotula," 170 and 176.

113. See Green, *Trotula*, 146–47: "Accipe gallas, rosas, sumac, plantaginem, consolidam maiorem, bolum armenicum, alumen, chimoleam . . ."

114. MS Bodley 682, fol. 186v. See Green, *Trotula*, 96–97, for the source recipe and translation, which recommends carrying the womb rather than a stone from the womb.

115. The *Florarium* full text is extant in London, Gray's Inn MS 4, and London, BL Royal MS 7. F. XI. Another copy lacking the opening and closing chapters survives in Cambridge University Library MS Mm. 2. 10. An abridgment of the whole work survives in Sion College, MS Sion Arc. L. 40. 2/L. 15. The chapter "De medicis" is extracted in BL MS Sloane 59, and BL MS Harley 106 contains notes from among the first ninety chapters, seemingly following the text of Gray's Inn MS 4 (Hartley and Aldridge, *Johannes de Mirfeld*, 169–74).

116. Hartley and Aldridge, *Johannes de Mirfeld*, 162–63.

117. A table of contents has been added to the manuscript in British Library MS Royal 7. F. XI (fols. 1–3). See Hartley and Aldridge, *Johannes de Mirfeld*, 135n4, and *Breviarium*, part XV, "De Regimine Sanitatis."

118. The systematic organization of diverse material "in an encyclopedic manner" was a new development in the fourteenth century (Von Nolcken, "Some Alphabetical Compendia," 271).

119. "Abstinentia" is the first heading in the *Manipulus florum* by Thomas Hibernicus (1306), John of Lathbury's *Alphabetum morale* (ca. 1356), and John of Grimestone's *Commonplace Book* (ca. 1372) (Von Nolcken, "Some Alphabetical Compendia," 284–85).

120. Von Nolcken, "Some Alphabetical Compendia," 272.

121. Cited from Hartley and Aldridge, *Johannes de Mirfeld*, 120–21.

122. Cited in ibid., 116–17. The editors use London, Gray's Inn, MS 4 as their base text for the edition. I have also consulted this manuscript for sections not included in the edition.

123. Ibid., 116–17.

124. Although the named addressee is a secular cleric, the fact that the title of the work includes Bartholomew could imply that the work was intended to be read within the religious community.

125. Hartley and Aldridge, *Johannes de Mirfeld*, 120–21.

126. Gray's Inn MS 4, fol. 3va. Here Mirfield seems to be summarizing from book 2 of St. Isidore's Sentences (PL 83:638C): "Libidinem abstinentia domat. Nam quantum corpus inedia frangitur, tantum mens ab illicito appetitu revocatur."

127. See Gregory the Great, *Homilia* 35, on Luke 15:1–10 (*PL* 76:1256C).

128. Hartley and Aldridge speculate that Mirfeld based this section on the work of the Dominican Humbert of Romans, whose sample sermons include

one directed to medical students beginning with the same biblical citation and continuing, as does Mirfield, "to treat of the duties of the physician from the point of view both of the body and of the soul" (Hartley and Aldridge, *Johannes de Mirfeld*, 106). See Humbert of Romans, *Sermones ad diversos status*, chap. 66.

129. Hartley and Aldridge, *Johannes de Mirfeld*, 122–23.

130. Ibid.

131. This passage from Bruno of Calabria is quoted in Green, *Making Women's Medicine*, 118–19. Green argues that it expresses the frustration inherent in "Bruno's paradox": the exclusion of women from learned medicine during the thirteenth and fourteenth centuries at the same time that physicians still needed their practical help in treating female patients. See Park, *Secrets of Women*, 85–87, on antifeminism in contemporary Italian medical writers, including Bruno. For an edition, see Hall, "*Cyrurgia Magna* of Brunus Longoburgensis," 4.

132. Comparison of this section with the "mulier" section in *Manipulus florum* reveals that even though certain authorities are favored, including Augustine and Isidore, there is virtually no overlap in the particular sources cited nor in their arrangements. See the Electronic *Manipulus florum* Project entry for "mulier" at https://manipulus-project.wlu.ca/MFedition/Mulier/index.html.

133. Gray's Inn MS 4, fol. 234ra. See Gratian, *Decretum*, 1:287, for the following statement: "Simul cum mulieribus sacerdotes habitare non licet."

134. Gray's Inn MS 4, fol. 234ra. Cited, e.g., by the canonist Hostiensis, *Summa Aurea*, liber 3, 856.

135. The origin of this passage is explained in Kellogg, "The Fraternal Kiss." The citation has not been found in Augustine's works but is attributed to him by Gregory the Great in *Epistola* 60 (*Ad Romanum*), 997.

136. Gray's Inn MS 4, fol. 236ra. This passage derives from a pseudo-Augustinian *Epistola* 17 (*PL* 33:1102).

137. Gray's Inn MS 4, fol. 234vb. For what may be Mirfield's source, see the *Excerptiones Patrum Collectanea* attributed to Bede (*PL* 94:542D). I am grateful to Michael G. Sargent for help with transcriptions and translations of this material.

138. Given Mirfield's sense, the term "noli" does not seem logical here; therefore, I have put it within brackets. It may be a vestige of his source, which he has clearly tinkered with. Some of these lines appear in a fifteenth-century German manuscript containing various verses: "Est res formosa mulier, quam tangere noli. / Si tangis, tangit; si tangit, cedere nescis. / Ergo fuge tactum, ne res procedat ad actum" (see Wattenbach, "Aus einer Halberstadter Handschrift," 348).

139. Gray's Inn MS 4, fol. 236ra. Mirfield has suppressed six lines from the full poem between the second and third lines quoted above. For the full text, see Neckham, *De vita monachorum*, 178.

THREE. Lay Reading in St. Bartholomew's Hospital Close

1. The rental is copied in SBHB/HC/2/1, fols. 7r–38r. The rental is translated and printed in Kerling, *Cartulary*, 153–74. For a detailed study of the residents and their relationships, see Barron, "People of the Parish." Barron's essay is accompanied by an annotated rental and a corresponding map of the close. Also see Sutton and Visser-Fuchs, "The Cult of Angels." I am indebted to Caroline Barron for sharing her essay with me before publication and for her generous help with research questions.

2. Barron, "People of the Parish," 359–63, surveys the residents and their professions.

3. For the latter type, see, e.g., Johanna Dursley, a resident widow who asked in her 1451 will to be buried in the hospital church, even though her husband was buried in St. Margaret Bridge Street alongside his first wife (Barron, "People of the Parish," 363–64).

4. Roger, "Blakberd's Treasure," 96n8: "Whether Wakeryng merely developed a pre-existing literary community in and around the hospital precinct, or was responsible for its creation, is uncertain." Sutton posits her subject, Alice Portaleyn, as a likely candidate to host a literary circle (Sutton, "Alice Domenyk-Markby-Shipley-Portaleyn," 53).

5. Barron, "People of the Parish," 358.

6. Guy Geltner, "Social Deviancy," 29–34. Note Orme and Webster's caveat about the marginal locations of hospitals. When in the fifteenth century hospitals and almshouses began to be incorporated into central locations, they were usually "almshouses for long-term infirm people suffering from age and poverty, not from repulsive diseases" (Orme and Webster, *Medieval Hospital*, 44).

7. See Connolly, *John Shirley*, 204, on Shirley's will. I thank Margaret Connolly for her thoughtful reading of this chapter and for suggestions during the revision process.

8. LMA DL/C/B/004/MS09171/005, fol. 166v. Vanessa Harding shows based on late medieval London wills that in-church burials were prestigious, especially in locations close to the altar where mass was celebrated. Testators also commonly requested burial near spouses. See Harding, "Burial Choice," 125–27.

9. "Item lego magistro dicti hospitalis xx s et cuilibet fratrum suorum ibidem iij s iiij d., et cuilibet sororum suarum ibidem vj s viij d ad orandum pro salute anime mee et omnium fidelium defunctorum" (I give to the master of the said hospital twenty shillings, and to each of the brothers three shillings four pence, and to each sister of the same six shillings eight pence to pray for the health of my soul) (LMA DL/C/B/004/MS09171/005, fol. 166v). I am grateful to

Michael G. Sargent for his generous help with transcribing this will and for suggesting translations.

10. "Item lego Mariote vxori michi Botiller infra hospitale predictum commorante iij s iiij d ad exorandum pro salute anime mee et omnium fidelium defunctorum. Item lego cuilibet pauperum viro et mulieri decrepitis infra ibidem hospitale iacenti iij d" (I give to Mariote the wife of Botiller within the foresaid hospital three shillings four pence to pray for the health of my soul. Also I give three pence to each pauper, man and woman, who lies ailing in the foresaid hospital). Mariota "was probably the wife of the Nicholas Botiller . . . who rented a shop three doors away from Gevendale in the part of the Close known as Paradys" (Barron, "People of the Parish," 371).

11. Barron's translation ("People of the Parish," 371, citing LMA DL/C/B/ 004/MS09171/005, fol. 167r). The Latin reads "illi capellano qui audit confessiones pauperem languentem infra hospitalem predictum et eisdem pauperibus sacramenta et sacramentalia tempore necessitatis ministrat."

12. LMA DL/C/B/004/MS09171/005, fol. 166v.

13. Barron, "People of the Parish," 369–70.

14. LMA DL/C/B/004/MS09171/006, fol. 188r.

15. Ibid.

16. LMA DL/C/B/004/MS09171/006, fol. 188r: "I bequeth to Harvy Dene son of Margaret Stones my dowghter xl s."

17. Sutton, "Alice Domenyk-Markby-Shipley-Portaleyn."

18. Sutton, "Alice Domenyk-Markby-Shipley-Portaleyn," 52–53.

19. Barron, "People of the Parish," 367. Elene Joynour's will is LMA DL/C /B/004/MS09171/003, fols. 262r–63v.

20. LMA DL/C/B/004/MS09171/003, fol. 262v. I am grateful to Maryanne Kowaleski for her generous help transcribing this will.

21. By 1449–50 Richard was apparently independent but still connected to the hospital, as he is recorded as renting one of the hospital properties (Kerling, *Cartulary*, 161). He seems to have gone on to become a prosperous grocer (Barron, "People of the Parish," 368n69).

22. LMA DL/C/B/004/MS09171/005, fol. 271r.

23. Sutton, "Alice Domenyk-Markby-Shipley-Portaleyn," 63. See LMA DL/ C/B/004/MS09171/006, fol. 283r.

24. LMA DL/C/B/004/MS09171/005, fol. 110r.

25. Sutton, "Alice Domenyk-Markby-Shipley-Portaleyn," 53.

26. Roger, "Blakberd's Treasure," 101.

27. Ibid., 89. See TNA, CP40/816, rot. 342.

28. Sutton, "Alice Domenyk-Markby-Shipley-Portaleyn," 63–65.

29. As Robert Meyer-Lee notes, Shirley made Lydgate's work available, and Lydgate's poetry provided the "cultural capital" that drew readers to Shirley's manuscripts (Meyer-Lee, *Poets and Power*, 53).

30. Stow, *Survey of London*, 2:24. Mentioned in Greenberg, "John Shirley," 373. Stow owned Shirley's anthology Trinity College Cambridge MS R. 3. 20 and must have worked with Ashmole 59 also, for he copied several of its texts into the manuscript that is now London, British Library, MS Harley 367 (see Connolly, *John Shirley*, 182–84).

31. Kathryn Veeman notes, "Shirley held the benefice of Roche, in Cornwall, as a non-resident incumbent for two brief periods beginning in the late 1390s" (Veeman, "Early Bureaucratic Career," 256). The benefice was rescinded because he did not enter the priesthood within a year of receiving it, as required by canon law (ibid., 257). Kerby-Fulton remarks upon Shirley's brief possession and rejection of the benefice, noting that he "still managed to sustain his career in the Exchequeur, as bureaucratic culture increasingly found ways other than the benefice to fund itself" (Kerby-Fulton, *Clerical Proletariat*, 31).

32. Veeman, "Early Bureaucratic Career," 259.

33. Connolly, *John Shirley*, 14–21.

34. Ibid., 52–54; also see 164. In 1432–33, Shirley held two positions at the Port of London: controller of the subsidy of tonnage and poundage, and controller of petty customs (ibid., 54, and Doyle, "More Light," 95).

35. Quoted phrases from Kerby-Fulton, *Clerical Proletariat*, 11 and 19, respectively.

36. Connolly, *John Shirley*, 27–40; see 30–31 for a table of the manuscript's composition and contents.

37. Cited in ibid., 206. Connolly transcribes the verse prefaces of BL MS Additional 16165 (fols. 2r–4v) and BL MS Additional 29729 (fols. 177v–79r) at 206–11.

38. Ibid., 47.

39. See ibid., 77, on the volume's dating. A missing section of this manuscript is now MS Sion Arc. L. 40. 2/E. 44. See Veeman, "Sende þis booke," 1–43, for detailed discussion of this manuscript.

40. See Connolly, *John Shirley*, 70–74, for a table of the manuscript's composition and contents. See Lydgate, *Mummings and Entertainments*, for editions of these performance texts.

41. Connolly, *John Shirley*, 192.

42. Veeman, "Sende þis booke," 3–4.

43. Connolly, *John Shirley*, 95.

44. Ibid., 58.

45. This personal connection might account for Shirley's move to the hospital (see Doyle, "More Light," 100).

46. SBHB/HC 2/1, fol. 7v.

47. Veeman thoughtfully speculates on Shirley's repeated but temporary possession of a benefice: "The fact that he held the same benefice twice, each time for a period of around one year, suggests that he may have struggled with the decision to become ordained, along with its concomitant vow of celibacy, for a number of years" (Veeman, "Early Bureaucratic Career," 257).

48. See Doyle, "More Light," 99–100; Greenberg, "John Shirley," 375–80. Also see Edwards, "John Shirley and the Emulation." Edwards suggests that Shirley's manuscripts make courtly culture available to bourgeois audiences, characterizing them as "attempts to replicate for a less socially defined audience the sort of things he wished to reassure them were read by the nobility" (316).

49. Edwards, "John Shirley, John Lydgate," 250. Edwards also points to Shirley's reference in BL Additional MSS 16165 and 29729 (copied by John Stow) to Lydgate's financial exigency as possible evidence that Shirley was writing with commercial intent (250–51). However, such references do not appear in the Ashmole volume. Kerby-Fulton suggests that in copying Lydgate's work, Shirley was promoting "a new voice for a newer generation" during a period in which monastic houses were assuming control of most benefices nationwide, and regular religious like Lydgate, Walton, Capgrave, and Bokenham were becoming more prominent authors (Kerby-Fulton, *Clerical Proletariat*, 30).

50. See Connolly, *John Shirley*, 170–82, on Shirley's lost manuscripts and on manuscripts, such as BL Additional 34360 and Harley 2251, that depend upon his collections for some of their texts. Veeman includes a useful summary of the debate over the nature and purposes of Shirley's book production (Veeman, "Sende þis booke," i–x).

51. Ibid., 195.

52. Boffey and Thompson note that if Shirley were running a business, it seems odd that his surviving volumes are "such unpolished artefacts." One explanation that would allow for private circulation and commercial production would be that Shirley shared his autograph copies either with friends or with would-be buyers who perused the volumes "to make their personal choice of contents for better-produced volumes of their own" (see Boffey and Thompson, "Anthologies and Miscellanies," 287).

53. Doyle, "More Light," 96. Also see Connolly, *John Shirley*, 58–59.

54. Roger, "Blakberd's Treasure," 96.

55. Shirley's will appears in LMA DL/C/B/004/MS09171/005, fol. 213r, and is printed in Connolly, *John Shirley*, 204–5.

56. Connolly, *John Shirley*, 158–61; citation at 161. Shirley may in some cases have been working with new exemplars, but in others he may have supplemented his originals.

57. Ibid., 164. Claire Sponsler also notes that Ashmole is the only volume that can be attributed to Shirley's residence in the hospital: she contends that Ashmole "assumes a different and broader audience" than his previous two collections (Sponsler, "Lydgate and London's Public Culture," 26).

58. See Connolly, *John Shirley*, 164–65. MS Ashmole 59, fols. 78r–83v (three prose texts attributed to Isidore and Augustine and verses following) are identical to British Library, MS Harley 1706, fols. 90r–93r and fols.140r–42v (where the same texts are repeated). The first part of Harley duplicates the whole of Oxford, Bodleian Library, MS Douce 322, a devotional anthology that William Baron commissioned for his niece, a nun at Dartford. Hence Douce was probably the exemplar for Harley, as first discussed in detail in Doyle, "Books Connected," 222 39. On Douce 322 as an ascetic collection, see Appleford, *Learning to Die*, 105–27.

59. Connolly, *John Shirley*, 165.

60. See the appendix to this chapter for a list of contents. Only fols. i–130r are in John Shirley's hand, followed by several folios of recipes and miscellaneous contents. Fols. 135r–84r contain an abbreviated text of John Lydgate's *Life of Our Lady* in a sixteenth-century hand, which was later bound with Shirley's book. For details on this arrangement, see Connolly, *John Shirley*, 145.

61. Connolly, *John Shirley*, 151. She notes a disruption between the third and fourth quire's texts, suggesting that Shirley first intended the second and third quire to be placed later in the volume. In contrast, Linne Mooney calls the volume a "miscellany" (see Mooney, "Shirley's Heirs," 182). Boffey and Thompson note that Shirley's manuscripts are generally not organized in any "coherent" way (Boffey and Thompson, "Anthologies and Miscellanies," 285). Derek Pearsall also considers most of Shirley's collections to be miscellaneous (Pearsall, "Whole Book," 22).

62. For a helpful reckoning with the terms and concepts of "miscellany" and "anthology," see Connolly and Radulescu, *Insular Books*, introduction.

63. Hardman, "Domestic Learning and Teaching," 18. The collections that she studies under this rubric include Edinburgh, National Library of Scotland, MS Advocates 19. 2. 1 (Auchinleck); Lincoln Cathedral Library, MS 91 (Thornton); Cambridge University Library, MS Ff. 2. 38; Edinburgh, National Library of Scotland, MS Advocates 19. 3. 1 (Heege); and Oxford, Bodleian Library, MS Ashmole 61 (Rate). The bibliography on these manuscripts is vast; see Hardman, "Domestic Learning and Teaching," 17n8, for a summary of work on Auchinleck and Thornton.

64. See Hardman, "Domestic Learning and Teaching," 21–24, on elementary religious content in the Auchinleck and Thornton manuscripts.

65. Caroline Barron notes the "great testamentary freedom" of widows (Barron, "Widow's World," xxxiii).

66. Anthony Bale, "Norfolk Gentlewoman," 266.

67. This phrase from Coleman, *Public Reading*, 133.

68. Burger, *Conduct Becoming*, 76.

69. Ibid., 15.

70. MS Ashmole 59, fol. 51v.

71. Somerset apparently did not reside in the hospital close but did live elsewhere in London. His name appears in a property deed for the Peter and Poule tavern together with hospital master Wakeryng and chaplain Fossard, among others (Roger, "Blakberd's Treasure," 97–98). Between 1443 and 1446 Somerset founded a chapel of St. Mary and the Nine Orders of Angels in Isleworth, a neighborhood where Alice Markby-Shipley-Portaleyn established a residence (Sutton, "Alice Domenyk-Markby-Shipley-Portaleyn," 54).

72. Excerpts of the "regimen sanitatis" appear in BL Sloane MS 3149; Additional MS 27582; Bodleian Digby MSS 29 and 36; and Bodley MS 58 (Hartley and Aldridge, *Johannes de Mirfeld*, 168). On Harley MS 59, see Hartley and Aldridge, *Johannes de Mirfeld*, 172–73. See Rawcliffe, "Fifteenth-Century *Medicus Politicus*," 101, for a mention of this manuscript, which Somerset lent to his student Roger Marchall, and later bequeathed to Peterhouse College, Cambridge. On Marchall's manuscripts, see Voigts, "A Doctor and His Books," where BL MS Sloane 59 is mentioned at 250, and 281 includes Marchall's description of its contents and his explicit noting Somerset's gift.

73. Rawcliffe, "Fifteenth-Century *Medicus Politicus*," 101. Also see Bonfield, "First Instrument of Medicine," which surveys several vernacular works derived from the *Secretum*.

74. Coleman, *Public Reading*, 79.

75. Ibid., 140.

76. Ibid., 96–97.

77. For discussion of Shirley's translations, see Connolly, *John Shirley*, 120–44.

78. Connolly, *John Shirley*, 130. Shirley calls the text "Decretum" in his colophon, "Et sic explicit Decretum Aristotelis," followed by his statement characterizing the collection as an "Abstracte Brevyarye."

79. As Connolly shows, canceled quire numbers running xiij–xxiij correspond to the extant quire markings i–xj (actually twelve quires). See Connolly, *John Shirley*, table 3 (146–50).

80. Ibid., 158. See MS Ashmole 59, fol. 13r. Boffey and Thompson note that this phase "would apply equally well to all of Shirley's collections," which do not

mark distinctions among authors or types of texts (Boffey and Thompson, "Anthologies and Miscellanies," 286).

81. Cited from Manzalaoui's edition of MS Ashmole 59 in *Secretum Secretorum*, 203 (emphasis added). Subsequent citations from the *Secretum* will be from this edition, followed by Manzalaoui's page numbers in parentheses.

82. The *Secretum* was even translated by Lydgate, as his final work, finished after his death by Burgh. See Lydgate and Burgh, *Secrees of Old Philisoffres*.

83. Barron, "People of the Parish," 362.

84. Veeman, "'Send þis booke,'" 147. On "Beware of Doublenesse," see Stavsky, "John Lydgate Reads": "Likewise couched in antiphrasis, and labeled so by the London book producer John Shirley, the poem 'Beware of Doubleness' adds another twist to the topos of false advice to women" (226).

85. Veeman, "Send þis booke," 147.

86. Ibid., 148.

87. Ibid.

88. Collette, *Performing Polity*, 12. Collette associates the valorization of prudence with the late medieval period and argues for the ascendency of obedience in the sixteenth century, as changing religious, medical, and marital regimes began to emphasize wifely subjection even more strongly than before.

89. MS Ashmole 59, fol. 38r. The text has been edited in Boffey and Edwards, "'Chaucer's Chronicle,'" 203. See ibid., 204–9, for discussion of Chaucer's possible authorship (MS Ashmole 59 offers the sole witness to this text).

90. All of the stanzas but one (the stanza of "Alceste," which actually recounts the story of Alcyone) recall the stories of Chaucer's *Legend*, and Philomena is omitted (Boffey and Edwards, "'Chaucer's Chronicle,'" 205).

91. MS Ashmole 59, fol. 39r.

92. Burger, *Conduct Becoming*, 25. He notes, "Since the conjoined body of the married estate brings the masculine and the feminine alongside each other in potentially troubling ways, this late medieval shift to a desiring system organized around husbands and good wives paradoxically depends upon the incitement of desire for counter-pleasure, that is, for a restrained lay conduct that both emulates and co-opts the benefits of monastic modes of ascesis" (ibid.)

93. Boffey and Edwards, "'Chaucer's Chronicle,'" 216 (fol. 38r) (underlining in original). On Chaucer's treatment of Lucrece, see Schwebel, "Livy and Augustine."

94. On Alice's rape and aftermath, see Sutton, "Alice Domenyk-Markby-Shipley-Portaleyn," 46–47.

95. Griffiths, "The Pursuit of Justice."

96. Barron, "People of the Parish," 364.

97. Shirley's copy of the poem in MS R. 3. 20 appears without the attribution to Lydgate. As Connolly notes, this omission could either indicate that he was unaware of the author or that he discreetly avoided Lydgate's name in a poem critical of the poet's patron. When Shirley copied Ashmole, Duke Humphrey was dead, so the need for discretion had passed (Connolly, *John Shirley*, 82).

98. Connolly gives these reasons to imply that Lydgate was probably the author (Connolly, *John Shirley*, 83). The poem is attributed to Lydgate without comment in *DIMEV* (item 159). Those who have questioned Lydgate's authorship include Pearsall (*John Lydgate*, 166), and Davenport ("Fifteenth-Century Complaints," 139–41).

99. Harker, "The Two Duchesses," 114. On Eleanor's history and her own poetic legacy, see Fumo, "Books of the Duchess."

100. Explicating this contrast in Lydgate's rhetoric is one of Harker's principal aims (see, esp., Harker, "The Two Duchesses," 120–23).

101. For an edition of this poem, see Lydgate, *Minor Poems*, 1:601–8.

102. MS Ashmole 59, fol. 57v.

103. The "Complaint" offers a good example of Shirley's tendency to amplify texts that he had previously copied in Trinity R. 3. 20. Here he extends almost every line with extra syllables. See Connolly, *John Shirley*, 157.

104. See Harker, "The Two Duchesses," 115–18, on Jacqueline's letters, in which she "simultaneously portrayed herself as a figure of pity and a voice of criticism" (116).

105. Riley, *Chronica Monasterii*, 1:20; cited in Harker, "Two Duchesses," 116. Also see Connolly, *John Shirley*, 82.

106. Harker, "Two Duchesses," 122.

107. MS Ashmole 59, fol. 58v.

108. Harker argues that one of Lydgate's main objectives in the poem was to villainize Eleanor in order to exculpate Duke Humphrey, who was, after all, his patron (Harker, "Two Duchesses," 122).

109. Bale, "Norfolk Gentlewoman," 267.

110. Ibid., 265. Bale speculates that since the poem appears just after a list of knights of the garter invested in 1416 (fol. 59v), which includes several men in Sibille's Norfolk social circle, the poem and the list might have to come to Shirley through a manuscript connected to Boys.

111. Connolly notes that the piece, like others such as "Stans puer," offers "a warning against idleness" (Connolly, *John Shirley*, 161). Stavsky observes that the poem is one of few in which Lydgate "unambiguously" praises a woman (Stavsky, "John Lydgate Reads," 239).

112. Bale, "Norfolk Gentlewoman," 266.

113. Ibid.

114. MS Ashmole 59, fol. 60r. The text is edited in Lydgate, *Minor Poems*, 1:14–18. I have followed McCracken's punctuation and silently emended a few transcription errors.

115. MS Ashmole 59, fol. 60r.

116. See the discussion of Chaucerian echoes in Bale, "Norfolk Gentlewoman," 266–67. He insightfully notes that Lydgate owes a debt to Chaucer's "ambivalent" use of the *mulier fortis* trope in portraits of Griselda, the Wife of Bath, and the wife of the Shipman's Tale (266).

117. Burger, *Conduct Becoming*, 19.

118. MS Ashmole 59, fol. 60v.

119. Ibid., fol. 60v (emphasis added). This line order follows McCracken's correction to what appears to be a copying mistake by Shirley, who (seemingly by accident) places the line "Which þat brought . . ." at the end of this passage, violating the rhyme scheme.

120. The *MED* definition of the verb "embracen" includes the literal meaning, 2(a) "To twist or wrap around (someone or something), to entwine or enfold; to put on (a girdle), gird; to put on (a close-fitting garment), to lace (a garment)"; and a figurative meaning associated with Providence: 5(a) "Of God or Providence: to encompass or pervade (all things); (b) to include as a part (of a larger whole)." Both seem to be in play here.

121. MS Ashmole 59, fol. 61r. Emphasis added.

122. See Bale, "Norfolk Gentlewoman," 262–63, on the considerable difficulties that Sibylle encountered in managing her estates, family, and relations with neighbors, and the gossip about her found in the Paston letters.

123. Burger, *Conduct Becoming*, 79.

124. MS Ashmole 59, fol. 51v.

125. Ibid., fol. 61r.

126. LMA DL/C/B/004/MS09171/006, fol. 188v.

127. Agnes, the sister of Avery Cornburgh, a royal civil servant who married Shirley's sister-in-law in 1460, became a nursing sister of Elsing Spital Cripplegate (Sutton, "Alice Domenyk-Markby-Shipley-Portaleyn," 52).

128. MS Ashmole 59, fols. 61r–v (emphasis added).

129. Sutton, "Alice Domenyk-Markby-Shipley-Portaleyn," 43 (emphasis added).

130. I thank Christopher Baswell for pointing out this implied transcendence of clerical authority.

131. Orme, "Children and Literature," 218.

132. Orme's four main (overlapping) categories in this survey include (1) works directed at children (e.g., nursery rhymes or didactic works on conduct); (2) narrative works (e.g., saints' lives or romances) intended for adults that

children might have encountered by reading or listening; (3) works intended for adults that could be used to educate children (e.g., primers); and (4) dramatic works that might have involved children in performance. See ibid., 219.

133. See ibid., 224–28, on educational reading and the household.

134. See Burger, *Conduct Becoming*, 6.

135. Orme, "Children and Literature," 239, notes these nongendered subjects. Also see ibid., 232, on the rather slim evidence for girls' reading. Orme cites a 1472 Paston letter in which the teenaged Anne Paston lends a copy of the "Sege of Thebes" (probably Lydgate's translation). He also notes the purported reading tastes of Jane Scrope, an orphaned knight's daughter described in John Skelton's *Philip Sparrow* (ca. 1502–9). Skelton credits Jane with reading numerous English romances and notes her familiarity with Lydgate and with "characters from biblical and classical history, characters whom she might have encountered in Lydgate's translation of Boccaccio's *Fall of Princes* or in Ranulf Higden's *Polychronicon*."

136. Connolly notes Shirley's preoccupation with authorities, especially in the volume's sixth and seventh quires (Connolly, *John Shirley*, 162). In addition to the citation of multiple authorities, including most proximately Chaucer, but also Boethius and others, Scogan's mention of "noble clerkis" as his source accords with Shirley's headings throughout that underline the venerable and authoritative sources of his information.

137. Wheatley, *Mastering Aesop*, 147.

138. Wheatley notes this idiosyncratic presentation (ibid., 128). In the two other copies of Lydgate's fables, the hound and the cheese appears last, framing the collection that starts with the cock and the jewel, a tale with a similar moral, i.e., that "covetousness destroys contentment" (ibid., 134).

139. MS Ashmole 59, fol. 24r. See Lydgate, *Minor Poems*, 2:598–99.

140. Wheatley, *Mastering Aesop*, 134.

141. As Orme notes, full collections of beast fables in the vernacular, such as those by Lydgate, later printed by Caxton (1484) seem to have been made more for adult readers than for children (Orme, "Children and Literature," 230).

142. Coleman, *Public Reading*, 133.

143. Headnote to "Scogan's Moral Balade," in Forni, *Chaucerian Apocrypha*. I have consulted Forni's edition of the text for punctuation guidelines but have retained Shirley's spellings, which Forni modernized.

144. This copy of the poem contains the text of Chaucer's "Gentillesse" (lines 105–25), which Shirley also copies as the next text in the Ashmole volume. See the brief discussion of Chaucer's appearance as "a moral advisor" in Langdell, "'What shal I call thee?,'" 262.

145. MS Ashmole 59, fols. 25v–26r (emphasis added).

146. Epstein, "Chaucer's Scogan," 14.

147. MS Ashmole 59, fol. 27v (emphasis added).

148. Ibid., fols. 26r–v.

149. Nightingale, *Medieval Mercantile Community,* 501.

150. MS Ashmole 59, fol. 29r. For the critical edition, see Lydgate, *Fall of Princes.*

151. MS Ashmole 59, fol. 29v.

152. Ibid.

153. Pearsall notes that the moral envoys from the *Fall of Princes* were frequently anthologized in miscellany manuscripts (Pearsall, "Whole Book," 21).

154. "Stans puer" appears on fols. 98r–99r.

155. For an edition of the full text, from MS R. 3. 20, see Lydgate, *Mummings and Entertainments,* 67–75. I have followed Sponsler's punctuation.

156. MS Ashmole 59, fol. 70v.

157. As Connolly observes, the first three stanzas are reversed, but the rubrics appear in their original order (Prudencia, Justicia, Temperancia). See Connolly, *John Shirley,* 162.

158. MS Ashmole 59, fol. 70v.

159. Ibid., fol. 71r (emphasis added).

160. This text is more coherent in Sponsler's edition: "God gave hym reson, / hys own doghter dere" (Lydgate, *Mummings and Entertainments,* 68, lines 46–51).

161. MS Ashmole 59, fols. 71r–v.

162. See Napierkowski, "*Summum Sapientiae,*" 50–53, on the *sententiae* as school texts. Napierkowski also notes the mainly secular nature of the work (57).

163. See Louis, "Manuscript Contexts," 228.

164. This is noted in ibid., 222.

165. Ibid., 229.

166. Nuttall, "Margaret of Anjou," 640.

167. Ibid., 643.

168. Napierkowski, "*Summum Sapientiae,*" 58–59.

169. MS Ashmole 59, fols. 85r–v (emphasis added). The final line reads, perhaps preferably, "So may ye atteine / honoure and desire" in Napierkowski's edition (base text BL MS Harley 7578), 90.

170. MS Ashmole 59, fol. 88r (emphasis added).

171. The term is "wrong" rather than "offte" in MS Harley 7578 (Napierkowski, "*Summum Sapientiae,*" 113).

172. MS Ashmole 59, fol. 85v (emphasis added).

173. On these topics, see fol. 90r (relations with neighbors), fol. 88v (on suspicion of "payntede wordes gaye," and fol. 88r (on avoiding covetousness), respectively.

174. MS Ashmole 59, fol. 88r (emphasis added).

175. Ibid., fol. 99v. "Stans puer ad mensam" is edited from Bodleian Library MS Laud Misc. 683 in Lydgate, *Minor Poems*, 2:739–49.

176. MS Ashmole 59, fol. 99v (emphasis added).

177. See Mitchell on the sequence of training that Lydgate imagined, beginning with his "Babees Book" and proceeding to "Stans puer" for the older child (Mitchell, *Becoming Human*, 147).

178. MS Ashmole 59, fol. 98r.

179. Fitzgerald has insightfully considered "Stans puer" in the context of a merchant's manuscript, Oxford Balliol MS 354, which collects a number of texts forming male children (Fitzgerald, "Compiling Mercantile Manhood"). One booklet of Hill's book contains "Stans puer" following *How the Wise Man Taught His Son*. The booklet also features Lydgate's fable of the "Churl and the Bird." Also see Fitzgerald, "Compiling Couplets," on the way in which the same group of "fungible couplets" was copied and replicated across several Middle English manuscripts, including Balliol 354, to create a larger "dramatic monologue of moral masculinity" (114–15).

180. The term is "langage" in MS Laud Misc. 683, but some form of "laughter" in all of the other texts that McCracken collated.

181. MS Ashmole 59, fol. 98r.

FOUR. Collaborative Devotional Reading<br>at St. Bartholomew's and St. Mark's

1. See Webber, "Latin Devotional Texts." Cok and Colman are briefly mentioned together as hospital scribes in Doyle, "Book Production by the Monastic Orders," 13. Also see Doyle, "Manuscripts with Marginalia," for discussion of Colman's productions.

2. Appleford, *Learning to Die in London*, 120.

3. Ibid., 104.

4. Ibid., 116.

5. See Rice, *Lay Piety and Religious Discipline*, esp. the introduction and chap. 1.

6. Appleford, *Learning to Die*, 142–43.

7. Ibid., 100.

8. Baswell, "Competing Archives," 641. Also see Kerby-Fulton's recent remarks on multilingualism as characteristic of the clerical proletariat and hence a notable feature in the resurgence of Middle English literature (*Clerical Proletariat*, xiii–xv).

9. Shirley's will is printed in Connolly, *John Shirley*, 204.

10. Judith Etherton notes, however, "There is no evidence in the London bishops' registers to confirm the description of Cok as a priest" (Etherton, "Cok [Coke], John," *ODNB*). Kerby-Fulton, *Clerical Proletariat*, 22, describes Cok as a "proletarian scribe-turned-writer" who attained "stability" when he joined the Augustinian Order at the hospital.

11. Connolly, *John Shirley*, 204 (emphasis added). Shirley also includes in this group Richard Caudrey, dean of St. Martin's; his mother-in-law, Alice Lynne; John Heyron, esquire of Lincoln; and Edward Norys, citizen and scrivener of London. His wife, Margaret, served as his executor.

12. Carole Rawcliffe, "Passports to Paradise," 19, briefly discusses Cok's institutional productions in. In addition to the volumes I discuss in this chapter, Cok annotated a Bible that survives as Wolfenbüttel, Herzog August Bibliothek, MS Extravagantes 25.1. He annotated the unique manuscript of the *Grail and Merlin*, written by the skinner Henry Lovelich, now Cambridge, Corpus Christi College, MS 80 (see Eddy, "Marginal Annotation," 273–337, and appendix C, 473–77). On the *Grail and Merlin*, see Radulescu, *Romance and Its Contexts*, chap. 3, esp. 95, 114–17, 143–48, on Cok's annotations. Pouzet locates Cok's scribal career at the interface between institutional and commercial book production: "The facets of Cok's scribal oeuvre reflect different destinations, distinct intentions of formality and various scribal times in his life" (Pouzet, "Book Production," 226).

13. Doyle, "More Light," 98.

14. Clark, "The Augustinians, History and Literature," 406.

15. This text, on fol. 183r, is a short proverb attributed to Chaucer. It begins, "Interrogacio Juventus: þis wordle is of so grete aspace / Hyt wolle not in my armes twayn," followed by "Responsio Sapientis: He þat alle þinge wolle embrace / Lytelle þinge may hym susteyn." For a detailed description of the manuscript, containing many helpful transcriptions, see Eddy, "Marginal Annotation," 451–72; proverb discussed and transcribed at 470–72.

16. The first extract, adapted from *Piers Plowman* C 16.182–201a, appears at p. 210. A much shorter passage on poverty, from *Piers Plowman* C 16.116, is copied into the margin of p. 87, below a passage on poverty from Rolle's *Emendatio vitae*. See Horobin, "John Cok and His Copy," 48–53. Horobin speculates that the book returned to the hospital after Shirley's death (54).

17. Horobin, "John Cok and His Copy," 48. Horobin's study focuses on the book's two excerpts from *Piers Plowman* C, one on free will (*liberum arbitrium*) and one on poverty (*paupertas*). Horobin hypothesizes that the additions, including the passages from *Piers* and a brief Pater Noster commentary copied onto the first leaf, were made after Shirley owned and used the book. In contrast, Kathryn Kerby-Fulton and Steven Justice suggest that Cok extracted the passages

from *Piers* for Shirley in response to his interest in the poem (Kerby-Fulton and Justice, "Langlandian Reading Circles," 67).

18. See description in Hanna, *English Manuscripts of Richard Rolle*, 6–8. For an introduction to the important Middle English Passion meditation included in the Caius volume, with links to manuscript descriptions, see West-phall, "Middle English *Meditationes de Passione Christi*."

19. Horobin, "John Cok and His Copy," 47.

20. Griffiths, "Newly Identified Manuscript," 91; Russell, "'As they read it,'" 184. John Bowers briefly mentions the Caius volume in Bowers, *Chaucer and Langland*, 129. In the context of studying the reception of *Piers Plowman* during a time of concern over lollardy, Bowers notes, "Cok selected a noncontroversial passage from *Piers* on free will which he rendered even more orthodox-looking by placing it under the heading 'nota bene de libero arbitrio secundum augustininum & ysidorum'" (ibid.). Also see Warner, *Myth of Piers Plowman*, 68–69.

21. Horobin, "John Cok and His Copy," 54. He hypothesizes that the marginal Latin additions were made after Shirley owned the book, and may thus have particular relevance to the hospital brothers, who would have formed a secondary audience for the book.

22. See my discussion of the *Form of Living* as a work for women religious in Rice, *Lay Piety and Religious Discipline*, 30–31. Rolle's Latin *Emendatio* survives in more than one hundred manuscripts; the Middle English *Emendatio* survives in sixteen manuscripts, in seven separate translations. For brief descriptions of the Latin manuscripts, see Rolle, *De emendatio vitae*, 25–85. On the English manuscripts, see Doyle and Hanna, *Hope Allen's Writings Ascribed*, 32–39.

23. Kempster, "*Emendatio Vitae*," lxxiii.

24. Marleen Cré's phrase in Cré, *Vernacular Mysticism*, 66; see 61 for an appraisal of Rolle's popularity. I briefly discuss the Latin *Emendatio vitae* in Cambridge Jesus College MS Q. D. 4, a priest's personal compilation; see Rice, "Lay Spiritual Texts," 161–63.

25. Cré, *Vernacular Mysticism*, 281.

26. MS 669*/646, p. 76.

27. Ibid., p. 81.

28. Ibid., p. 91.

29. Ibid., p. 98.

30. Watson, *Richard Rolle*, 213–14.

31. MS 669*/646, p. 118.

32. Ibid., p. 130.

33. Pouzet, "Book Production," 227.

34. Etherton, "Cok [Coke], John," *ODNB*. For these remarks by Cok, see Kerling, ed., *Cartulary*, 166. See Barron, "People of the Parish," 355–56, on Lamport.

35. See Webber, "Devotional Texts," on *Speculum peccatoris* (28) and on the *Soliloquium* as attested in Augustinian libraries (35). Thurgarton possessed a copy of *Speculum peccatoris* (Webber and Watson, *Libraries*, 417); Leicester owned multiple copies of *De arrha anime* (Webber and Watson, *Libraries*, 172, 186, 187).

36. Harry, "Monastic Devotion," 106; the influence of the *Meditaciones* on *De interiori domo* (68); the *Speculum peccatoris* as a fellow traveler in manuscripts (102).

37. Visitation records of 1364, from TNA C 270/20, m. 2.

38. Barron, "People of the Parish," 371.

39. Cok adds this phrase at the end of copying stints on fols. 140r and 178r also.

40. Eddy, "Marginal Annotation," 456.

41. On the Gregorian scheme of seven cardinal sins and its elaboration in connection with the high medieval regime of confession, see Bloomfield, *Seven Deadly Sins*, 70–103; see 123–32 on the treatment of the sins in the great theological summae of the thirteenth century.

42. Wenzel, "Preaching," 156. For examination of a contemporary macaronic sermon that relates the sins to diseases and shows them being "cured" by Christ, see Johnson, "Fifteenth-Century Sermon."

43. McCann, *Soul-Health*, 60.

44. On the work's dissemination in French, see Chesney, "Notes on Some Treatises," 32–38. See Jolliffe, *Check-List*, 81, on the Middle English manuscript witnesses. Shirley may have encountered this text in English in BL MS Harley 1706, a volume connected to William Baron, possibly the source for several texts in MS Ashmole 59.

45. MS Additional 10392, fol. 47v. I am grateful to Michael G. Sargent for generous help with deciphering passages and translating difficult passages. For a printed edition of *Speculum peccatoris*, see *PL* 40:983–92.

46. MS Additional 10392, fol. 48r.

47. MS Additional 10392, fol. 51r. Cok adds emphasis by elongating the ascender of the "V" in "Velox" and filling in the letter with yellow.

48. See Verheijen, *La Règle de Saint Augustin*, 1:148 (emphasis added). This sentence, "Ante omnia . . . nobis data," opens the short version of the Rule (*Ordo monasterium* or *Regula Secunda*), and many medieval versions of the *Praeceptum* (*Regula Tertia*) begin with this sentence, then proceed with the longer version, as in Oxford, St. John's College MS 173, Colman's book. Although we do not know which version of the Rule Cok and his brothers followed, it is likely that it began with this sentence.

49. On the popularity of the *Fifteen Oes*, see Duffy, *Stripping of the Altars*, 249–56. Duffy characterizes the Oes as a devotion that bridges learned and

popular modes: "Despite their immense popularity, these are learned prayers, with roots in Patristic and early medieval theology, as well as the writings of Rolle and the affective tradition" (250).

50. See Barron, "People of the Parish," 369n76.

51. In the two other examples that I have examined, British Library MS Harley 2985 (a book of hours made in the southern Netherlands for the English market) and Morgan Library MS 150, a fragment of a book of hours, there are no such annotations, despite ample room in the marginal space.

52. Duffy, *Stripping of the Altars*, 250.

53. Ibid.

54. MS Additional 10392, fol. 113r.

55. Krug, "Jesus' Voice," 112. I am grateful to Becky Krug for her suggestions via email on this point.

56. MS Additional 10392, fol. 114r.

57. They share some features of the meditative hands described by Geneviève Hasenohr (especially to those in BL MS Harley 4987, which is almost certainly Augustinian, given the presence of the Augustinian Rule together with the *Expositio*). See Hasenohr, "Méditation et mnémotechnique," 373–75.

58. These read "quid, quare, quantum, quomodo, quamdiu"; see Hasenohr, "Méditation et mnémotechnique," 373.

59. McCann, *Soul-Health*, 84, citing Augustine, *In Epistolam Joannis ad Parthos*, tract 9.4 (*PL* 35:2048).

60. BL MS Harley 4987, fol. 121r.

61. These images are discussed in Marks, "Picturing Image and Text," 187. These images also feature considerable Latin writing, which Marks notes "must have demanded considerable powers of comprehension by its readers; yet their presence in parish churches suggests that this was not beyond the abilities of some at least of the laity." He also observes the parallel with devotional diagrams in books (ibid.). I thank Marlene V. Hennessy for this reference.

62. Shirley and Colman also both owned copies of Rolle's *Expositio super novem lectiones mortuorum* (hereafter *Super novem*), his commentary on the nine readings from Job used in matins for the Office of the Dead. In chapter 6, I consider the significance of this text, which survives in Bodleian MS Lyell 38, for the life of St. Mark's Hospital. Shirley's copy of the *Super novem* survives as the only text in Yale University, Beinecke MS Osborn a29. *Emendatio* and *Super novem*, the only Latin works of Rolle that medieval readers considered "canonical," frequently appear together in manuscripts (Hanna, "Circulation," 319). Andrew Kraebel, whose critical edition of *Super novem* is forthcoming, has recently counted nineteen collocations of the two texts (personal communication). Also see Kraebel, *Biblical Commentary and Translation*, chap. 3 on Rolle.

63. Both Haulle and Colman are listed as present at an episcopal visitation of the house in 1498. See Morton's *Register*, 2:130, number 464. Referenced in Erler, "Reading at the Gaunts," 71n4. Haulle's later life is obscure: he is not mentioned as one of the remaining brothers in the suppression document of 1539.

64. See Ross, *Cartulary*, for translation (7) and for the Latin (168).

65. See Barker, *Mayor's Chapel*, 51.

66. See Ralph, *Great White Book*, 60. The context is a dispute between St. Augustine's Abbey and the mayor of Bristol, in which Tiler gave a deposition. Also cited in Doyle, "Books with Marginalia," 179.

67. Doyle, "Books with Marginalia," 178 and 184.

68. Jessica Lamothe found a previously unremarked inscription on MS 6, fol. 1r: "sic incipitur in xiii° die mensis Augusti anno domini 1502 per Willelmum Haulle," identifying Haulle as the scribe (Lamothe, "An Edition of the Latin," 88). I am very grateful to my reader for alerting me to this discovery. Haulle's later history is unknown, for he was not named as one of the remaining brothers at the house's suppression.

69. Doyle, "Books with Marginalia," 184.

70. St. Mark's Hospital Cartulary (BA MS 3301/1, fol. 33v); translation from Ross, *Cartulary*, 47.

71. BA MS 3301/1, fols. 34r–v; translation from Ross, *Cartulary*, 48.

72. Sacks, *Widening Gate*, 24.

73. Translation from Ross, *Cartulary*, 117. The document founding a perpetual chantry for the wealthy benefactor John le Strete credits his donations for "increasing its opportunities to perform the blessed commerce of changing the earthly into the celestial and the transitory into the divine." The Latin reads, "sic amplificauit facultates vt terrena in celestia et transitoria in eterna felici comercio transerant" (MS 3301/1, fol. 92v).

74. Also see Skeeters, *Community and Clergy*, 15, for a brief discussion of Sywarde's will.

75. His will is TNA, PROB 11/11/75. I am very grateful to Esther Lewis for directing me to this reference and the following one and for providing me with photographs of the documents.

76. Will of Walter Wralltesley is TNA, PROB 11/13/389. This information is taken from the Hockaday abstract of his will (Gloucestershire Archives, D3439/1 /441). Wralltesley's bequest is noted in Doyle, "Books with Marginalia," 188n5.

77. There may be a connection between Colman and St. Ewen's, for a "Sir John Colman, parson" is noted as having given "two bokes of sermon matters" to that church in 1501–2. However, that date is long before our John Colman was ordained in 1516, so perhaps this Colman was an older relative. Noted in Doyle, "Books with Marginalia," 190n17. See Maclean, "Notes on the Accounts," 155.

78. Skeeters, *Community and Clergy*, 163.

79. A detailed description is found in De la Mare, *Catalogue*, 105–7.

80. Doyle, "Books with Marginalia," 179.

81. Doyle's comment is noted in the manuscript description by De la Mare, *Catalogue*, 106. Doyle, "Books with Marginalia," seeks the sources for Colman's marginal comments in several manuscripts. Spahl's critical edition of the *Emendatio vitae* constructs a stemma for the manuscripts and concludes that MS Lyell 38 is descended, like BL MS Additional 24661, from Dublin, Trinity College MS 281. See Rolle, *De emendatio vitae*, 115–17.

82. Oxford, Bodleian Lyell MS 38, fol. 4r.

83. Spahl's base text (CUL MS Dd. 4. 54) and most other witnesses read "desideranda": other readings include "devitanda" and "desiderata" (Rolle, *De emendatio vitae*, 168–69).

84. Oxford, St. John's College, MS 173, fol. 87r. (Cf. *PL* 176:884A.)

85. Lyell MS 38, fol. 5r.

86. Ibid., fol. 15v.

87. Ibid., fol. 16v.

88. St. John's College MS 173, fol. 107r. The manuscript reading "corripere" is unusual: most manuscripts read "corrigere." See critical text in Verheijen, *La Règle de Saint Augustin*, 426–27; translation by Robert Russell, OSA, at http://faculty.georgetown.edu/jod/augustine/ruleaug.html.

89. Lyell MS 38, fol. 17r.

90. Ibid., fol. 17v.

91. Ibid., fol. 17v.

92. Ibid., fol. 18r.

93. Erler, "Reading at the Gaunts," 52.

94. For a detailed description of this manuscript, see Hanna, *Descriptive Catalogue*, 240–43.

95. The *Expositio* is commonly attested in Augustinian houses: Leicester's Abbey of St. Mary owned at least four copies. See Webber and Watson, *Libraries*, 182, 185.

96. Erler, "Reading at the Gaunts," 58–61.

97. Leicester Abbey also possessed a large miscellany of theological, penitential, and meditative texts containing part of the *Institutio monialis* and the *Sermo ad fratres* 56 (Webber and Watson, *Libraries*, 154–57).

98. Ibid., 61.

99. Latin itself was not a monolithic language, for different cultural and religious settings (from grammar schools to secular and ecclesiastical courts) produced vastly different skills and competencies. See Somerset, "'Al þe comonys,'" 112–14.

100. On the link between women and the vernacular as a cultural commonplace, and the greater availability of English writings to women in later medieval England, see Dearnley, "'Women of oure Tunge,'" 261–62. On the underestimation of women's abilities in Latin, see the introduction to Churchill, Brown, and Jeffrey, *Women Writing Latin*, 2.

101. Meale, "... 'all the bokes that I haue,'" 138.

102. Erler, *Women, Reading, and Piety*, 57.

103. Ibid.

104. For a bilingual manuscript (Paris, Bibliothèque Nationale MS fr. 24766) in which the Latin text is surrounded by translation and commentary, see Wogan-Browne, "Time to Read." The thirteenth-century Augustinian Angier of St. Frideswide created a French translation and commentary on Gregory the Great's *Dialogues* explicitly for a mixed lay and clerical audience, whom he envisaged as "an audience of hearers and readers" (ibid., 66). For a mid-fifteenth-century bilingual medical manuscript that groups English and Latin texts on similar subjects, see Honkapohja, "Multilingualism," esp. 32–33.

105. Erler, "Reading at the Gaunts," 55.

106. TNA PROB 11/16/443.

107. Erler, "Reading at the Gaunts," 57. The possibility of female patronage is raised and detailed analysis of the paintings undertaken in Gill and Howard, "Glimpses of Glory."

108. Oxford, St. John's College MS 173, fol. 33r.

109. This letter is dated to 1059/60. The identity of Countess Blanca is unknown, but Peter refers to her in three other letters. Some have speculated that "Blanca" was Empress Agnes, to whom Peter wrote six known letters (Damian, Letter 66, 40).

110. Ibid., 41. The Latin text is edited in Reindel, *Die Briefe*, 2:247–79.

111. This section frequently circulated independently in manuscripts without mention of its source (Damian, Letter 66, 50).

112. MS 173, fol. 27r. Translation from Damian, Letter 66, 50.

113. Ibid. Translation from Damian, Letter 66, 51.

114. These four notes are extracts, respectively, from Bernard, Sermon 52 "De misericordiis," 40–41; Bernard, Sermon 51 on the Song of Songs, 2:87; Augustine, *De libere arbitrio*, 19 (bk. 1 sec. 61); Bernard, Sermon 4 on "Qui habitat," 4:398.

115. John Scahill makes this point in reference to homiletic texts attributed to Bernard of Clairvaux that appear in Latin, followed by English, in Cambridge, Trinity College, MS B. 14. 39. See Scahill, "Trilingualism," 21.

116. MS 173, fol. 28v. See Bernard, Sermon "De misericordiis," 41.

117. MS 173, fol. 29r. English translation adapted from Augustine, *Sermons 341–400*, 107.

118. See *PL* 39:1533. I have omitted "my brothers and sisters," which appears in the translation, because this form of address does not occur in the manuscript.

119. MS 173, fol. 29v. Translation from Augustine, *Sermons 341–400*, 108.

120. MS 173, fol. 30r. Translation from Augustine, *Sermons 341–400*, 108.

121. Ibid. (emphasis added). Translation from Augustine, *Sermons 341–400*, 108.

122. The other possible Anna would be the mother of the Virgin Mary, also a pious widow.

123. Leicester Abbey probably owned a copy of Sermon 350, listed as "Sermo . . . de laude caritatis" (Webber and Watson, *Libraries*, 289), and Sermon 56 (155–56). Thurgarton Priory records a book containing *Sermones ad fratres in eremo*, but it is not clear which sermons are included (see Webber and Watson, *Libraries*, 421).

124. Saak, *Creating Augustine*, 58; see 81–117 for an account of the collection's complex textual history.

125. MS 173, fol. 31v. See *PL* 40:1339 (cf. Psalm 118). Colman has placed a "nota bene" mark in the margin here.

126. This text is listed as I.6 under the category "General Positive Teaching" in Jolliffe, *Check-List*, 105.

127. MS 173, fols. 33v–34r.

128. Ibid., fol. 34r.

129. Copies of Hugh of Fouilloy's *De claustro animae*, the Latin predecessor to the *Abbey*, are attested in the booklist of Leicester Abbey (see Webber and Watson, *Libraries*, 186–87).

130. MS 173, fols. 34r–34v.

131. Ibid., fol. 34v (emphasis added).

132. Ibid., fol. 34v.

133. Erler, "Reading at the Gaunts," 60.

134. Erler notes (citing a 2005 communication from Ian Doyle) that this text is a variant on the "six profits of tribulation" printed in Horstmann, *Yorkshire Writers*, 2:389–90 (Erler, "Reading at the Gaunts," 60). Webber notes that Peter of Blois' text on the twelve profits of tribulation is attested in the Thurgarton library (Webber, "Latin Devotional Texts," 28). Also see Webber and Watson, *Libraries*, 192 and 269–70, for copies of Peter of Blois' text at Leicester.

135. Bristol PL MS 6, fol. 119v. See Jolliffe, *Check-List*, J.14 (119).

136. MS 6, fols. 120r–v.

137. Appleford, *Learning to Die*, 111.

138. This text is a version of the "nine points pleasing to God" that circulated widely in both Latin and English. See Jolliffe, *Check-List*, I.12 (106–8). One of the English versions is printed in Horstmann, *Yorkshire Writers*, 1:110–12.

139. MS 6, fol. 120v.

140. Ibid., fol. 121r.

141. These are detailed in William Flete's *Remedia*, copied in MS 6, fols. 121v–27v. See Erler, "Reading in the Gaunts," 60, on the Flete text, which is often attested in manuscripts owned by women. This text is also found in BL MS Harley 1706, which has connections to St. Bartholomew's Hospital via William Baron.

### FIVE.  Poverty, Charity, and Poetry

1. McIntosh, *Poor Relief*, 117–21 (quotations from 121).

2. In this discussion I use "lollard" rather than "Lollard" in accordance with Fiona Somerset's model, to suggest a flexible, descriptive use of the term rather than "implying that 'Lollards' are a distinctive, cohesive social group" (Somerset, *Feeling Like Saints*, 16).

3. Aston, "'Caim's Castles,'" 61.

4. Orme and Webster, *English Hospital*, 135.

5. Hudson, *Selections*, 26 (emphasis added).

6. For a helpful discussion on lollard views of predestination and salvation, see Somerset, *Feeling Like Saints*, 30–32.

7. Hudson, *Selections*, 26.

8. Ibid., 136–37.

9. Hudson, *Premature Reformation*, 114.

10. Hudson, *Selections*, 135 (emphasis added). The "statut made at Cambrigge" is the 1388 law requiring the poor who cannot work to return to their hometowns. See Aston, "'Caim's Castles,'" 57, on the specifics of the law, which accorded with provisions of the 1349 Statute of Laborers.

11. The proposal notes near the end, "And yitt have we nat touched of colages, of chauntres, of White Canons, of cathederall chirches with her temperaltes, and chirches with here temperaltes, and chirches appropred into houses of monkes, of Charterhouses, and ne of Frenche monkes, ne of glebes, ne of Bonehommes, ne of spytells, ne ermytages, ne of Crouched Freres" (Hudson, *Selections*, 137).

12. See discussion of this petition, with a translation appended, in Rawcliffe, "Crisis of Confidence," 93–94.

13. *Rotuli Parliamentorum*, 4:19; translation from Rawcliffe, "Crisis of Confidence," 107. This list of unfortunates largely repeats but augments the lists of St. Bartholomew's hospital patients found in the decrees of Edward III and Henry VI (see chapter 2 herein).

14. *Rotuli Parliamentorum*, 4:19; translation from Rawcliffe, "Crisis of Confidence," 108.

15. *Rotuli Parliamentorum*, 4:20. This despite another petition of 1414, part of a larger set of "Articuli de reformatione ecclesiae" supposedly originating from Oxford, which called for the reform of hospitals and other institutions, such as "abbatiis prioratibus, et ecclesiis collegiatis, quibus multae possessiones et praedia conferuntur" (abbeys, priories and collegiate churches which have possessions to distribute to the poor and destitute). Cited from *Concilia Magna Britanniae* 3:365; translation from Orme and Webster, *English Hospital*, 136.

16. *Rotuli Parliamentorum*, 4:81.

17. Rawcliffe, "Crisis of Confidence," 94.

18. Quotation from Carlin, *Medieval Southwark*, 80.

19. Rawcliffe, "Crisis of Confidence," 95.

20. Ibid., 98. Rawcliffe takes the quoted phrase from the list of churches in BL MS Egerton 1995, which I cited in chapter 2. She draws particular attention to the successful career of John Wakeryng, St. Bartholomew's master in the later fifteenth century.

21. Barron, *London in the Later Middle Ages*, 292.

22. McIntosh, *Poor Relief*, chap. 3, "Late Medieval Hospitals and Almshouses," esp. 71–78 on "the residents on hospitals and almshouses." Also see Nicholls, *Almshouses*, 90–137.

23. Barron, *London in the Later Middle Ages*, 276. The city of London issued a proclamation in 1359 requiring beggars able to work to leave the city, while making alms available to "poor folks, lepers, the blind, the halt, and persons oppressed with old age and other maladies" (ibid.).

24. Rubin, "Imagining Medieval Hospitals," 22–23.

25. See Sweetinburgh, *Role of the Hospital*, 60–67: "The new houses in Warwickshire and Wiltshire rarely provided shelter for the sick or poor travellers; instead, founders and patrons directed their benevolence towards the local poor or their elderly servants and retainers" (63). Also see Barron, *London in the Later Middle Ages*, 267, on the foundation of almshouses in London starting in the early fifteenth century.

26. Rawcliffe, "Crisis of Confidence," 99.

27. Richmond, "Victorian Values," 229. Also see Rosenthal, *Purchase of Paradise*, on Ewelme (71–72). Rosenthal discusses Ewelme and other newly founded

hospitals as demonstrating a larger philanthropic "shift in concern from regular to secular branches of the ecclesiastical structure" among the nobility (ibid., 128).

28. Richmond, "Victorian Values," 234.

29. Ibid., 229–30.

30. Orme and Webster, *English Hospital*, 55. Marjorie McIntosh observes, "Donors of an endowed charity gained spiritual reward, not only through the gift itself but through the ongoing prayers of the beneficiaries, just as strong a feature of Protestant almshouses as of Catholic hospitals" (McIntosh, "Poverty, Charity, and Coercion," 467). Dyer, "Poverty and Its Relief," 7, makes a similar point.

31. Orme and Webster, *English Hospital*, 52–53.

32. Fisher, *English Works of John Fisher*, 240.

33. Rawcliffe, "Crisis of Confidence," 101.

34. Slack, "Hospitals, Workhouses," 230.

35. Somerville, *Savoy*, 24–25. These survive in two manuscripts: BL MS Cotton Cleopatra C. V and Harvard Law School Library, MS 11.

36. Somerville, *Savoy*, 29–33. For a translation of Santa Maria Nuova's statutes and comparison to the Savoy's, see Park and Henderson, "First Hospital among Christians"; "The Savoy appears to have been less communally and more hierarchically organized, and its statutes devote relatively more space to issues of moral and religious discipline and less to medical procedures and record-keeping" (168).

37. After its dissolution, the Savoy was refounded in 1556, but it foundered administratively and was in receivership by 1570 (Somerville, *Savoy*, 44).

38. Rawcliffe, "Crisis of Confidence," 101–2; quotation from the bill at 109.

39. McIntosh, *Poor Relief*, 117–18.

40. Rawcliffe, "Crisis of Confidence," 106.

41. Marshall argues that the "radicalism" and the "intense contemporary interest" that the *Supplication* provoked have been underappreciated by modern scholars (Marshall, *Beliefs and the Dead*, 49).

42. Fish, *Supplicacyon*, 412.

43. Ibid.

44. Hudson, *Premature Reformation*, 501–2. Also see Orme and Webster, *English Hospital*, 151, on Fish.

45. Fish, *Supplicacyon*, 419.

46. Ibid., 422.

47. Ibid.

48. Ibid.

49. Ibid.

50. Ingram, *Carnal Knowledge*, 266.

51. Ibid.

52. W. G. Moore was the first to identify Balsac's poem as the source for the second half of the *Hye Way*. See Moore, "Robert Copland."

53. Erler, "*The maner*," 229.

54. Orme and Webster, *English Hospital*, 154.

55. See Erler's excellent introductory discussion in her edition (Copland, *Poems*, 221–24). She notes of the *Hye Way*, "If it conveys the anxiety and to some extent the helplessness produced by these social problems, a profound concern for personal failures in charity also underlies its rueful jocularity" (ibid., 223).

56. Daly, "Hospitals of London," 54; Orme and Webster, *English Hospital*, 154.

57. Orme and Webster, *English Hospital*, 154–55.

58. Dionne, "Fashioning Outlaws," 52. Likewise Paolo Pugliatti calls the *Hye Way* "the first autochthonous English literary account of beggars" (Pugliatti, *Beggary and Theatre*, 132).

59. Karen Helfand Bix uses the quoted phrase to characterize early vagabond texts, in Bix, "'Masters of Their Occupation,'" 172.

60. *Hye Way*, in Copland, *Poems*, ed. Erler, lines 44–45. All quotations from the *Hye Way* are taken from this edition. Further line numbers will appear in parentheses within the main text.

61. Erler notes that much the same list appears in *Piers Plowman* C text 10.175–81 (Copland, *Poems*, 230).

62. Martine Van Elk contends that counterfeiting becomes constitutive of vagrancy in this literature. "We see early modern rogue literature rehearse over and over again that many vagrants who beg pretend to be ill, impotent, lame, dumb, or in another form unable to take on regular employment, thus attempting, falsely, to place themselves in the category of the deserving poor" (Van Elk, "Counterfeit Vagrant," 128).

63. For the first passage, see Moore, "Robert Copland," 418; for the second, see Coldiron, "Translation's Challenge," 328. For the third, see Orme and Webster, *English Hospital*, 154.

64. Van Elk, "Counterfeit Vagrant," 125, emphasizes, "'Counterfeiting' is central to the rogue's mobility in the rogue literature."

65. See Copland, *Poems*, 234.

66. The full passage (*Piers Plowman* C-Text, V.44–52) reads:

And so y leue yn London and opelond bothe;
The lomes [tools] þat y labore with and lyflode deserue
Is *pater-noster* and my prymer, *placebo* and *dirige*,
And my sauter som tyme and my seuene psalmes.
This y segge for here soules of suche as me helpeth,

And tho þat fynden me my fode fouchen-saf, y trowe,
To be welcome when y come, oþer-while in a monthe,
Now with hym, now with here; on this wyse y begge
Withoute bagge or botel but my wombe one.

Kerby-Fulton cites this passage, which some view as autobiographical, as a key locus for Langland's expression of "vocational crisis" among the clerical proletariat (see Kerby-Fulton, *Clerical Proletariat*, 79–83). I find the resemblance between the two passages striking, but I am not asserting that Copland was consciously citing Langland.

67. For the phrase "labouring psalms," see Kerby-Fulton, *Clerical Proletariat*, 83.

68. As Erler notes, "Aue regina" is an antiphon, and "Quem terra ponthus" and "Ave maris stella" are both hymns (Copland, *Poems*, 234).

69. A few hospitals existed specifically for retired or infirm priests, such as the hospital at Clyst Gabriel near Exeter, founded in the early fourteenth century by Bishop Walter Stapledon (Orme, "A Medieval Almshouse").

70. On the commonplace of rogue fraternity, see Dionne, "Fashioning Outlaws," 48–49.

71. The name "Pappey" comes from the church of St. Augustine's de Papey, which was appropriated to the fraternity (Hugo, "The Hospital," 187). Also see discussion of the fraternity in Erler, *Reading and Writing*, 16, 25. The institution is referred to as a "hospital" in Cardinal Pole's 1556 Pension Book (Hugo, "The Hospital," 218).

72. For a transcription of Henry VI's Latin letter patent, see Hugo, "The Hospital," 214, and 189 for translation. I have expanded abbreviations.

73. BL MS Egerton 1995, fols. 84r–v. Cited in Gairdner, *Historical Collections*, viii.

74. Hugo, "The Hospital," 210. Hugo does not provide a transcription for this regulation (VIII).

75. Ibid., 214, and translation at 190.

76. For a list of masters and wardens up to 1548, see Hugo, "The Hospital," 198–202. For details of the house's property at the Dissolution, see ibid., 203–5, 217.

77. See Copland, *Poems*, 235.

78. Copland's *Secrete of Secretes* includes an extensive discussion of physiognomy, introducing the subject as follows: "a noble and meruaylous scyence that is called physonomy by the which thou shalt knowe the nature and condycyon of people"; see Copland, *The Secrete of Secretes*, 31.

79. *Statutes of the Realm*, 3:330 (emphasis added).

80. Hartley and Aldridge, *Johannes de Mirfeld*, 132–33.

81. Moore, "Robert Copland," 418.

82. Bix, "'Masters of Their Occupation,'" 173. She notes that the rogue's "unreformable" quality is one of his most constant in the literature.

83. "Ceux qui par faulte de reparation qu'ilz feroint bien laissent cheoir une maison" (cited in Moore, "Robert Copland," 412, as an example of an adapted passage).

84. See Erler's discussion in Copland, *Poems*, 242. She notes that swearing is a "characteristic late medieval inclusion."

85. See *MED*, s.v. disese, n., for this range of meanings.

86. Coldiron, "Translation's Challenge," 326.

SIX. Dissolution, Disappearance, and Refoundation

1. These phrases from Marshall, *Beliefs and the Dead*, 107. Marshall is referring not to hospitals but rather to the wider crisis over purgatory, yet I find his terms helpful for characterizing hospital concerns.

2. See Orme and Webster, *English Hospital*, 147–65; Daly, "Hospitals of London," 91–111.

3. Marshall asserts, "There is no doubt that the authors of the dissolution policy were aware of the perceived link with purgatory and intercession, but there is no direct evidence for the assertion that the intention to seize monastic assets was a primary motivation for the increasing radicalization of the king's attitude toward purgatory" (Marshall, *Beliefs and the Dead*, 83).

4. Orme and Webster, *English Hospital*, 156.

5. Ibid.

6. Cranmer, "Confutation of Unwritten Verities," 16.

7. Orme and Webster, *English Hospital*, 157. They call the new cathedral almsmen "the most positive achievement of Henry VIII's regime with regard to hospitals and almshouses" (159). The Chantry Act of 1545, intended to ensure that any remaining intercessory institutions should revert to the Crown, similarly outlined a program of reforming institutions "for more godly and virtuous purposes" (ibid.)

8. Slack, "Hospitals, Workhouses," 229.

9. Magnus surrendered the house in return for personal benefits, including a pension, an on-site dwelling, a Yorkshire grange, and other goods. For the

surrender document, see Brewer et al., *Letters and Papers*, 14.2:227, and *ODNB* entry "Magnus, Thomas (1463/4–1550)." The visitations, which focused on monastic possessions, adherence to monastic rules, and sexual conduct, reported that they found at St. Leonard's only one sodomite and two brothers seeking release from their vows. See Brewer et al., *Letters and Papers*, 10:141.

10. See Cullum, "Hospitals and Charitable Provision," 49.

11. TNA, MS C 66/626, m. 1. The grant is calendared in Brewer et al., *Letters and Papers*, 1.2:30. I am grateful to Michael G. Sargent for help with transcribing and translating this document.

12. Ibid.

13. See Raine, *Mediaeval York*, 115.

14. See *Cartulary of St. Leonard's*, 2:608, 914–16 on the lands in Newton, and 922 on the church of Newton.

15. YML MS M/2/6/e, fol. 49v. The following will in the register, that of laborer Robert Godson, leaves the same amount to the hospital (ibid., fol. 50r).

16. See Rice and Pappano, *Civic Cycles*, 74, on the suppression of Corpus Christi. The procession resumed for several years under the brief reign of Queen Mary (1553–58). See ibid., 74–81, for discussion of this new beginning. For the order suppressing the Death, Assumption, and Coronation of the Virgin pageants, see *REED: York*, 1:291–92.

17. The entire cycle was suspended because of plague in 1550 and 1552. There are two substitutions on record: in 1535 the Creed play was performed instead of the Corpus Christi play, and in 1536 the Pater Noster play was performed as an alternative to the Corpus Christi play. See discussion of the cycle's final 1569 performance in Rice and Pappano, *Civic Cycles*, 220–27.

18. Another financial challenge was the hospital's struggle throughout the fifteenth century to secure its traditional right to the Petercorn, a thrave of wheat from every ploughland in the diocese. After a 1469 revolt in the East Riding, partially inspired by resentment over this imposition, King Edward IV abolished the Petercorn, but the hospital was never remunerated as the king had promised. See Orme and Webster, *English Hospital*, 103–4.

19. Only the seventh and ninth stations, at forty pence each, were cheaper.

20. See *REED: York*, 1:85 (1454), 1:101 (1468), 1:180 (1499). For the 1516 reference, see 1:213. Quotation from Beadle, *York Plays*, 2:138.

21. For this 1399 petition by the commons to limit the number of stations to twelve, see *REED: York*, 1:11; translation 2:268.

22. See *REED: York*, 1:15 for Latin and 2:701 for translation.

23. *REED: York*, 1:42–43 for Latin and 2:728 for translation.

24. *REED: York*, 1:268.

25. In late 1538 the six priories surrendered (St. Andrew's, Holy Trinity, and the four orders of friars), while St. Mary's Abbey surrendered in November 1539, quickly followed by St. Leonard's (Palliser, *Tudor York*, 235).

26. *REED: York*, 1:283 (emphasis added).

27. Moran, *Growth of English Schooling*, 96.

28. Ibid., 167–68.

29. Palliser, *Reformation in York*, 16. Palliser claims (17) that York had no functioning grammar school from 1539 to 1546, but Moran's evidence of smaller lay-founded schools that had sprung up in the sixteenth century would seem to complicate this argument. See Moran's appendix B of York schools in Moran, *Growth of English Schooling*, 278–79.

30. YML MS M/2/6/e, fol. 43v.

31. Moran, *Growth of English Schooling*, 75. See Raine, ed., *York Civic Records*, 2:71–73.

32. *Valor Ecclesiasticus* transcript in Carpenter, *Cartulary*, 2:924–28 (927).

33. Moran, *Education and Learning*, 9.

34. On Magnus's foundation, see *ODNB* entry on Magnus, and Moran, *Growth of English Schooling*, 33.

35. Wynter was appointed in 1528 and resigned in 1529, succeeded by Magnus.

36. Brewer et al., *Letters and Papers*, 4.2:1365.

37. This figure, like all of the *Valor*'s numbers, was probably an underestimate (Cullum, "Hospitals and Charitable Provision," 414).

38. For the number of poor supported, see *Valor* transcript in Carpenter, *Cartulary*, 2:925.

39. Cullum, "Hospitals and Charitable Provision," 390–91.

40. See Hoyle, *Pilgrimage of Grace*, 83–84.

41. Ibid., 88.

42. The examination, in which Aske responds to questions from Cromwell, is dated April 15, 1537 (see Bateson and Crumwell, "Aske's Examination," 561; emphasis added).

43. Hoyle emphasizes that Aske's "monastophilia" may not have been shared by all: "Monasteries may well have been a familiar and valued part of the fabric of early sixteenth-century northern society, but the risings of 1536 were not primarily about their defence" (Hoyle, *Pilgrimage of Grace*, 49).

44. Palliser, *Tudor York*, 235.

45. Only a portion of the laymen put on trial were executed, yet all of the twenty accused clerics were put to death, suggesting Henry's extreme antipathy toward the religious orders (Hoyle, *Pilgrimage of Grace*, 453).

46. Palliser, *Tudor York*, 237.

47. This rhetorical emphasis is noted by Palliser (*Tudor York*, 236) and Hoyle (*Pilgrimage of Grace*, 74). In the event, Darcy declined the offer in favor of several other former monastic properties (Hoyle, *Pilgrimage of Grace*, 79).

48. Brewer et al., *Letters and Papers*, 14.2:227.

49. For a transcription and expansion of the 1535 *Valor Ecclesiasticus* report on St. Leonard's, see Carpenter, *Cartulary*, 2:924–27; 925 for "Distributionibus elemosinarum . . . pro sustentatione sexaginta pauperum infra firmarium."

50. Quotation from the Commissioners of the North in their letter to Thomas Cromwell, December 8, 1539 (Wright, *Three Chapters of Letters Relating to the Suppression*, 166).

51. Brewer et al., *Letters and Papers*, 14.2: 227.

52. For a 1541 lease to Henry Thwaytes of York of several hospital properties, see Brewer et al., *Letters and Papers*, 16:724. For a 1542 grant of the hospital's manor of Bramhope, Yorkshire, see ibid., 17:159.

53. Cullum, "Hospitals and Charitable Provision," 427–28.

54. *REED: York*, 1:274–75. The event is planned and described in the House Books (see ibid., 270–74).

55. Badir, "'The whole past,'" 21.

56. Ibid.

57. Both possibilities are suggested by Cullum, "Hospitals and Charitable Provision," 446, and Palliser, *Tudor York*, 238.

58. See discussion of the Trinity Hospital's Reformation history in Rice and Pappano, *Civic Cycles*, 220–27.

59. See York Explore Y/COU/2/1/5, the 1478 indenture detailing the terms by which the hospital would be governed jointly by the guild members and the hospital's master, brothers, and sisters.

60. York Explore Y/Soc/3/1/2 (pp. 1–2).

61. York Explore Y/COU/1/1/20, fol. 102r. Printed in Raine, *York Civic Records*, 5:75.

62. Hall, "York's Medieval Infrastructure," 83.

63. York Explore Y/COU/1/1/21, fol. 116v. Printed in Raine, *York Civic Records*, 5:137.

64. Daly, "Hospitals of London," offers an excellent discussion of the hospital's fortunes from the 1540s through circa 1570. See esp. 91–190 on threats to the hospital and its refoundation process.

65. Ingram, *Carnal Knowledge*, 267–68.

66. Ibid., 237.

67. Moore, *History of St. Bartholomew's Hospital*, 2:125–26. Daly agrees that it seems to have continued to function (Daly, "Hospitals of London," 67).

68. "Petition of the Mayor, Aldermen, and Commonalty of the City of *London* to King *Henry* the Eighth; 1538," in Firth, *Memoranda, References and Documents,* appendix 1, 1. I have silently expanded abbreviations. Further citations from this edition will appear in parentheses in the main text.

69. See brief discussion of this traditional piety in Slack, "Hospitals, Workhouses," 230.

70. "Translation of Letters Patent containing the Grant and Establishment of St. Bartholomew's Hospital; 1544," in Firth, *Memoranda,* appendix 1, 5. This is a translation with additions of Latin, where decipherable, from the damaged copy of the document preserved at the hospital (SBHB/HC/1/2000).

71. "Translation of Letters Patent containing the Grant and Establishment of St. Bartholomew's Hospital; 1544," in Firth, *Memoranda,* appendix 1, 5.

72. Henry leaves the detailed reenvisioning of the hospital to the citizens responsible for it. B. G. Gale suggests that the city's recent assistance in supplying men and funding for Henry's wars in Scotland and France had "shifted the advantage in bargaining from the King to the City," perhaps making him willing to cede control over the functioning of the hospital (Gale, "Dissolution and the Revolution," 93–94).

73. In April 1546 he gives the hospital 500 marks per year to endow the institution, provided that the citizens raise another 500 on their own (Daly, "Hospitals," 149).

74. Daly, "Hospitals of London," 149; see 149–59 for the details of negotiations in 1546–47.

75. "Deed of Covenant between King Henry VIII and the Mayor, Commonalty, and Citizens of London, respecting the Hospitals," in Firth, *Memoranda,* appendix , 12.

76. Again the Savoy statutes, which require a matron, vice-matron, and twelve nurses, may have served as inspiration. See the 1523 Savoy statutes in Harvard Law School MS 11, pp. 51–59, detailing the nurses' duties, clothing, and responsibilities, including detailed rules stipulating punishment for sexual infractions.

77. "Deed of Covenant between King Henry VIII and the Mayor, Commonalty, and Citizens of London, respecting the Hospitals," in Firth, *Memoranda,* 16.

78. See Daly, "Hospitals of London," 160–71, for details on the long, difficult process of securing funding.

79. Ibid., 171.

80. As Barron has noted, the influence of the Savoy statutes is also felt in the royal regulations issued in 1557 to St. Thomas's, Bridewell, St. Bartholomew's, and Christ's hospitals (Barron, *London in the Later Middle Ages,* 293). These are printed in Firth, *Memoranda,* appendix 1, 83–107.

81. Daly, "Hospitals of London," 175.

82. Brigden, *London and the Reformation*, 478.

83. Slack, "Social Policy," 108.

84. A minute from the Court of Aldermen's February 1552 meeting reported that "the boke that Thomas Vycars barbour-surgeon hath devysed for the relcif of the pore" should be printed by Grafton (Branch, *Faith and Fraternity*, 96, citing LMA, Repertory 12/2, fol. 449). As ordinances tended to be written collectively, Vicary probably appeared on behalf of the hospital governors "rather than as the sole author" (ibid.). Grafton's authorship of the preface is asserted in Kingdon, *Richard Grafton*, 54. For the phrase "clearly Edwardian," see Branch, *Faith and Fraternity*, 97. Grafton served as governor of St. Thomas's Hospital in Southwark when it was acquired by the city in 1551, and he later served as governor of the city's hospitals (Ferguson, "Grafton, Richard," 2). See Sisson, "Grafton and the London Grey Friars," on Grafton's residence at the house of the Grey Friars and establishment of his press there in 1539.

85. The production of the Great Bible (so called because of its large format) had begun in Paris under printer François Regnault, but after an edict was passed to suppress its production, the printing materials were transported to London, where Grafton used them to print the Bible at Grey Friars (Ferguson, "Grafton, Richard," 1–2).

86. Brigden, *London and the Reformation*, 345. Quotation from Kingdon, *Richard Grafton*, 91. Grafton had also printed the authorized English primer of 1545 (see Butterworth, *English Primers*, 256–75).

87. On Grafton's two editions of Hardyng's *Chronicle*, see Devereux, "Empty Tuns," 35–38.

88. See Manchester, "Chronicling the English Reformation," on Grafton's later historical works, including *The Chronicle at Large* (1569), in which Grafton drew from earlier chronicles while augmenting his sources with enthusiasm for reformed theology and distaste for Catholicism.

89. *The Ordre of the Hospital*, 1552, A2r. The text is also printed in *Anatomie of the Bodie of Man*, 289–336. Subsequent references will cite from the original 1552 edition with page numbers noted in the main text.

90. Daly, "Hospitals of London," 182, calls this a "counterblast against criticisms of the hospital."

91. See Judith 13:17–10. I am grateful to Kathryn Smith for identifying this image.

92. Latimer, *Sermons*, 378, "Fourth Lenten Sermon." See discussion of Judith's popularity as a Reformation symbol in Stocker, *Judith*, 46–66.

93. Ingram, Carnal Knowledge, 195.

94. Brooks, Law, Politics and Society, 394.

95. This is the charge to the matron, and such phrasing is virtually identical among the different officers' charges.

96. For example, the Savoy regulations charge the hospital's doorkeeper to admit the "honesti" while keeping out the "infames and suspecti" (Harvard Law School MS 11, p. 42).

97. This claim is mentioned by Slack, "Social Policy," 108.

98. See Siena, "The Clean and the Foul."

99. It is worth noting the connection between York's Trinity Hospital, run by the Mercers Company, and the Last Judgment pageant that they sponsored, in which the works of mercy feature as the preeminent signs of charity by the blessed souls. See Rice and Pappano, *The Civic Cycles*, 209–27.

100. See the similar promises made to the surveyors, who will for their labors receive "rest and pleasure in heauen" (B8v) and the stewards/butlers, who like the governors are exhorted to view their duties to the poor as the same as to God: any negligence in running the house, "either with excesse prices, or not makyng your prouision in due tyme, the same damage and hurt you do unto GOD whose members the poore are, and therefore ye ought the rather to study to serue in this house with feare of GOD, and conscience, as one that manifestly and plainly walketh before the face of God, who perfectlie seeth and beholdeth the very thoughtes of your herte" (D6v–7r).

101. Daly, "Hospitals of London," 173, notes that the governors are imbued with "an aura of spiritual authority." See also Branch, *Faith and Fraternity*, 98.

102. See Harvard LS MS 11, p. 33. The Savoy *hospitularius* was charged with supervising the admission and care of the poor as well as the activities of the other staff members.

103. The Savoy Hospital statutes also indicate the importance of keeping records safe. See, e.g., Harvard LS MS 11, p. 78, describing the "secundum scrinium" to hold the hospital's original ordinances and statutes, along with documents testifying to the house's possessions and grants.

104. See Van Elk, "Counterfeit Vagrant," 126, on the importance of naming and labeling vagrants in legal records.

105. The Hospital Museum has on display a large triple-locked chest that may be the chest mentioned here, but it may be a "parish chest" for the newly created St. Bartholomew the Less (*Nine Centuries of Health Care*, 15).

106. For description of this type of "passport," see McIntosh, *Poor Relief*, 58.

107. See the brief discussion of these books in Ramsay and Willoughby, *Hospitals, Towns and the Professions*, 79–80, with particular attention to the provision and keeping of books at the refounded house.

108. Quoted phrase from Rawcliffe, "Hospital Nurses," 64.

109. See Pelling, "Nurses and Nursekeepers," 192.

110. Cabré, "Women or Healers?," 24.

111. The office of matron may derive from the 1546 covenant via the Savoy Hospital's definition of this role as the head nurse of twelve women who pledge obedience to her. See Harvard LS MS 11, p. 51 and 52.

112. Pelling, "Nurses and Nursekeepers," 190. In the seventeenth century, the Royal College of Physicians cited a matron of St. Bartholomew's acting as an "irregular practictioner" of medical care (Pelling and White, *Medical Conflicts*, 153).

113. Daly, "Hospitals of London," 200. She was courted by St. Katherine's by the Tower and by St. Thomas's.

114. This language too is probably borrowed from the Savoy statutes, which emulated Santa Maria Nuova in directing the washing and delousing of patients and their clothes (see Harvard LS MS 11, p. 56). Pelling notes the persistent connection between nursing patients and washing laundry (Pelling, "Nurses and Nursekeepers," 192).

115. See Harvard LS MS 11, pp. 58–59.

116. Pollock, "Childbearing and Female Bonding," 298.

117. See McIntosh, *Poor Relief*, 116–18. Pelling and Webster note that in the period between 1550 and 1600, London parishes commonly paid women to care for orphans and take in the sick poor (Pelling and Webster, "Medical Practitioners," 187).

118. SBHB/HB/1/1, fol. 105r (emphasis added).

119. Other rewards on the same folio included, e.g., "to Alice Wright one of the susters in rewarde for one monethe service don in the last new made chambres for disseased persons."

120. SBHB/HB/1/1, fol. 141r. Also mentioned in Daly, "Hospitals of London," 186.

121. SBHB/HB/1/1, fol. 239v.

122. Daly has found other references to "Mother Hall" in the records for treating children: this may be the same woman (Daly, "Hospitals of London," 186).

123. SBHB/HA/1/1, fol. 181v.

124. Vicary had lived in the hospital since 1551. In January 1552 he was nominated as "one of the assistants" to the hospital for a lifetime term (Daly, "Hospitals of London," 198).

125. SBHB/HA/1/1, fol. 196r, a later record, notes that one of the poor, Elizabeth Hamlyn, is to be dismissed because she is with child. Perhaps the unnamed woman found herself in a similar situation.

126. Ibid., fol. 238v.

127. Ibid., fol. 240r. This affliction and "bleach" were "ill-defined skin diseases," according to Forbes, "By what disease or casualty," 130.

128. See Power, "Notes on the Bibliography," 91–92, and Branch, *Faith and Fraternity*, 98.

129. Hickman, "From Catholic to Protestant," 126.

130. Both quotations from ibid., 133.

131. The Litany was the first vernacular service to be officially authorized, published in 1544 (Cummings, *Book of Common Prayer*, 705).

132. Barker, *Mayor's Chapel*, 65.

133. Henry's letter patent of 1541 grants the hospital's properties to the mayor and city corporation. See BA, CC/1/33 (charter with seal intact) and *Bristol Charters*, 84–92, for a transcript of the text.

134. Cranmer's 1534 order is printed in Cranmer, *Miscellaneous Writings and Letters*, 460–61. Also see Skeeters, *Community and Clergy*, 38–46, on the Latimer controversy.

135. Marshall, *Beliefs and the Dead*, 65.

136. Skeeters, *Community and Clergy*, 57–66. Also see the discussion of Edgworth's preaching, which connected Bristol's port location to the importation of evangelical ideas (and to venereal disease), in MacCulloch, *Tudor Church Militant*, 114.

137. Skeeters, *Community and Clergy*, 73.

138. Ibid., 67. Skeeters notes that the among the clergy, the friars were the only order that protested their dissolution.

139. Ibid., 74.

140. Noting that rules had to be passed in the 1420s requiring local guild members to participate in the yearly Corpus Christi procession, Sacks argues that "by the 1530s this rejection of the cult of the saints was very general in Bristol" (Sacks, *Widening Gate*, 157).

141. Green, *Letters of Royal and Illustrious Ladies*, 2:160 (emphasis added).

142. Erler, "Reading at the Gaunts," 66.

143. Smith, *Mayor of Bristowe is Kalendar*, 55.

144. On the transition from monastery to cathedral, see Bettey, "Conversion of St. Augustine's."

145. Latham, *Bristol Charters*, 86. The Latin reads, "tam ob sinceram affeccionem quam erga villam nostram Bristollie gerimus quam mille librarum sterlingorum." Also see Smith, *Mayor of Bristowe is Kalender*, 56, for a record of this grant.

146. Smith, *Mayor of Bristowe is Kalendar*, 54.

147. Barrett, *History and Antiquities*, 373 (emphasis added).

148. BRO, F/Au/1/2, p. 205. See Barker, *Mayor's Chapel*, 58–59.

149. BRO, F/Au/1/2, p. 208. See Barker, *Mayor's Chapel*, 59.

150. Barker, *Mayor's Chapel*, 59.

151. Ibid., 60.

## Epilogue

1. If he had declined the position, he would have received a smaller pension: "if he refuse thenne to have but vj li" (Barker, *Mayor's Chapel*, 50).

2. Ibid., 61. See information on Ellis's biography in Skeeters, *Community and Clergy*, 167.

3. Barker, *Mayor's Chapel*, 60.

4. Erler, *Reading and Writing*, 53. She cites the ex-canon Thomas Hikkelyn, who after the dissolution of St. Bartholomew's Hospital became the first vicar of St. Bartholomew the Less.

5. Of St. Mark's chapel in the seventeenth century, Jonathan Harlow notes, "As a chapel, St Mark's might of course be used for services including baptisms, marriages and funerals, so there were registers but there were no churchwardens, no vestry and certainly no separate parish" (Harlow, *Religious Ministry in Bristol*, 36). I assume that the same held true from the beginning of its establishment as a chapel.

6. Andrew Kraebel's critical edition of *Super novem* is forthcoming.

7. See Butterworth, *English Primers*, 47–117 on the primers of 1534–35, and 181–99 on the primer of 1539. For printed editions of the primers of 1535, 1539, and 1545, see *Three Primers*.

8. See discussion in Duffy, *Stripping of the Altars*, 444–45.

9. Cited from *Manuall of Prayers*, n.p. See *Three Primers*, 414, for modernized text.

10. 1 Corinthians 15:51–54. *Manuall of Prayers*, n.p. See *Three Primers*, 417, for modernized text.

11. A transcription of Fechett's will appears in McGrath and Williams, *Bristol Wills*, 1–3.

12. See Barker, *Mayor's Chapel*, 53, for his pension (£6 13d 4s), and see Skeeters, *Clergy and Community*, 168, for the available biographical information on Fechett.

13. McGrath and Williams, *Bristol Wills*, 1. These ( ) are present in the transcriptions. I have unfortunately not been able to examine the original document.

14. Ibid.

15. Ibid.

16. Ibid. (emphasis added).

17. Ibid. (emphasis added).

18. Ibid., 2–3 (emphasis added).

19. Bodleian MS Lyell 38, fol. 76v. Translation by Michael G. Sargent.

20. Ibid. See Moyes, *Expositio*, 2:209. Moyes comments at ibid., 1:86, on Colman's tendency to annotate the text.

21. Many thanks to Michael G. Sargent for help deciphering this marginal note.

22. Bodleian MS Lyell 38, fol. 79r. See Moyes, *Expositio*, 2:213.

23. Marshall, *Beliefs and the Dead*, 94.

24. Bodleian Lyell MS 38, fol. 82r. See Moyes, *Expositio*, 2:218.

25. Ibid.

26. Marshall, *Beliefs and the Dead*, 108. In 1553, article 23 of the Forty-Two Articles would decree, "The Doctrine of School authors concerning purgatory, pardons, worshipping and adoration as well of images as of relics, and also invocation of Saints, is a fond thing, vainly feigned, and grounded upon no warrant of scripture, but rather repugnant to the word of God" (Ketley, ed., *The Two Liturgies*, 532).

27. See Duffy, *Stripping of the Altars*, 467.

28. Tyacke, "Introduction: Rethinking the English Reformation," in Tyacke, ed., *England's Long Reformation*, 13.

29. Marshall also notes that changes in the Communion service reflected the rupture between the living and the dead: "The prayer for 'the whole state of Christ's Church' now carried the important qualifier 'militant here in earth', and the commendation of the departed was now entirely omitted" (Marshall, *Beliefs and the Dead*, 111).

30. Burial of the Dead, 1549, in Cummings, *Book of Common Prayer*, 82.

31. Ibid.

32. Ibid., and see discussion of the hymn at 717.

33. Ibid., 82.

34. Dickens, ed., "Robert Parkyn's Narrative," 76.

35. Ibid., 58.

36. See Marshall, *Beliefs and the Dead*, 117–18.

37. Barker, *Mayor's Chapel*, 65 and 66.

38. Duffy, *Stripping of the Altars*, 495: "The surprising failure of the Marian laity in many regions to re-establish the cult of the dead on anything like its former footing is probably less to do with any scepticism about doctrine that with the loss of this vital dimension of continuity." Sacks, *Widening Gate*, 133, makes a similar point.

39. Transcribed in Fleming, *Maire of Bristowe is Kalendar*, 16.

40. Barrett, *Histories and Antiquities*, 376.

41. Vicary, *Anatomie of the Bodie of Man*, 11. The *Anatomie* was first issued in 1548 and reprinted in this edition of 1577.

42. Simpson, *Reform and Cultural Revolution*, 1.

# BIBLIOGRAPHY

## PRIMARY SOURCES

### Manuscripts

*Bristol*
Bristol Archives
    BA 3301/1
    BA CC/1/33
    BA F/Au/1/2
Bristol Public Library
    BPL MS 6

*Cambridge, MA*
Harvard Law School Library
    HLS MS 11

*Cambridge, UK*
Gonville and Caius College Library
    Gonville and Caius MS 669*/646
Trinity College Library
    TCC MS R. 3. 20

*Gloucester*
Gloucestershire Archives
    MS D349/1/441

*Kew*
National Archives
    TNA C 66/626
    TNA C 270/20
    TNA PCC Prob. 11/11/75
    TNA PCC Prob. 11/13/389
    TNA PCC Prob. 11/16/443

*London*
Barts Health NHS Trust Archives and Museums
    SBHB/HA/1/1
    SBHB/HB/1/1
    SBHB/HC/1/2000
    SBHB/HC/2/1
British Library
    BL MS Additional 5467
    BL MS Additional 10392
    BL MS Cotton Vespasian B. IX
    BL MS Egerton 1995
    BL MS Harley 3
    BL MS Harley 2378
    BL MS Harley 2985
    BL MS Harley 4987
    BL MS Royal 7. F. XI
    BL MS Royal 10. E. IV
Gray's Inn Library
    Gray's Inn MS 4
London Metropolitan Archives
    LMA DL/C/B/004/MS09171/003
    LMA DL/C/B/004/MS09171/005
    LMA DL/C/B/004/MS09171/006

*New York*
Pierpont Morgan Library
    Morgan MS 150

*Oxford*
Bodleian Library
    MS Ashmole 59
    MS Bodley 682
    MS Lyell 38
Pembroke College Library
    Pembroke College MS 2
St. John's College Library
    St. John's College MS 173

*York*
York Minster Library
    YML MS M 2/6/e

York Explore Library (City Archives)
   Y/Soc/3/1/2
   Y/COU/1/1/21
   Y/COU/1/1/20
   Y/COU/2/1/5

Early Printed Books

*London*
British Library
   Copland, Robert. *The Hye Way to the Spyttell Hous.* C.57.b.30
   *The Ordre of the Hospital Of St. Bartholomewes in Westsmythfielde.*
      C.58.a.21(2)

Published Primary Sources

Alain de Lille. *Liber Poenitentialis.* Edited by Jean Longère. Analecta Mediaevalia
   Namurcensia 17. Louvain/Lille: Nauwelaerts/Librairie Girard, 1965.
Anderson, J. J., ed. *Records of Early English Drama: Newcastle-Upon-Tyne.* Toronto:
   University of Toronto Press, 1982.
Augustine. *De libere arbitrio libri tres.* Edited by William M. Green. Corpus Scripto-
   rum Ecclesiasticorum Latinorum 74. Vienna: Hoelder-Pichler-Tempsky, 1956.
———. Augustine. *Sermons 341–400.* Translated by Edmund Hill, O.P. Hyde Park,
   NY: New City Press, 1995.
Baker, Donald C., John L. Murphy, and Louis B. Hall Jr., eds. *The Late Medieval
   Religious Plays of Bodleian MSS Digby 133 and E Museo 160.* EETS OS 283.
   Oxford: Oxford University Press, 1982.
Baldwin, Elizabeth, Lawrence M. Clopper, and David Mills, eds. *Records of Early
   English Drama: Cheshire Including Chester.* 2 vols. Toronto: University of To-
   ronto Press, 2007.
Balsac, Robert de. *Le Droict Chemin de L'Opital.* In *La Nef des Princes et des Ba-
   tailles de Noblesse avec le Chemin Pour Aller a L'Ospital et Aultres Enseigne-
   ments.* Paris, 1502.
Barrett, William. *The History and Antiquities of the City of Bristol.* Bristol: Wil-
   liam Pine, 1789.
Bateson, Mary, and Thomas Crumwell, eds. "Aske's Examination." *English Historical Review* 5, no. 19 (1890): 550–73.
Beadle, Richard, ed. *The York Plays: A Critical Edition of the York Corpus Christi
   Play as Recorded in British Library MS Additional 35290.* 2 vols. EETS SS
   23–24. Oxford: Oxford University Press, 2009 and 2013.

Beadle, Richard, and Peter Meredith, eds. *The York Play: A Facsimile of British Library MS Additional 35290; Together with a Facsimile of the "Ordo Paginarum" Section of the A/Y Memorandum Book.* Leeds: University of Leeds Press, 1983.

Bernard of Clairvaux. Sermon "De misericordiis." In *Sancti Bernardi Opera Omnia*, edited by Jean Leclercq, C. H. Talbot, and Henri Rochais, 6.1:40–43. Rome: Editions Cistercienses, 1970.

———. Sermon 4 on "Qui habitat." In *Sancti Bernardi Opera Omnia*, edited by Jean Leclercq, C. H. Talbot, and Henri Rochais, 4:397–401. Rome: Editions Cistercienses, 1966.

———. Sermon 51 on the Song of Songs. In *Sancti Bernardi Opera Omnia*, edited by Jean Leclercq, C. H. Talbot, and Henri Rochais, 2:83–89. Rome: Editions Cistercienses, 1957.

*The Book of the Foundation of St. Bartholomew's Church in London.* Edited by Sir Norman Moore. EETS OS 163. London: Oxford University Press, 1923.

Brewer, J. S., et al., eds. *Letters and Papers Foreign and Domestic of the Reign of Henry VIII.* 21 vols. London: Longman, Green, 1862–1932.

Burton, Edward, ed. *Three Primers Put Forth in the Reign of Henry VIII.* Oxford: Oxford University Press, 1843.

*Calendar of the Patent Rolls: Henry IV, Vol. 1, A.D. 1399–1401.* London: H. M. Stationery Office, 1903.

*Calendar of the Patent Rolls: 15 Henry VI, Vol. 3, A.D. 1436–1441.* London: H. M. Stationery Office, 1907.

Carpenter, David X., ed. *The Cartulary of St. Leonard's Hospital, York, Rawlinson Volume.* Record Series 163. Borthwick Texts and Studies 42. Woodbridge: The Boydell Press, 2015.

Copland, Robert. *The Hye Way to the Spyttell Hous.* In Copland, *Poems*, 187–245.

———. *Poems.* Edited by Mary C. Erler. Toronto: University of Toronto Press, 1993.

———. *The Secrete of Secretes.* London, 1528.

Cranmer, Thomas. "The Confutation of Unwritten Verities." In *Miscellaneous Writings and Letters of Thomas Cranmer*, 1–67.

———. *Miscellaneous Writings and Letters of Thomas Cranmer, Archbishop of Canterbury, Martyr.* Edited by John Edmund Cox. Cambridge: Cambridge University Press, 1846.

Cummings, Brian, ed., *The Book of Common Prayer: The Texts of 1549, 1559, and 1662.* Oxford: Oxford University Press, 2011.

Damian, Peter. Letter 66. In *Die Briefe des Petrus Damian*, edited by Kurt Reindel, 2:247–79. Munich: Monumenta Germania Historiae, 1988.

———. Letter 66. In *Letters 61–90*, translated by Owen J. Blum, 40–69. Washington, DC: Catholic University of America Press, 1992.

Davis, Norman, ed. *Non-Cycle Plays and Fragments.* EETS SS 1. Oxford: Oxford University Press, 1970.

Dickens, A. G., ed. "Robert Parkyn's Narrative of the Reformation." *English Historical Review* 62, no. 242 (1947): 58–83.

Dugdale, William, ed. *Monasticon Anglicanum: A History of the Abbies and Other Monasteries, Hospitals, Frieries, and Cathedral and Collegiate Churches, with their Dependencies, in England and Wales.* 6 vols. London: Bohn, 1846.

Elliott, J. J., ed. *The Apocryphal New Testament.* Oxford: Oxford University Press, 1993.

Firth, James, ed. *Memoranda, References and Documents Relating to the Royal Hospitals of London.* 2nd ed. London: Benjamin Pardon, 1863.

Fish, Simon. *A Supplicacyon for the Beggers.* In *The Complete Works of Sir Thomas More,* edited by Frank Manley, Richard Marius, Germain Marc'hadour, and Clarence H. Miller, 7:409–22. New Haven, CT: Yale University Press, 1990.

Fisher, John. *The English Works of John Fisher.* Edited by John E. B. Mayor. EETS ES 27. London, 1876.

Fleming, Peter, ed. *The Maire of Bristowe is Kalendar.* Bristol: Bristol Record Society, 2015.

Forni, Kathleen, ed. *The Chaucerian Apocrypha: A Selection.* Kalamazoo, MI: TEAMS, 2005.

Gairdner, James, ed. *The Historical Collections of a Citizen of London in the Fifteenth Century.* London: Camden Society, 1876.

Gilbertus Anglicus. *Compendium Medicine Gilberti Anglici tam Morborum Universalium Quam Particularium Nondum Medicis sed et Cyrurgis Utilissimum.* Lyons, 1510.

Gratian. *Decretum Gratiani Emendatum et notatione.* Venice, 1600.

Green, Mary Anne Everett, ed. *Letters of Royal and Illustrious Ladies of Great Britain.* 3 vols. London: Henry Colman, 1846.

Green, Monica, ed. *The Trotula: A Medieval Compendium of Women's Medicine.* Philadelphia: University of Pennsylvania Press, 2001.

Green, Monica H., and Linne R. Mooney, eds. *The Sickness of Women.* In *Sex, Aging, and Death in a Medieval Compendium: Trinity College Cambridge MS R.14.52, Its Texts, Language, and Scribe,* edited by M. Teresa Tavormina, 2:455–568. Tempe: Arizona Center for Medieval and Renaissance Studies, 2006.

Gregory the Great. Epistola 60 (*Ad Romanum*). In *PL* 77:996–97.

———. *Homilia* 35. In *PL* 76:1259–65.

Harper-Bill, Christopher, ed. *The Register of John Morton, Archbishop of Canterbury 1486–1500.* 3 vols. Canterbury & York Society 78. Woodbridge: Boydell & Brewer, 1991.

Hartley, Sir Percival Horton-Smith, and Harold Richard Aldridge, eds. *Johannes de Mirfeld of St. Bartholomew's, Smithfield: His Life and Works.* Cambridge: Cambridge University Press, 1936.

Henderson, W. G., ed. *Manuale et Processionale ad Usum Ecclesiae Eboracensis.* Surtees Society 63. Durham: Surtees Society, 1875.

———, ed. *Missale ad usum insignis Ecclesiae Eboracensis.* Durham: Andrew & Co., 1874.

Henry of Grosmont. *Le Livre de Seyntz Medicines (The Book of Holy Medicines).* Translated and edited by Catherine Batt. Tempe: Arizona Center for Medieval and Renaissance Studies, 2014.

Horstmann, Carl, ed. *Yorkshire Writers: Richard Rolle of Hampole, An English Father of the Church, and His Followers.* 2 vols. London: Swan Sonnenschein, 1895.

Hudson, Anne, ed. *Selections from English Wycliffite Writings.* Toronto: University of Toronto Press, 1997.

Humbert of Romans. *Sermones ad Diversos Status. Cum Epistola Ejusdem.* Haguenau: Gran, Heinrich, 1508.

Humphries, K. W., ed. *The Friars' Libraries.* London: The British Library, 1990.

"Index of Wills from St. Leonard's Hospital, York 1410–1533." *Yorkshire Archaeological Society Records Series* 60 (1920): 191–93.

Johnston, Alexandra, and Margaret Rogerson, eds. *Records of Early English Drama: York.* 2 vols. Toronto: University of Toronto Press, 1979.

Kerling, Nellie, ed. *Cartulary of St. Bartholomew's Hospital.* London: Lund Humphries, 1973.

Ketley, Joseph, ed. *The Two Liturgies, A.D. 1549, and A.D. 1552: with Other Documents Set Forth by Authority in the Reign of King Edward VI.* Cambridge: Cambridge University Press, 1844.

King, Pamela M., and Clifford Davidson, eds. *The Coventry Corpus Christi Plays.* Kalamazoo, MI: Medieval Institute, 2000.

Lancashire, Ian, ed. *Dramatic Texts and Records of Britain: A Chronological Topography to 1558.* Toronto: University of Toronto Press, 1984.

Lang, Sheila, and Margaret McGregor, eds. *Tudor Wills Proved in Bristol 1546–1603.* Bristol: Bristol Record Society, 1993.

Langland, William. *Piers Plowman: The C-Text.* Edited by Derek Pearsall. Exeter: University of Exeter Press, 1994.

Latham, R. C., ed. *Bristol Charters, 1509–1899.* Bristol: Bristol Record Society, 1947.

Latimer, Hugh. *Sermons.* Edited by G. E. Corrie. Cambridge: Cambridge University Press, 1844.

Le Grand, Léon, ed. *Statuts d'Hotels-Dieu et de Léproseries: Recueil de Textes du XIIe au XIVe Siècle.* Paris: Alphonse Picard, 1901.

Lumiansky, R. M., and David Mills, eds. *The Chester Mystery Cycle*. 2 vols. EETS SS 3, 9. London: Oxford University Press, 1974.

Lydgate, John. *The Fall of Princes*. Edited by Harry Bergen. EETS OS 121. London: Oxford University Press, 1967.

———. *The Minor Poems of Lydgate*. Edited by H. M. McCracken. Part I. EETS ES 107. Oxford: Oxford University Press, 1911.

———. *Mummings and Entertainments*. Edited by Claire Sponsler. Kalamazoo, MI: Medieval Institute, 2010.

Lydgate, John, and Benedict Burgh. *Lydgate and Burgh's "Secrees of Old Philisofres": A Version of the "Secreta Secretorum."* Edited by Robert Steele. EETS OS 66. London: Paul, Trench, Trübner, 1894.

Manzalaoui, M. A., ed. *Secretum Secretorum: Nine English Versions*. EETS OS 276. Oxford: Oxford University Press, 1977.

Matheson, Lister, ed. *Death and Dissent: Two Fifteenth-Century Chronicles*. Cambridge: The Boydell Press, 1999.

McGrath, Patrick, and Mary E. Williams, eds. *Bristol Wills, 1546–1593*. Bristol: University of Bristol, Department of Extra-Mural Studies, 1975.

McHardy, A. K. *The Church in London, 1375–1392*. London: London Record Society, 1977.

Mirk, John. *John Mirk's Festial, Edited from British Library MS Cotton Claudius A.II*. Edited by Susan Powell. 2 vols. EETS OS 334, 335. Oxford: Oxford University Press, 2009 and 2011.

Mowat, J. L. G., ed. *Sinonoma Bartholomei, a Glossary From a Fourteenth-Century Manuscript in the Library of Pembroke College, Oxford*. Oxford: Clarendon, 1880.

Neckham, Alexander. *De vita monachorum*. In *The Anglo-Latin Satirical Poets and Epigrammatists of the Twelfth Century*, edited by Thomas Wright, 2:175–200. London: Longman, 1872.

Nicholaus of Salernitanum. *Antidotarium*. Venice: N. Jenson, 1471.

Raine, Angelo, ed. *York Civic Records*. 8 vols. Wakefield: Yorkshire Archaeological Society Record Series, 1939–53.

Raine, James, and J. W. Clay, eds. *Testamenta Eboracensia*. 6 vols. Durham: J. B. Nichols and Son, 1830–96.

Ralph, Elizabeth, ed. *The Great White Book of Bristol*. Bristol: Bristol Record Society, 1979

Ramsay, Nigel, and James M. W. Willoughby, eds. *Hospitals, Towns, and the Professions*. Corpus of British Medieval Library Catalogues 14. London: The British Library, 2009.

Riley, Henry Thomas., ed. *Chronica Monasterii S. Albani*. Rolls Series 28. 12 vols. London: Longman, 1863–76.

Rolle, Richard. *De emendatio vitae: Eine kritische Ausgabe des lateinischen Textes von Richard Rolle.* Edited by Rüdiger Spahl. Bonn: Bonn University Press, 2009.

———. *Expositio Super Novem Lectiones Mortuorum.* 2 vols. Edited by Malcolm Robert Moyes. Salzburg Studies in English Literature 92:12. Salzburg: Institut für Anglistik und Amerinistik, 1988.

Ross, C. D., ed. *The Cartulary of St. Mark's Hospital, Bristol.* Bristol: Bristol Record Society, 1959.

*Rotuli Parliamentorum ut et Placita in Parliamento.* Edited by John Strachey and Richard Blyke. London, 1767.

Smith, Lucy Toulmin, ed. *"The Mayor of Bristowe is Kalender" by Robert Ricard, the Town Clerk of Bristol 18 Edward IV.* London: Camden Society, n.s., 5 (1872).

*The Statutes of the Realm, Printed by Command of His Majesty King George the Third, in Pursuance of an Address of the House of Commons of Great Britain. From Original Records and Authentic Manuscripts.* Edited by Alexander Luders and others. 11 vols. London: London, Dawsons, 1810–1828.

Stow, John. *A Survey of London.* Edited by Charles Lethbridge Kingsford. Oxford: Clarendon, 1908.

Sugano, Douglas, ed. *The N-Town Plays.* Kalamazoo, MI: Medieval Institute, 2007.

Tanner, Norman P., ed. *Decrees of the Ecumenical Councils.* London: Sheed and Ward, 1989.

Tolhurst, J. B. L. ed. *The Ordinale and Customary of the Abbey of Saint Mary York.* Cambridge: Henry Bradshaw Society, 1936.

Verheijen, Luc, ed. *La Règle de Saint Augustin.* 2 vols. Paris: Études Augustiniennes, 1967.

Vicary, Thomas. *The Anatomie of the Bodie of Man.* Edited by Frederick J. Furnivall. EETS ES 53. London: N. Trübner, 1888.

*Vita S. Leonardi.* In *Acta Sanctorum,* edited by Hippolyte Delehaye et al., 66 (November, part 3):150–55. Brussels: Société des Bollandistes, 1910.

Webb, E. A., ed. *The Records of St. Bartholomew's Priory and St. Bartholomew the Great, West Smithfield: Volume 1.* Oxford: Oxford University Press, 1921.

Wilkins, David, ed. *Concilia Magnae Britanniae et Hiberniae.* 4 vols. London: R. Gosling, 1737.

Wright, Thomas, ed. *The Anglo-Latin Satirical Poets and Epigrammatists of the Twelfth Century.* London: Longman, 1872.

———. *Three Chapters of Letters Relating to the Suppression of the Monasteries.* Durham: Surtees Society, 1843.

Young, Karl. *The Drama of the Medieval Church.* 2 vols. Oxford: Clarendon, 1933.

## SECONDARY SOURCES

Alakas, Brandon. "Seniority and Mastery: The Politics of Ageism in the Coventry Cycle." *Early Theatre* 9 (2006): 15–36.

Appleford, Amy. *Learning to Die in London, 1380–1540*. Philadelphia: University of Pennsylvania Press, 2014.

Arbesmann, Rudolph. "The Concept of the *Christus Medicus* in St Augustine." *Traditio* 10 (1954): 1–28.

Ashley, Kathleen. "Sponsorship, Reflexivity, and Resistance: A Cultural Reading of the York Cycle Plays." In *The Performance of Middle English Culture*, edited by Lawrence Clopper, James Paxson, and Sylvia Tomasch, 9–24. Cambridge: Boydell and Brewer, 1998.

Aston, Margaret. "'Caim's Castles': Poverty, Politics and Disendowment." In *The Church, Politics and Patronage in the Fifteenth Century*, edited by R. B. Dobson, 45–81. Gloucester: Palgrave, 1984.

Badir, Patricia. "'The whole past, the whole time': Untimely Matter and the Playing Spaces of York." In *Performing Environments: Site-Specificity in Medieval and Early Modern English Drama*, edited by Susan Bennett and Mary Polito, 17–35. London: Palgrave Macmillan, 2014.

Bale, Anthony. "A Norfolk Gentlewoman and Lydgatian Patronage: Lady Sibylle Boys and Her Cultural Environment." *Medium Aevum* 78, no. 2 (2009): 261–80.

Barker, W. R. *St. Mark's, or the Mayor's Chapel, Bristol*. Bristol: W. C. Hemmons, 1892.

Barron, Caroline. "Introduction: The Widow's World in Later Medieval London." In *Medieval London Widows, 1300–1500*, edited by Caroline Barron and Anne Sutton, xiii–xxxiv. London: Hambledon, 1994.

———. *London in the Later Middle Ages: Government and People, 1200–1500*. Oxford: Oxford University Press, 2004.

———. "The People of the Parish." In *Harlaxton Medieval Studies*, Vol. 29, *The Urban Church in Late Medieval England*, edited by David Harry and Christian Steer, 353–79. Donington: Shaun Tyas, 2019.

Barron, Caroline, and Anne F. Sutton, eds. *Medieval London Widows, 1300–1500*. London: Hambledon, 1994.

Baswell, Christopher. "Competing Archives, Competing Histories: French and Its Cultural Location in Late-Medieval England." *Speculum* 90, no. 3 (2015): 635–41.

Beadle, Richard. "Nicholas Lancaster, Richard of Gloucester and the York Corpus Christi Play." In *The York Mystery Plays: Performance in the City*, edited by Margaret Rogerson, 31–52. York: York Medieval Press, 2011.

Becquet, Jean. "Chanoines réguliers et érémitisme clérical." *Revue d'histoire de la spiritualité: Revue d'ascétique et de mystique* 48 (1972): 361–70.

Bettey, Joseph. "The Conversion of St. Augustine's, Bristol to a Cathedral." In *The Medieval Art, Architecture and History of Bristol Cathedral: An Enigma Explored*, edited by Jon Cannon and Beth Williamson, 263–76. Woodbridge: The Boydell Press, 2011.

Biddle, M., H. T. Lambrick, and J. N. L. Myres. "The Early History of Abingdon, Berkshire, and its Abbey." *Medieval Archaeology* 12, no. 1 (1968): 26–69.

Bix, Karen Helfand. "'Masters of Their Occupation': Labor and Fellowship in the Cony-Catching Pamphlets." In *Rogues and Early Modern English Culture*, edited by Craig Dionne and Steve Mentz, 171–92. Ann Arbor: University of Michigan Press, 2004.

Bloomfield, M. W. *The Seven Deadly Sins: An Introduction to the History of a Religious Concept, with Special Reference to Medieval English Literature*. East Lansing: Michigan State Press, 1967.

Boffey, Julia, and A. S. G. Edwards. "'Chaucer's Chronicle,' John Shirley, and the Canon of Chaucer's Shorter Poems." *Studies in the Age of Chaucer* 20 (1998): 201–18.

Boffey, Julia, and John Thompson. "Anthologies and Miscellanies: Production and Choice of Texts." In *Book Production and Publishing in Britain, 1375–1475*, edited by Jeremy Griffiths and Derek Pearsall, 279–315. Cambridge: Cambridge University Press, 1989.

Bonfield, Christopher. "The First Instrument of Medicine: Diet and Regimens of Health in Late Medieval England." In *A Very Parfit Praktisour: Essays Presented to Carole Rawcliffe*, edited by Linda Clark and Elizabeth Danbury, 99–119. Cambridge: Boydell & Brewer, 2017.

———. "The *Regimen Sanitatis* and Its Dissemination in England, *c.* 1348–1550." D. Phil thesis, University of East Anglia, 2006.

Bovey, Alixe. "Communion and Community: Eucharistic Narratives and Their Audience in the Smithfield Decretals." In *The Social Life of Illumination: Manuscripts, Images and Communities in the Late Middle Ages*, edited by Joyce Coleman, Mark Cruse, and Kathryn Smith, 53–82. Turnhout: Brepols, 2013.

Bowers, John. *Chaucer and Langland: The Antagonistic Tradition*. Notre Dame, IN: Notre Dame University Press, 2007.

Branch, Laura. *Faith and Fraternity: London Livery Companies and the Reformation 1510–1603*. Leiden: Brill, 2017.

Brigden, Susan. *London and the Reformation*. Oxford: Clarendon, 1989.

Brooks, C. W. *Law, Politics and Society in Early Modern England*. Cambridge: Cambridge University Press, 2009.

Brown, Sarah. *Stained Glass at York Minster.* York: Scala Arts Publishers, 2017.

Bullough, Vern. "A Note on Medical Care in Medieval English Hospitals." *Bulletin of the History of Medicine* 35 (1961): 74–77.

Burger, Glenn. *Conduct Becoming: Good Wives and Husbands in the Later Middle Ages.* Philadelphia: University of Pennsylvania Press, 2017.

Burgess, Clive. *The Right Ordering of Souls: The Parish of All Saints' Bristol on the Eve of the Reformation.* Woodbridge, Suffolk: The Boydell Press, 2018.

Butterworth, Charles. *The English Primers, 1529–1545: Their Publication and Connection with the English Bible and the Reformation in England.* Philadelphia: University of Pennsylvania Press, 1953.

Bynum, Caroline Walker. "The Spirituality of Regular Canons in the Twelfth Century." In *Jesus as Mother: Studies in the Spirituality of the High Middle Ages,* 22–58. Berkeley: University of California Press, 1982.

Cabré, Montserrat. "Women or Healers? Household Practices and the Categories of Health Care in Late Medieval Iberia." *Bulletin of the History of Medicine* 82, no. 1 (2008): 18–51.

Caciola, Nancy M. *Discerning Spirits: Divine and Demonic Possession in the Middle Ages* Ithaca, NY: Cornell University Press, 2003.

Cadden, Joan. *The Meanings of Sex Differences in the Middle Ages.* Cambridge: Cambridge University Press, 1993.

———. *Nothing Natural Is Shameful: Sodomy and Science in Late Medieval Europe.* Philadelphia: University of Pennsylvania Press, 2013.

Carlin, Martha. "Medieval English Hospitals." In *The Hospital in History,* edited by Lindsay Granshaw and Roy Porter, 21–40. London: Routledge, 1989.

———. *Medieval Southwark.* London: Hambledon Press, 1996.

Chesney, Kathleen. "Notes on Some Treatises of Devotion Intended for Mary of York." *Medium Aevum* 20 (1951): 11–39.

Christie, Sheila. "Bridging the Jurisdictional Divide: The Masons and the York Corpus Christi Play." In *The York Mystery Plays: Performance in the City,* edited by Margaret Rogerson, 53–74. York: York Medieval Press, 2011.

Churchill, Laurie J., Phyllis R. Brown, and Jane E. Jeffrey, eds. *Women Writing Latin: Medieval and Early Modern Women Writing Latin.* London: Routledge, 2002.

Citrome, Jeremy J. *The Surgeon in Medieval English Literature.* New York: Palgrave Macmillan, 2016.

Clark, James G. "The Augustinians, History and Literature in Late Medieval England." In *The Regular Canons in the Medieval British Isles,* edited by Janet Burton and Karen Stöber, 403–16. Turnhout: Brepols, 2011.

Coldiron, A. E. B. "Translation's Challenge to Critical Categories: Verses from French in the Early English Renaissance." *Yale Journal of Criticism* 16, no. 2 (2003): 315–44.

Coleman, Joyce. *Public Reading and the Reading Public in Late Medieval England and France.* Cambridge: Cambridge University Press, 1996.

Coletti, Theresa. "Genealogy, Sexuality, and Sacred Power: The Saint Anne Dedication of the Digby Candelmas Day and the Killing of the Children of Israel." *Journal of Medieval and Early Modern Studies* 29 (1999): 25–59.

———. *Mary Magdalene and the Drama of Saints.* Philadelphia: University of Pennsylvania, 2004.

———. "Social Contexts of the East Anglian Saint Play: The Digby *Mary Magdalene* and the Late Medieval Hospital?" In *Medieval East Anglia*, edited by Christopher Harper-Bill, 287–301. Woodbridge: Boydell and Brewer, 2005.

Collette, Carolyn. *Performing Polity: Women and Agency in the Anglo-French Tradition, 1385–1620.* Turnhout: Brepols, 2006.

Collier, Richard J. *Poetry and Drama in the York Corpus Christi Play.* Hamden: Archon, 1978.

Connolly, Margaret. *John Shirley: Book Production and the Noble Household.* Aldershot: Ashgate, 1998.

Connolly, Margaret, and Raluca Radulescu, eds. *Insular Books: Vernacular Manuscript Miscellanies in Late Medieval Britain.* Oxford: Oxford University Press, 2015.

Coster, William. "Purity, Profanation, and Puritanism: The Churching of Women, 1500–1700." In *Women in the Church: Papers Read at the 1989 Summer Meeting and the 1990 Winter Meeting of the Ecclesiastical History Society*, edited by W. J. Sheils and Diana Wood, 377–87. Studies in Church History 27. Oxford: Blackwell, 1990.

Cré, Marleen. *Vernacular Mysticism in the Charterhouse: A Study of London, British Library, MS Additional 37790.* Turnhout: Brepols, 2006.

Cressy, David. *Birth, Marriage, and Death: Ritual, Religion, and the Life-Cycle in Tudor and Stuart England.* Oxford: Oxford University Press, 1997.

Crislip, Andrew. *From Monastery to Hospital.* Ann Arbor: University of Michigan Press, 2005.

Cullum, P. H. "'And Hir Name Was Charite': Charitable Giving by and for Women in Late Medieval Yorkshire." In *Woman Is a Worthy Wight: Women in English Society c. 1200–1500*, edited by P. J. P. Goldberg, 182–211. Stroud: Sutton, 1992.

———. *Cremetts and Corrodies: Care of the Poor and Sick at St. Leonard's Hospital, York in the Middle Ages.* Borthwick Paper 79. York: University of York, 1991.

———. "'For Pore Peple Harberles': What Was the Function of the Maisondieu?" In *Trade, Devotion and Governance: Papers in Late Medieval History*, edited by Dorothy J. Clay, Richard G. Danes, and Peter McNiven, 36–54. Stroud: Sutton, 1994.

———. "Hospitals and Charitable Provision in Medieval Yorkshire, 936–1547." D. Phil thesis, University of York, 1989.

———. "St Leonard's York: The Spatial and Social Analysis of an Augustinian Hospital." In *Advances in Monastic Archaeology*, edited by Roberta Gilchrist and Harold Mytum, 11–18. British Archaeological Reports, British Series 227. Oxford: BAR, 1993.

———. "Vowcsscs and Lay Female Piety in the Province of York, 1300–1530." *Northern History* 23 (1996): 21–41.

Daly, Christopher. "The Hospitals of London: Administration, Refoundation, and Benefaction, c. 1500–1572." D. Phil thesis, University of Oxford, 1993.

Davenport, Tony. "Fifteenth-century Complaints and Duke Humfrey's Wives. " In *Nation, Court and Culture: New Essays on Fifteenth-century English Poetry*, edited by Helen Cooney, 129–52. Dublin: Four Courts, Press, 2001.

Davidson, Clifford. *Festivals and Plays in Late Medieval Britain*. Aldershot: Ashgate, 2007.

Davis, Adam. *The Medieval Economy of Salvation: Charity, Commerce and the Rise of the Hospital*. Ithaca, NY: Cornell University Press, 2019.

Dearnley, Elisabeth. " 'Women of oure Tunge Cunne Bettir Reede and Vnderstonde This Langage': Women and Vernacular Translation in Later Medieval England." In *Multilingualism in Medieval Britain (c. 1066–1520)*, edited by Judith A. Jefferson and Ad Putter, 259–72. Turnhout: Brepols, 2013.

De la Mare, Albinia. *Catalogue of the Collection of Medieval Manuscripts Bequeathed to the Bodleian Library Oxford by James P. R. Lyell*. Oxford: Clarendon, 1971.

Devereux, E. J. "Empty Tuns and Unfruitful Grafts: Richard Grafton's Historical Publications." *Sixteenth Century Journal* 21, no. 1 (1990): 33–56.

Dickinson, J. C. *The Origins of the Austin Canons and Their Introduction in England*. London: SPCK, 1950.

Dinkova-Bruun, Greti. "The Book of Job in Latin Biblical Poetry of the Later Middle Ages." In *A Companion to Job in the Middle Ages*, edited by Franklin Harkins and Aaron Canty, 324–53. Leiden: Brill, 2016.

———. "Notes on Poetic Composition in the Theological Schools ca. 1200 and The Latin Poetic Anthology from Ms. Harley 956: A Critical Edition." *Sacris Erudiri* 43 (2004): 299–391.

Dionne, Craig. "Fashioning Outlaws: The Early Modern Rogue and Urban Culture." In *Rogues and Early Modern English Culture*, edited by Craig Dionne and Steve Mentz, 33–61. Ann Arbor: University of Michigan Press, 2004.

Dobson, R. B. "Craft Guilds and City: The Historical Origins of the York Mystery Plays Reassessed." In *The Stage as Mirror: Civic Theatre in Late Medieval Europe*, edited by Alan E. Knight, 91–105. Cambridge: Boydell and Brewer, 1997.

Doyle, A. I. "Books Connected with the Vere Family and Barking Abbey." *Transactions of the Essex Archaeological Society*, n.s., 25 (1955/60): 222–43.

———. "Books with Marginalia from St. Mark's Hospital, Bristol." In *New Directions in Medieval Manuscript Studies and Reading Practices: Essays in Honor of Derek Pearsall*, edited by Kathryn Kerby-Fulton, John J. Thompson, and Sarah Baechle, 177–91. Notre Dame, IN: University of Notre Dame Press, 2014.

———. "More Light on John Shirley." *Medium Aevum* 30 (1961): 93–101.

Doyle, A. I., and Ralph Hanna, eds. *Hope Allen's Writings Ascribed to Richard Rolle: A Corrected List of Copies*. Publications of the Journal of Medieval Latin 13. Turnhout: Brepols, 2019.

Duffy, Eamon. "Holy Maydens, Holy Wyfes: The Cult of Women Saints in Fifteenth- and Sixteenth-Century England." In *Women in the Church: Papers Read at the 1989 Summer Meeting and the 1990 Winter Meeting of the Ecclesiastical History Society*, ed. W. J. Sheils and Diana Wood, 175–96. Studies in Church History 27. Oxford: Blackwell, 1990.

———. *The Stripping of the Altars: Traditional Religion in England, 1400–1580*. New Haven, CT: Yale University Press, 1992.

Dyer, Christopher. "Poverty and Its Relief in Late Medieval England," *Past and Present* 21 (August 2010): 41–78.

Eddy, Nicole. "Marginal Annotation in Medieval Romance Manuscripts: Understanding the Contemporary Reception of the Genre." PhD diss., University of Notre Dame, 2012.

Edwards, A. S. G. "John Shirley and the Emulation of Courtly Culture." In *The Court and Cultural Diversity*, edited by E. Mullaly and J. Thompson, 309–17. Cambridge: D. S. Brewer, 1997.

———. "John Shirley, John Lydgate, and the Motives of Compilation." *Studies in the Age of Chaucer* 38 (2016): 245–54.

Eldredge, L. M. *The Index of Middle English Prose Handlist IX: Manuscripts in the Ashmole Collection, Bodleian Library, Oxford*. Woodbridge, Suffolk: D. S. Brewer, 1992.

Elliott, Dyan. *Fallen Bodies*. Philadelphia: University of Pennsylvania Press, 1999.

Epstein, Robert. "Chaucer's Scogan and Scogan's Chaucer." *Studies in Philology* 96, no. 1 (1999): 1–21.

Erler, Mary C. "*The maner to Lyue well* and the Coming of English in François Regnault's Primers of the 1520s and 1530s." *The Library* 6, no. 3 (1984): 229–43.

———. *Reading and Writing during the Dissolution*. Cambridge: Cambridge University Press, 2013.

———. "Three Fifteenth-Century Vowesses." In *Medieval London Widows, 1300–1500*, ed. Caroline Barron and Anne Sutton, 165–83. London: Bloomsbury Academic, 1994.

———. "Widows in Retirement: Region, Patronage, Spirituality, Reading at the Gaunts, Bristol." *Religion and Literature* 37, no. 2 (2005): 51–75.

———. *Women, Reading, and Piety in Later Medieval England.* Cambridge: Cambridge University Press, 2002.

Evans, Ruth. "When a Body Meets a Body: Fergus and Mary in the York Cycle." *New Medieval Literatures* 1 (1997): 193–212.

Ferguson, Meraud Grant. "Grafton, Richard (1506/7–1573)." In *ODNB.*

Fitzgerald, Christina M. "Compiling Couplets: Performing Masculinity in Middle English Moral Poetry." *Exemplaria* 32, no. 2 (2021): 107–29.

———. "Compiling Mercantile Manhood in Richard Hill's Book (Oxford Balliol College MS 354)." Paper presented at the Annual Meeting of the Modern Language Association, 2019.

———. *The Drama of Masculinity and Medieval English Guild Culture.* New York: Palgrave, 2007.

Forbes, Thomas R. "By What Disease or Casualty: The Changing Face of Death in London." *Journal of the History of Medicine and Allied Sciences* 31, no. 4 (1976): 395–420.

Forde, Simon. "The Educational Organization of the Augustinian Canons in England and Wales, and Their University Life at Oxford, 1325–1448." *History of Universities* 13 (1994): 21–60.

French, Katherine. "Maidens' Lights and Wives' Stores: Women's Parish Guilds in Late Medieval England." *Sixteenth Century Journal* 29 (1998): 399–425.

———. "The Material Culture of Childbirth in Late Medieval London and Its Suburbs." *Journal of Women's History* 28 (2016): 126–48.

Gale, B. G. "The Dissolution and the Revolution in London Hospital Facilities." *Medical History* 11, no. 1 (1967): 91–96.

Geltner, Guy. "Social Deviancy: A Medieval Approach," In *Why the Middle Ages Matter: Medieval Light on Modern Injustice,* edited by Celia Chazelle et al., 29–40. London: Taylor and Francis, 2011.

Getz, Faye M. "John Mirfield and the *Breviarium Bartholomei*: The Medical Writings of a Clerk at St. Bartholomew's Hospital in the Later Fourteenth Century." *Society for the Social History of Medicine Bulletin* 37 (1985): 24–26.

———. *Medicine in the English Middle Ages.* Princeton, NJ: Princeton University Press, 1998.

Gibson, Gail M. "Blessing from Sun and Moon: Churching as Women's Theater." In *Bodies and Disciplines: Intersections of Literature and History in Fifteenth-Century England,* edited by Barbara Hanawalt and David Wallace, 139–54. Minneapolis: University of Minnesota Press, 1996.

———. "Manuscript as Sacred Object: Robert Hegge's N-Town Plays." *Journal of Medieval and Early Modern Studies* 44 (2014): 503–29.

———. *Theater of Devotion: East Anglian Drama and Society in the Late Middle Ages.* Chicago: University of Chicago Press, 1989.

Gilchrist, Roberta. "Christian Bodies and Souls: The Archaeology of Life and Death in Later Medieval Hospitals." In *Death in Towns: Urban Responses to the Dying and the Dead, 100–1600*, edited by Steven Bassett, 101–18. Leicester: Leicester University Press, 1992.

———. *Sacred Heritage: Monastic Archaeology, Identities, Beliefs.* Cambridge: Cambridge University Press, 2019.

Gill, Miriam, and Helen Howard, "Glimpses of Glory: Paintings from St. Mark's Hospital, Bristol." In *Almost the Richest City: Bristol in the Later Middle Ages*, edited by Laurence Keen, 97–106. Bristol Archeological Society Transactions 19. London: Routledge,1997.

Goldberg, P. J. P. "Craft Guilds, the Corpus Christi Play and Civic Government." In *The Government of Medieval York: Essays in Commemoration of the 1396 Royal Charter*, edited by Sarah Rees Jones, 141–63. York: University of York, 1997.

———. "From Tableaux to Text: The York Corpus Christi Play ca. 1378–1428." *Viator* 43 (2012): 247–76.

———. "Performing the Word of God: Corpus Christi Drama in the Northern Province." In *Life and Thought in the Northern Church, c. 1100–c. 1700*, edited by Diana Wood, 145–70. Woodbridge: Boydell and Brewer, 1999.

———. *Women, Work, and Life Cycle in a Medieval Economy: Women in York and Yorkshire c. 1300–1520.* Oxford: Oxford University Press, 1992.

Gottfried, Robert S. *Doctors and Medicine in Medieval England.* Princeton, NJ: Princeton University Press, 1986.

Green, Monica H. "The Development of the Trotula." *Revue d'Histoire des Textes* 26 (1996): 119–203.

———. "Flowers, Poisons and Men: Menstruation in Medieval Western Europe." In *Menstruation: A Cultural History*, edited by Andrew Shail and Gillian Howie, 51–64. New York: Palgrave Macmillan, 2005.

———. "From 'Diseases of Women' to 'Secrets of Women': The Transformation of Gynecological Literature in the Later Middle Ages." *Journal of Medieval and Early Modern Studies* 30, no. 1 (2000): 5–39.

———. *Making Women's Medicine Masculine.* Oxford: Oxford University Press, 2008.

Greenberg, Cheryl. "John Shirley and the English Book Trade." *The Library*, 6th ser., 4, no. 4 (1982): 369–80.

Gregg, W. W. *"The Trial and Flagellation": With Other Studies in the Chester Cycle.* Oxford: Malone Society, 1935.

Griffiths, Jeremy. "A Newly Identified Manuscript Inscribed by John Shirley." *The Library* 14, no. 2 (1992): 83–92.

Griffiths, Ralph. "The Pursuit of Justice and Inheritance from Marcher Lordships to Parliament: The Implications of Margaret Malefaunt's Abduction in Gower in 1438." In *The Fifteenth Century XIV: Essays Presented to Michael Hicks*, edited by Linda Clark, 77–90. Woodbridge: Boydell & Brewer, 2015.

Hall, Derek. "'Unto yone hospital at the tounis end': The Scottish Medieval Hospital." *Tayside and Fife Archaeological Journal* 12 (2006): 89–105.

Hall, Richard A. "York's Medieval Infrastructure." In *Lübecker Kolloquium zur Stadtarchäologie im Hanseraum IV: Die Infrastruktur*, edited by Manfred Gläser, 75–86. Lübeck: Schmidt-Römhild, 2004.

Hall, Susan P. "The *Cyrurgia Magna* of Brunus Longoburgensis: A Critical Edition." D. Phil thesis, Oxford University, 1957.

Hanna, Ralph III. "Augustinian Canons and Middle English Literature." In *The English Medieval Book: Studies in Memory of Jeremy Griffiths*, edited by A. S. G. Edwards, 27–42. London: The British Library, 2000.

———. *The English Manuscripts of Richard Rolle: A Descriptive Catalogue*. Exeter: University of Exeter Press, 2010.

———. "The Transmission of Richard Rolle's Latin Works." *The Library* 14 (2013): 313–33.

Hanna, Ralph, III, using material collected by the late Jeremy Griffiths. *A Descriptive Catalogue of the Western Manuscripts of St. John's College Oxford*. Oxford: Oxford University Press, 2002.

Harding, Vanessa. "Burial Choice and Burial Location in Later Medieval London." In *Death in Towns: Urban Responses to the Dying and the Dead, 100–1600*, edited by Steven Bassett, 119–35. Leicester: Leicester University Press, 1992.

Hardman, Phillipa. "Domestic Learning and Teaching: Investigating Evidence for the Role of 'Household Miscellanies' in Late-Medieval England." In *Women and Writing, c.1340–c.1650: The Domestication of Print Culture*, edited by Anne Lawrence-Mathers and Phillipa Hardman, 15–33. Woodbridge, UK: Boydell & Brewer, 2010.

Harker, C. Marie. "The Two Duchesses of Gloucester and the Rhetoric of the Feminine." *Historical Reflections/Réflexions Historiques* 30, no. 1 (2004): 109–25.

Harlow, Jonathan. *Religious Ministry in Bristol 1603–1689: Uniformity to Dissent*. Bristol: Bristol Record Society, 2017.

Harry, David. "Monastic Devotion and the Making of Lay Piety in Late Medieval England." D. Phil thesis, University of Bristol, 2013.

Hasenohr, Geneviève. "Méditation et mnémotechnique: Un témoignage figuré ancien (XIII–XIVe s)." In *Clio et son regard: Mélanges d'histoire d'art et d'archéologie offerts à Jacques Stiennon à l'occasion de ses vint-cinq ans d'enseignement*, edited by Rita Lejeune and Joseph Deckers, 365–82. Liège: P. Mardaga, 1982.

Henderson, John. *The Renaissance Hospital: Healing the Body and Healing the Soul.* New Haven, CT: Yale University Press, 2006.

Hickman, David. "From Catholic to Protestant: The Changing Meaning of Testamentary Religious Provisions in Elizabethan London." In *England's Long Reformation, 1500–1800,* ed. Nicholas Tyacke, 117–39. London: UCL Press, 1998.

Honkapohja, Alpo. "Multilingualism in Trinity College Cambridge Manuscript O.1.77." In *Foreign Influences on Medieval English,* edited by Jacek Fisiak and Magdalena Bator, 26–45. Frankfurt: Peter Lang, 2011.

Horden, Peregrine. *Cultures of Healing: Medieval and After.* Aldershot: Ashgate, 2019.

———. "A Discipline of Relevance: The Historiography of the Later Medieval Hospital." *Social History of Medicine* 1, no. 3 (1988): 359–74.

———. *Hospitals and Healing from Antiquity to the Later Middle Ages.* Aldershot: Ashgate, 2008.

Horobin, Simon. "John Cok and His Copy of *Piers Plowman.*" *Yearbook of Langland Studies* 27 (2013): 45–59.

"Hospitals: York." In *A History of the County of York,* edited by William Page, 3:336–52. London: Institute of Historical Research, 1974. http://www .british-history.ac.uk/vch/yorks/vol3/pp336-352.

Hoyle, R. W. *The Pilgrimage of Grace and the Politics of the 1530s.* Oxford: Oxford University Press, 2002.

Hudson, Anne. *The Premature Reformation.* Oxford: Clarendon, 1987.

Hugo, Thomas. "The Hospital of Le Papey, in the City of London." *Transactions of the London and Middlesex Archaeological Society* 5, no. 2 (1877): 183–221.

Hunt, Tony. *Popular Medicine in Thirteenth-Century England.* Cambridge: D. S. Brewer, 1990.

Imray, Jean. *The Charity of Richard Whittington.* London: Athlone Press, 1968.

Ingram, Martin. *Carnal Knowledge: Regulating Sex in England, 1470–1600.* Cambridge: Cambridge University Press, 2017.

Johnson, Holly. "A Fifteenth-Century Sermon Enacts the Seven Deadly Sins." In *Sin in Medieval and Early Modern Culture,* edited by Richard Newhauser and Susan Ridyard, 107–31. Woodbridge: Boydell and Brewer, 2012.

Johnston, Alexandra. "Cycle Drama in the Sixteenth Century: Texts and Contexts." In *Early Drama to 1600,* edited by Albert H. Tricomi, 1–15. Binghamton: University of New York, 1987.

———. "The *York Cycle* and the Libraries of York." In *The Church and Learning in Later Medieval Society: Essays in Honour of R. B. Dobson: Proceedings of the 1999 Harlaxton Symposium,* edited by Caroline M. Barron and Jenny Stratford, 355–70. Donington: Shaun Tyas, 2002.

Jolliffe, P. S. *A Check-list of Middle English Prose Writings of Spiritual Guidance.* Toronto: Pontifical Institute of Mediaeval Studies, 1974.

Kaplan, M. Lindsay, ed. *The Culture of Slander in Early Modern England.* Cambridge: Cambridge University Press, 1997.

Karras, Ruth Mazo. *Common Women: Prostitution and Sexuality in Medieval England.* Oxford: Oxford University Press, 1998.

———. "The Regulation of Brothels in Late Medieval England." *Signs* 14, no. 2 (1989): 399–433.

Kealey, Edward J. *Medieval Medicus: A Social History of Anglo-Norman Medicine.* Baltimore: Johns Hopkins University Press, 1981.

Kellogg, Alfred. "The Fraternal Kiss in Chaucer's 'Summoner's Tale.'" *Scriptorium* 7, no. 1 (1953): 115.

Kempster, Hugh. "*Emendatio Vitae: Amendinge of Lyf,* A Middle English Translation, Edited from Dublin, Trinity College, MS 432." D. Phil thesis, University of Waikato, 2007.

Kerby-Fulton, Kathryn. *The Clerical Proletariat and the Resurgence of Middle English Poetry.* Philadelphia: University of Pennsylvania Press, 2021.

Kerby-Fulton, Kathryn, and Steven Justice. "Langlandian Reading Circles and the Civil Service in London and Dublin, 1380–1427." *New Medieval Literatures* 1 (1998): 59–83.

Kerling, Nellie J. M. "The Foundation of St. Bartholomew's Hospital in West Smithfield, London." *The Guildhall Miscellany* 4, no. 3 (1972): 137–48.

King, Pamela M. "*Civitas* versus *Templum.*" *Medieval English Theatre* 25 (2003): 84–97.

———. *The York Mystery Cycle and the Worship of the City.* Westfield Medieval Studies 1. Woodbridge: Boydell and Brewer, 2006.

Kingdon, J. A. *Richard Grafton, Citizen and Grocer of London.* London: Rixon and Arnold, 1901.

Knowles, David, and R. Neville Hadcock, *Medieval Religious Houses: England and Wales.* New York: Macmillan, 1971.

Kosmin, Jennifer. "Midwifery Anatomized: Vesalius, Dissection, and Reproductive Authority in Early Modern Italy." *Journal of Medieval and Early Modern Studies* 48, no. 1 (2018): 79–104.

Kraebel, Andrew. *Biblical Commentary and Translation in Later Medieval England: Experiments in Interpretation.* Cambridge: Cambridge University Press, 2020.

Krug, Rebecca. "Jesus' Voice: Dialogue and Late-Medieval Readers." In *Form and Reform: Reading across the Fifteenth Century,* edited by S. Gayk and K. Tonry, 110–29. Columbus: Ohio State University Press, 2011.

Kumler, Aden. "*Imitatio rerum:* Sacred Objects in the St. Giles Hospital Processional." *Journal of Medieval and Early Modern Studies* 43, no. 4 (2014): 469–502.

Lamothe, Jessica. "An Edition of the Latin and Four Middle English Versions of William Flete's *De remediis contra temptaciones*." D. Phil thesis, University of York, 2017.

Lang, S. L. "The *Philomena* of John Bradmore and Its Middle English Derivative: A Perspective on Surgery in Late Medieval England." D. Phil thesis, University of St. Andrews, 1998.

Langdell, Sebastian. " 'What shal I call thee? What is thy name?' Thomas Hoccleve and the Making of 'Chaucer.' " *New Medieval Literatures* 16 (2016): 250–76.

Lee, Becky R. "Men's Recollections of a Woman's Rite: Medieval English Men's Recollections Regarding the Rite of the Purification of Women after Childbirth." *Gender and History* 14 (2002): 224–41.

———. " 'Women Ben Purifyid of Her Childeryn': The Purification of Women after Childbirth in Medieval England." PhD diss., University of Toronto, 1998.

L'Estrange, Elizabeth. *Holy Motherhood: Gender, Dynasty and Visual Culture in the Later Middle Ages*. Manchester: Manchester University Press, 2008.

Louis, Cameron. "Manuscript Contexts of Middle English Proverb Literature." *Mediaeval Studies* 20 (1998): 219–38.

MacCulloch, Diarmaid. *Tudor Church Militant: Edward VI and the Protestant Reformation*. London: Penguin, 1999.

Maclean, John. "Notes on the Accounts of the Procurators, or Churchwardens, of the Parish of St. Ewen's, Bristol." *Transactions of the Bristol & Gloucestershire Archaeological Society* 15 (1890–91): 139–82.

Manchester, Andrea. "Chronicling the English Reformation: The Historical Works of Richard Grafton." PhD diss., Kent State University, 2007.

Marks, Richard. *Image and Devotion in Late Medieval England*. Phoenix Mill: Sutton, 2004.

———. "Picturing Image and Text in the Late Medieval Parish Church." In *Image, Text and Church, 1380–1600: Essays for Margaret Aston*, edited by L. Clark, M. Jurkowski, and C. Richmond, 162–202. Toronto: University of Toronto, 2009.

Marshall, Peter. *Beliefs and the Dead in Reformation England*. Oxford: Oxford University Press, 2002.

Matthews, Kate. "Textual Spaces/Playing Places: An Exploration of Convent Drama in the Abbey of Origny-Ste-Benoîte." *European Medieval Drama* 7 (2003): 69–86.

McCann, Daniel. *Soul-Health: Therapeutic Reading in Late Medieval England*. Cardiff: University of Wales Press, 2018.

McIntosh, Marjorie K. *Poor Relief in England, 1350–1600*. Oxford: Oxford University Press, 2012.

———. "Poverty, Charity, and Coercion in Elizabethan England." *Journal of Interdisciplinary History* 25, no. 3 (2005): 457–79.

Meale, Carole M. ". . . 'all the bokes that I haue of latyn, englisch and french': Laywomen and Their Books in Late Medieval England." In *Women and Literature in Britain, 1150–1500*, edited by Carole M. Meale, 126–58. Cambridge: Cambridge University Press, 1993.

Meyer-Lee, Robert. *Poets and Power from Chaucer to Wyatt*. Cambridge: Cambridge University Press, 2007.

Mitchell, J. Allan. *Becoming Human: The Matter of the Medieval Child*. Minneapolis: University of Minnesota Press, 2014.

Mooney, Linne. "Shirley's Heirs." *Yearbook of English Studies* 33 (2003): 182–98.

Moran, Joann Hoeppner. *Education and Learning in the City of York 1300–1560*. Borthwick Paper 55. York: St. Anthony's Press, 1979.

———. *The Growth of English Schooling, 1340–1548*. Princeton, NJ: Princeton University Press, 1985.

Moore, Norman. *The History of St. Bartholomew's Hospital*. 2 vols. London, C. A. Pearson Ltd., 1918.

Moore, W. G. "Robert Copland and His *Hye Way*." *Review of English Studies* 7 (1931): 406–18.

Napierkowski, Thomas Joseph. "A Critical Edition of the *Summum Sapientiae*." PhD diss., University of Colorado at Boulder, 1971.

Nicholls, Angela. *Almshouses in Early Modern England: Charitable Housing in the Mixed Economy of Welfare, 1550–1725*. Woodbridge: Boydell, 2017.

Niebrzydowski, Sue. *Bonoure and Buxum: A Study of Wives in Late Medieval English Literature*. Bern: Peter Lang, 2006.

———. "Secular Women and Late-Medieval Marian Drama." *Yearbook of English Studies* 43 (2013): 121–39.

Nightingale, Pamela. *Medieval Mercantile Community: The Grocers' Company and the Politics and Trade of London, 1000–1485*. New Haven, CT: Yale University Press, 1995.

*Nine Centuries of Health Care*. London: Barts Health NHS Trust, n.d.

Normington, Katie. *Gender and Medieval Drama*. Cambridge: Boydell and Brewer, 2004.

Nuttall, Jenni. "Margaret of Anjou as Patron of English Verse? The *Liber Proverbiorum* and the *Romans of Partenay*." *Review of English Studies*, n.s., 67, no. 281 (2016): 636–59.

Orlemanski, Julie. *Symptomatic Subjects: Bodies, Medicine, and Causation in the Literature of Late Medieval England*. Philadelphia: University of Pennsylvania Press, 2019.

Orme, Nicholas. "Children and Literature in Medieval England." *Medium Aevum* 58 (1999): 218–46.

———. "A Medieval Almshouse for the Clergy: Clyst Gabriel Hospital near Exeter." *Journal of Ecclesiastical History* 39, no. 1 (1988): 1–15.

Orme, Nicholas, and Margaret Webster. *The English Hospital, 1070–1570.* New Haven, CT: Yale University Press, 1995.

Palliser, D. M. *The Reformation in York, 1534–1553.* Borthwick Paper 40. York: St. Anthony's Press, 1971.

———. *Tudor York.* Oxford: Oxford University Press, 1979.

Palmer, Barbara. "Recycling 'The Wakefield Cycle': The Records." *Research Opportunities in Renaissance Drama* 41 (2002): 88–130.

Pantin, W. A. *The English Church in the Fourteenth Century.* Cambridge: Cambridge University Press, 1955.

Park, Katharine. *Secrets of Women: Gender, Generation, and the Origins of Human Dissection.* New York: Zone Books, 2006.

Park, Katharine, and John Henderson. "The First Hospital among Christians: The Ospedale di Santa Maria Nuova in Sixteenth-Century Florence." *Medical History* 35 (1991): 164–88.

Pearsall, Derek. *John Lydgate.* London: Routledge, 1970.

———. "The Whole Book: Late Medieval Manuscript Miscellanies and Their Modern Interpreters." In *Imagining the Book,* edited by Stephen Kelly and Ryan Perry, 17–29. Turnhout: Brepols, 2005.

Pelling, Margaret. "Healing the Sick Poor: Social Policy and Disability in Norwich, 1550–1640." *Medical History* 29 (1985): 115–37.

———. "Nurses and Nursekeepers: Problems of Identification in the Early Modern Period." In *The Common Lot: Sickness, Medical Occupations and the Urban Poor in Early Modern England,* edited by Margaret Pelling, 179–202. London: Longman, 1998.

Pelling, Margaret, and Charles Webster. "Medical Practitioners." In *Health, Medicine and Mortality in the Sixteenth Century,* edited by Charles Webster, 165–235. Cambridge: Cambridge University Press, 1979.

Pelling, Margaret, and Frances White. *Medical Conflicts in Early Modern London: Patronage, Physicians, and Irregular Practitioners, 1550–1640.* Oxford: Clarendon, 2003.

Phillips, Kim. "Desiring Virgins: Maidens, Martyrs and Femininity in Late Medieval England." In *Youth in the Middle Ages,* edited by P. J. P. Goldberg and Felicity Riddy, 45–59. Cambridge: Boydell & Brewer, 2004.

———. "Maidenhood as the Perfect Age of Women's Life." In *Young Medieval Women,* edited by Katherine J. Lewis, Noël James Menuge, and Kim M. Phillips, 1–24. New York: St. Martin's Press, 1999.

Pollock, Linda A. "Childbearing and Female Bonding in Early Modern England." *Social History* 22, no. 3 (1997): 286–306.

Post, J. B. "A Fifteenth-Century Customary of the Southwark Stews." *Journal of the Society of Archivists* 5, no. 7 (1977): 418–28.

Pouzet, Jean-Pascal. "Book Production outside Commercial Contexts." In *The Production of Books in England 1350–1500*, edited by Alexandra Gillespie and Daniel Wakelin, 212–38. Cambridge: Cambridge University Press, 2011.

———. "Quelques aspects de l'influence des chanoines augustins sur la production and la transmission littéraire vernaculaire en Angleterre (XIIIe–XVe siècles)." *Comptes rendus des séances de l'Académie des Inscriptions et Belles-Lettres*, 148e année, no. 1 (2004): 169–213.

Power, D'Arcy. "Notes on the Bibliography of Three Sixteenth-Century English Books Connected with the London Hospitals." *The Library*, 4th ser. (1921): 73–94.

Pugliatti, Paolo. *Beggary and Theatre in Early Modern England* Aldershot: Ashgate, 2003.

Radulescu, Raluca. *Romance and Its Contexts in Fifteenth-Century England: Politics, Piety and Penitence.* Cambridge: Boydell & Brewer, 2013.

Ragab, Ahmed. *The Medieval Islamic Hospital: Medicine, Religion, and Charity.* Cambridge: Cambridge University Press, 2015.

Raine, Angelo. *Mediaeval York: A Topographical Study Based on Original Sources.* London: Murray, 1955.

Rawcliffe, Carole. "Christ the Physician Walks the Wards: Celestial Therapeutics in the Medieval Hospital." In *London and the Kingdom: Essays in Honour of Caroline M. Barron, Proceedings of the 2004 Harlaxton Symposium*, edited by Matthew Davies and Andrew Prescott, 78–97. Donington: Shaun Tyas, 2008.

———. "Communities of the Living and of the Dead: Hospital Confraternities in the Later Middle Ages." In *Hospitals and Communities, 1100–1960*, ed. Christopher Bonfield, Jonathan Reinarz, and Teresa Huguet-Termes, 125–54. Oxford: Peter Lang, 2013.

———. "A Crisis of Confidence? Parliament and the Demand for Hospital Reform in Early-15th and Early-16th Century England." *Parliamentary History* 35, no. 2 (2016): 85–110.

———. "The Eighth Comfortable Work: Education and the Medieval English Hospital." In *The Church and Learning in Later Medieval Society: Essays in Honour of R. B. Dobson, Proceedings of the 1999 Harlaxton Symposium*, ed. Caroline M. Barron and Jenny Stratford, 371–98. Donington: Shaun Tyas, 2002.

———. "A Fifteenth-Century *Medicus Politicus*: John Somerset, Physician to Henry VI." In *The Fifteenth Century X: Parliament, Personalities, and Power,*

*Papers Presented to Linda S. Clark*, edited by Hannes Kleinecke, 97–120. Cambridge: Boydell & Brewer, 2011.

———. "Hospital Nurses and Their Work." In *Daily Life in the Late Middle Ages*, edited by Richard Britnell, 43–64. Stroud: Sutton, 1998.

———. "The Hospitals of Later Medieval London." *Medical History* 28.1 (January 1984): 1–21.

———. *Medicine and Society in Later Medieval England*. Stroud: Alan Sutton, 1995.

———. *Medicine for the Soul: The Life, Death and Resurrection of an English Medieval Hospital, St Giles's, Norwich, c. 1292–1550*. Stroud: Sutton, 1999.

———. "Medicine for the Soul: The Medieval English Hospital and the Quest for Spiritual Health." In *Religion, Health and Suffering: A Cross-Cultural Study of Attitudes to Suffering and the Implications for Medicine in a Multi-Religious Society*, edited by Roy Porter, 316–38. London: Routledge, 1999.

———. "Passports to Paradise: How Medieval Hospitals and Almshouses Kept their Archives." *Archives* 27, no. 106 (2002): 2–22.

———. A Word from Our Sponsor: Advertising the Patron in the Medieval Hospital." In *The Impact of Hospitals, 300–2000*, edited by John Henderson, Peregrine Horden, and Alessandro Pastore, 167–93. Oxford: Peter Lang, 2007.

———. "Written in the Book of Life: Building the Libraries of Medieval English Hospitals and Almshouses." *The Library* 3, no. 2 (2002): 127–62.

Reddan, M. "St. Bartholomew's Hospital." In *The Religious Houses of London and Middlesex*, edited by Caroline M. Barron and Matthew Davies, 149–54. London: Centre for Metropolitan History and Victoria County History, 2007.

Reinke, Darrel F. "'Austin's Labour': Patterns of Governance in Medieval Augustinian Monasticism." *Church History* 56 (1987): 157–71.

Rice, Nicole R. *Lay Piety and Religious Discipline in Middle English Literature*. Cambridge: Cambridge University Press, 2008.

———. "Lay Spiritual Texts and Pastoral Care in Two Fifteenth-Century Priests' Collections." In *Middle English Religious Writing in Practice: Texts, Readers, and Transformations*, edited by Nicole R. Rice, 149–77. Turnhout: Brepols, 2013.

Rice, Nicole R., and Margaret Aziza Pappano. *The Civic Cycles: Artisan Drama and Identity in Premodern England*. Notre Dame, IN: University of Notre Dame Press, 2015.

Richmond, Colin. "Victorian Values in Fifteenth-Century England: The Ewelme Almshouse Statutes." In *Pragmatic Utopias: Ideals and Communities, 1200–1630*, edited by Rosemary Horrox and Sarah Rees-Jones, 224–41. Cambridge: Cambridge University Press, 2001.

Riddle, John M. "Theory and Practice in Medieval Medicine." *Viator* 5 (1974): 157–84.

Rieder, Paula M. *On the Purification of Women: Churching in Northern France, 1100–1500.* New York: Palgrave, 2006.

Ritchey, Sara. *Acts of Care: Recovering Women in Late Medieval Healthcare.* Ithaca, NY: Cornell University Press, 2021.

Roffey, Simon. "Medieval Leper Hospitals in England: An Archaeological Perspective." *Medieval Archaeology* 56 (2012): 203–33.

Roger, Euan C. "Blakberd's Treasure: A Study in Fifteenth-Century Administration at St. Bartholomew's Hospital, London." In *The Fifteenth Century XIII: Exploring the Evidence; Commemoration, Administration, and the Economy,* edited by Linda Clark, 81–107. Cambridge: Boydell Press, 2014.

Rosenthal, Joel T. *The Purchase of Paradise: Gift Giving and the Aristocracy, 1307–1485.* London: Routledge & Kegan Paul, 1972.

Rubin, Miri. *Charity and Community in Medieval Cambridge.* Cambridge: Cambridge University Press, 1987.

———. "Development and Change in English Hospitals, 1100–1500." In *The Hospital in History,* edited by Lindsay Granhouse and Roy Porter, 41–60. London: Routledge, 1989.

———. "Imagining Medieval Hospitals: Considerations on the Cultural Meaning of Institutional Change." In *Medicine and Charity before the Welfare State,* edited by Jonathan Barry and Colin Jones, 14–25. London: Routledge, 1991.

Russell, G. H. "'As they read it': Some Notes on Early Responses to the C-Version of *Piers Plowman.*" *Leeds Studies in English* 29 (1989): 173–89.

Ryan, Denise. "Playing the Midwife's Part in the English Nativity Plays." *Review of English Studies* 54, no. 216 (2003): 435–48.

Saak, Eric. *Creating Augustine: Interpreting Augustine and Augustinianism in the Later Middle Ages.* Oxford: Oxford University Press, 2012.

———. *High Way to Heaven: The Augustinian Platform between Reform and Reformation, 1292–1524.* Leiden: Brill, 2002.

Sacks, David Harris. *The Widening Gate: Bristol and the Atlantic Economy, 1450–1700.* Berkeley: University of California Press, 1991.

Scahill, John. "Trilingualism in Early Middle English Miscellanies: Languages and Literature." *Yearbook of English Studies* 33 (2003): 18–32.

Schorr, Dorothy C. "The Iconographic Development of the Presentation in the Temple." *Art Bulletin* 28 (1946): 17–32.

Schwebel, Leah. "Livy and Augustine as Negative Models in the *Legend of Lucrece.*" *Chaucer Review* 52, no. 1 (2017): 29–45.

Sergi, Matthew. *Practical Cues and Social Spectacle in the Chester Plays.* Chicago: University of Chicago Press, 2020.

———. "Un-dating the Chester Plays: A Reassessment of Lawrence Clopper's 'History and Development' and MS Peniarth 399." In *Early British Drama in Manuscript,* edited by Tamara Atkin and Laura Estil, 71–102. Turnhout: Brepols, 2019.

Siena, Kevin. "The Clean and the Foul: Paupers and the Pox in London Hospitals, c.1550–c.1700." In *Sins of the Flesh: Responding to Sexual Disease in Early Modern Europe,* edited by Kevin Siena, 261–84. Toronto: University of Toronto Press, 2005.

Signori, Gabriella. "Veil, Hat or Hair? Reflections on an Asymmetrical Relationship." *Medieval History Journal* 8, no. 1 (2005): 25–47.

Simpson, James. *The Oxford English Literary History,* Vol. 2, *Reform and Cultural Revolution.* Oxford: Oxford University Press, 2002.

Sisson, Charles J. "Grafton and the London Grey Friars." *The Library,* 4th ser., 11, no. 2 (1930): 121–49.

Skeeters, Martha C. *Community and Clergy: Bristol and the Reformation, c. 1530–c. 1570.* Oxford: Clarendon, 1993.

Slack, Paul. "Hospitals, Workhouses and the Relief of the Poor in Early Modern London." In *Health Care and Poor Relief in Protestant Europe 1500–1700,* edited by Andrew Cunningham and Ole Peter Grell, 229–46. London: Routledge, 1997.

———. "Social Policy and the Constraints of Government, 1547–58." In *The Mid-Tudor Polity,* edited by Jennifer Loach and Robert Tittler, 94–115. London: Macmillan, 1980.

Solberg, Emma Maggie. "Madonna, Whore: Mary's Sexuality in the N-Town Plays." *Comparative Drama* 48 (2014): 191–219.

———. *Virgin Whore.* Ithaca, NY: Cornell University Press, 2018.

Somerset, Fiona. "'Al þe comonys with o voys atonys': Multilingual Latin and Vernacular Voice in *Piers Plowman.*" *Yearbook of Langland Studies* 19 (2005): 107–36.

———. *Feeling Like Saints: Lollard Writings After Wyclif.* Ithaca: Cornell University Press, 2014.

Somerville, Robert. *The Savoy: Manor, Hospital, Chapel.* London: Duchy of Lancaster, 1960.

Spahl, Rudiger. "Richard and William, or to Whom Was Richard Rolle's *Emendatio vitae* Dedicated?" *Revue d'histoire des textes* 32 (2003): 301–12.

Sperling, Jutta Gisela. *Queer Lactations: The Roman Charity in Early Modern Visual Culture.* Bielefeld: transcript-Verlag, 2016.

Sponsler, Claire. "Lydgate and London's Public Culture." In *Lydgate Matters*, edited by Lisa H. Cooper and Andrea B. Denny-Brown, 13–33. New York: Palgrave, 2008.

Stavsky, Jonathan. "John Lydgate Reads the Clerk's Tale." *Studies in the Age of Chaucer* 34 (2012): 209–46.

Stocker, Margarita. *Judith, Sexual Warrior: Women and Power in Western Culture.* New Haven, CT: Yale University Press, 1998.

Stoertz, Fiona Harris. "Suffering and Survival in Medieval English Childbirth." In *Medieval Family Roles: A Book of Essays*, edited by Cathy Jorgensen Itnyre, 101–20. New York: Taylor & Francis Group, 1999.

Stokes, James. "Women and Mimesis in Medieval and Renaissance Somerset (and Beyond)." *Comparative Drama* 27, no. 2 (1993): 176–96.

———. "Women and Performance in Medieval and Early Modern Suffolk." *Early Theatre* 15 (2012): 27–43.

Sumpter, Guy. "Lady Chapels and the Manifestation of Devotion to Our Lady in Medieval England." D. Phil thesis, University of Leicester, 2008.

Sutton, Anne F. "Alice Domenyk-Markby-Shipley-Portaleyn of St Bartholomew's Close and Isleworth: The Inheritance, Life and Tribulations of an Heiress." *The Ricardian* 20 (2010): 23–65.

Sutton, Anne, and Livia Visser-Fuchs. "The Cult of Angels in Late Fifteenth-Century England." In *Women and the Book: Assessing the Visual Evidence*, edited by J. H. M. Taylor and Lesley Smith, 230–65. London: The British Library, 1996.

Swann, Alaya. "'By Expresse Experiment': The Doubting Midwife Salome in Late Medieval England." *Bulletin of the History of Medicine* 89 (2015): 1–24.

Swanson, Heather. *Medieval Artisans: An Urban Class in Late Medieval England.* Oxford: Blackwell, 1989.

Sweetinburgh, Sheila. *The Role of the Hospital in Medieval England: Gift-Giving and the Spiritual Economy.* Dublin: Four Courts Press, 2004.

Taylor, Andrew. *Textual Situations: Three Medieval Manuscripts and Their Readers.* Philadelphia: University of Pennsylvania Press, 2002.

Trease, G. E., and J. H. Hodson. "The Inventory of John Hexham, a Fifteenth-Century Apothecary." *Medical History* 9 (1965): 76–81.

Twycross, Meg. "Forget the 4:30 am Start: Recovering a Palimpsest in the York *Ordo paginarum*." *Medieval Theatre* 25 (2003): 98–152.

———. "The *Ordo paginarum* Revisited, with a Digital Camera." In *"Bring Furth the Pagants": Essays in Early English Drama Presented to Alexandra F. Johnston*, edited by David N. Klausner and Karen Sawyer Marsalek, 105–31. Toronto: University of Toronto Press, 2007.

Tyacke, Nicholas, ed. *England's Long Reformation, 1500–1800.* London: UCL Press, 1998.

Veeman, Kathryn. "John Shirley's Early Bureaucratic Career." *Studies in the Age of Chaucer* 38 (2016): 255–63.

———. " 'Send þis Booke Ageyn Hoome To Shirley': John Shirley and the Circulation Of Manuscripts in Fifteenth-Century England." PhD diss., University of Notre Dame, 2010.

Van Elk, Martine. "The Counterfeit Vagrant: The Dynamic of Deviance in the Bridewell Court Records and the Literature of Roguery." In *Rogues and Early Modern English Culture*, edited by Craig Dionne and Steve Mentz, 120–39. Ann Arbor: University of Michigan Press, 2004.

Varnam, Laura. "*The Book of the Foundation of St Bartholomew's Church*: Consecration, Restoration, and Translation." In *Sacred Text—Sacred Space: Architectural, Spiritual and Literary Convergences in England and Wales*, edited by Joseph Sterrett and Peter Thomas, 57–75. Leiden: Brill, 2011.

Voigts, Linda E. "A Doctor and His Books: The Manuscripts of Roger Marchall." In *New Science out of Old Books*, edited by Richard Beadle and A. J. Piper, 249–315. Aldershot: Scolar Press, 1995.

Von Nolcken, Christina. "Some Alphabetical Compendia and How Preachers Used Them in Fourteenth-Century England." *Viator* 12 (1981): 271–88.

Waller, Gary. *The Virgin Mary in Late Medieval and Early Modern English Literature and Popular Culture.* Cambridge: Cambridge University Press, 2011.

Warner, Lawrence. *The Myth of "Piers Plowman."* Cambridge: Cambridge University Press, 2014.

Watson, A. G. "Christopher and William Carye, Collectors of Monastic Manuscripts, and 'John Carye.'" *The Library*, 5th ser., 20 (1965): 135–42.

Watson, Nicholas. *Richard Rolle and the Invention of Authority.* Cambridge: Cambridge University Press, 1991.

Watson, Sethina. "City as Charter: Charity and the Lordship of English Towns, 1170–1250." In *Cities, Texts and Social Networks, 400–1500: Experiences and Perceptions of Medieval Urban Space*, edited by Caroline Goodson, Anne E. Lester, and Carol Symes, 235–62. Aldershot: Ashgate, 2010.

———. "A Mother's Past and her Children's Futures: Female Inheritance, Family and Dynastic Hospitals in the Thirteenth Century." In *Motherhood, Religion and Society in Medieval Europe, 400–1400: Essays Presented to Henrietta Leyser*, edited by Conrad Leyser and Lesley Smith, 213–49. Farnham: Ashgate, 2011.

———. *On Hospitals: Welfare, Law, and Christianity in Western Europe, 400–1320.* Oxford: Oxford University Press, 2020.

———. "The Origins of the English Hospital." *Transactions of the Royal Historical Society*, 6th ser., 16 (2006): 75–94.

Wattenbach, W. "Aus einer Halberstadter Handschrift." *Anzeiger fur Kunde Der Deutschen Vorzeit* 11 (1878): 345–50.

Webber, Teresa. "Latin Devotional Texts and the Books of the Augustinian Canons of Thurgarton Priory and Leicester Abbey in the Late Middle Ages." In *Books and Collectors 1200–1700: Essays Presented to Andrew Watson*, edited by James P. Carley and Colin G. C. Tite, 27–41. London: The British Library, 1997.

Webber, Teresa, and A. G. Watson. *The Libraries of the Augustinian Canons*. Corpus of British Medieval Library Catalogues 6. London: British Library, 1998.

Wenzel, Siegfried. "Preaching the Seven Deadly Sins." In *In the Garden of Evil: The Vices and Culture in the Middle Ages*, edited by Richard Newhauser, 145–69. Toronto: Pontifical Institute, 1998.

Westphall, Alan F. "Middle English *Meditationes de Passione Christi*." Available at *Geographies of Orthodoxy: Mapping Middle English Pseudo-Bonaventuran Lives of Christ, 1350–1550*. https://geographies-of-orthodoxy.qub.ac.uk/resources/?section=corpus&id=9.

Wheatley, Edward. *Mastering Aesop: Medieval Education, Chaucer, and His Followers*. Gainesville: University Press of Florida, 2000.

Wilmer, Harry A., and Richard E. Scammon. "Neuropsychiatric Patients Reported Cured at St. Bartholomew's Hospital in The Twelfth Century." *Journal of Nervous and Mental Disease* 119, no. 1 (1954): 1–22.

Wogan-Browne, Jocelyn. "Time to Read: Pastoral Care, Vernacular Access and the Case of Angier of St. Frideswide." In *Texts and Traditions of Medieval Pastoral Care*, edited by Cate Gunn and Catherine Innes-Parker, 62–77. Woodbridge: Boydell & Brewer, 2009.

Woolf, Rosemary. *English Mystery Plays*. London: Routledge & Kegan Paul, 1972.

Wright, Laura. "On Medieval Wills and the Rise of Written Monolingual English." In *Approaches to Middle English: Variation, Contact and Change*, ed. Juan Camilo Conde-Silvestre and Javier Calle-Martín, 35–54. Frankfurt am Main: Peter Lang, 2015.

Wyatt, Diana. "Play Titles without Play Texts: What Can They Tell Us, and How? An Investigation of the Evidence for the Beverley Corpus Christi Play." In *Staging Scripture: Biblical Drama, 1350–1600*, edited by Peter Happé and Wim Hüsken, 68–91. Leiden: Brill, 2016.

# Manuscripts Index

N I C O L E   R .   R I C E
is professor of English at St. John's University, author of a number of
books and essays, and co-author of *The Civic Cycles: Artisan Drama and
Identity in Premodern England* (University of Notre Dame Press, 2015).

Milton Keynes UK
Ingram Content Group UK Ltd.
UKHW050624220224
438108UK00010B/26